MANUAL OF INFECTION CONTROL
PROCEDURES

2nd Edition

To my wife Laila, and my children Numair and Namiz for
their abiding love, understanding and encouragement

MANUAL OF INFECTION CONTROL PROCEDURES

2nd Edition

Dr N. N. DAMANI

MSc (Lond.), MBBS, FRCPath, FRCPI

Clinical Director Pathology & Laboratory Services
Consultant Microbiologist & Infection Control Doctor
Craigavon Area Hospital Group Trust, Portadown, UK

Honorary Lecturer
Department of Medical Microbiology
Queens University, Belfast, UK

Treasurer, International Federation of Infection Control

Foreword by
Professor A. M. Emmerson

OBE, FRCP, FRCPath, FMedSci, DipHIC
Emeritus Professor of Microbiology
Division of Microbiology and Infectious Diseases
University Hospital
Queen's Medical Centre
Nottingham, UK

CAMBRIDGE
UNIVERSITY PRESS

CAMBRIDGE UNIVERSITY PRESS
Cambridge, New York, Melbourne, Madrid, Cape Town, Singapore, São Paulo

Cambridge University Press
The Edinburgh Building, Cambridge CB2 2RU, UK

Published in the United States of America by Cambridge University Press, New York

www.cambridge.org
Information on this title: www.cambridge.org/9780521687010

First published 1997
Second Edition Published 2003
Digitally reprinted by Cambridge University Press 2006

A catalogue record for this publication is available from the British Library

ISBN-13 978-0-521-68701-0 paperback
ISBN-10 0-521-68701-2 paperback

What, will these hands ne'er be clean?

WILLIAM SHAKESPEARE
Macbeth

Foreword to the Second Edition

When Professor Graham Ayliffe wrote the foreword to the first edition of this manual in 1997, he said *'this manual contains a wealth of practical advice, a number of useful tables, diagrams, definitions and essential references.'* He also said that the policies were detailed enough and provided enough instruction to allow health care workers (HCWs) to carry out individual procedures. In this respect, the second edition of this manual fulfils these requirements and will appeal to both medical and nursing practitioners in infection control and to nurse educators whose job it is to provide first-hand practical advice to those responsible for the provision of a safe environment for patients and staff alike.

This second edition has been revised and updated and the reader eager to find out what is new and different from the first edition will be pleasantly surprised. New sections include the *Principles of Infection Control, Design and Management of Health Care Facilities, Surveillance and Outbreak Control, Epidemiology and Biostatistics* and not least a section on *Infection Control Information Resources.* This latter section, together with the updated and easily accessible reading lists which are highlighted at strategic points in the text and at the end of each section provides a wealth of information for the inquisitive reader. In this respect, as much evidence-based information as there is available has been presented.

Infection control is a quality improvement activity that focuses on improving the care of patients and protecting the health of staff, and yet, despite advances in modern medicine and surgery, 5–10% of patients admitted to hospital subsequently acquire an infection of varying degrees of severity. Because of the need to discharge patients to the community with the shortest possible length of stay in hospital, some patients may not manifest their hospital-acquired infection (HAI) until some time later. Post-discharge surveillance is still in its infancy but some record of its occurrence will need to be taken into account before the true cost of HAIs can be measured. Unfortunately, the incidence of HAI is as high today as it has been for many years, but there are many reasons for this. Improvements in supportive care have led to more aggressive medical and surgical therapy and seriously ill patients with several underlying risk factors are often highly susceptible to infection.

This manual addresses the need for patient care and recognises that the factors involved in HAI are complex and that cost-effective measures to combat them are needed which are based on evidence-based guidelines. Reliable comparisons of infection rates between units, hospitals and countries are difficult without ongoing monitoring with risk factor adjustment and benchmarking. The new section on *Epidemiology and Biostatistics* will facilitate worthwhile comparison and make benchmarking a challenge, not a threat.

The control of infection in hospitals has greatly improved in recent years; we have many more professional staff, who are better trained, and more resources are being set aside for infection control since the acknowledgement by management that infection control is part of the quality improvement process required of health care services. However, the free movement of patients between hospitals and the community, by breaking down invisible barriers, will always remain a challenge for HCWs. We still lack sufficient isolation facilities to contain the major problems of patients with antibiotic-resistant strains of bacteria such as multi-drug resistant tuberculosis (MDR-TB), methicillin-resistant *Staphylococcus aureus* (MRSA) and gylcopeptide resistant enterococci (GRE). A combined approach of prudent antibiotic prescribing, effective surveillance and good infection control practices is essential if antibiotic resistance is to be contained. This is a worldwide problem, and the spread of infection is a major problem in the developed world, but the principles of effective control are the same throughout the world.

In the developed world, people are having longer and more 'adventurous' surgery and transplantation is being carried out in hospitals in the face of emerging new diseases and newly-identified micro-organisms which are difficult to treat. There is a sharp increase in the use of minimally invasive surgery, with the widespread use of expensive, heat-labile equipment like endoscopes, which require a high quality system for decontamination. This manual contains most of the procedures necessary to carry out such a service, but the author has not forgotten that basic hand washing is generally considered to be the most important single measure in the control of hospital infection and is dealt with in detail in this manual.

I have enjoyed reading this manual and commend it to all health care workers involved in the prevention and control of infection.

M. Emmerson
London
November, 2002

Foreword to the First Edition

Hospital-acquired (nosocomial) infection is a major problem in the hospitals of most countries and despite improvements in control methods, the prevalence of infection remains at 5–10%. Infections are mainly of surgical wounds, the respiratory and urinary tracts, and the skin. The important risk factors for the acquisition of infection are invasive procedures which include operative surgery, intravascular and urinary catheterization and mechanical ventilation of the respiratory tract. Other risk factors include traumatic injuries, burns, age (elderly and neonates), immunosuppression and existing disease.

Many infections are endogenous (i.e. acquired from the patient's own microbial flora) and are not necessarily preventable, although infection can be kept to a minimum by good aseptic techniques. The spread of infection from patient to patient is often difficult to prevent, particularly in overcrowded hospitals with staff shortages and limited facilities. The prevention of cross-infection with highly antibiotic-resistant organisms, such as epidemic methicillin-resistant *Staphylococcus aureus* (MRSA) can be difficult and often requires considerable resources. Vancomycin-resistant enterococcal infections may be untreatable with currently available antibiotics and Gram-negative bacilli resistant to the quinolones and the third generation cephalosporins frequently cause therapeutic problems. Cross-infection can be considerably reduced by a few basic measures, for example handwashing or disinfection correctly performed at the right time. Handwashing is generally considered to be the most important single measure in infection control and is dealt with in detail in this manual. Although prevention of transmission is of major importance, the rational use of antibiotics and restriction of certain agents is necessary to achieve a long-term effect. Other organisms which have emerged in hospitals in recent years include *Clostridium difficile*, causing outbreaks in the elderly, and legionella associated with cooling towers and contaminated water supplies. Food poisoning is mainly a problem in the community, but epidemics occur in hospitals. *Escherichia coli* 0157:H7 has recently been responsible for large outbreaks of severe gastroenteritis and occasional deaths from renal failure.

The potential hazards of blood-borne viruses (hepatitis B (HBV) and C (HCV) and human immunodeficiency virus (HIV)), particularly from injuries due to sharp instruments, cause considerable anxiety to staff. Policies for the safe disposal of clinical waste, especially needles, must be correctly implemented. Spread of these blood-borne infections to patients from contaminated medical equipment is also a potential hazard and the production of safe decontamination policies is a major responsibility of infection control teams. Although decontamination of equipment by heat is the optimal method, many items are heat-labile and chemical disinfection is required. Flexible endoscopes fall into this category and are difficult to clean and disinfect. The nature of surgery is also changing and minimal access surgery is often replacing conventional surgery, but the equipment is often heat-labile and difficult to clean. All of these problems have been well addressed in this manual.

Litigation for negligence is becoming increasingly common and often involves possible deficiences in control of infection procedures. This further emphasises the importance of having well-defined procedures and ensuring that they are implemented by training of staff and audit.

The prevention of infection is one of the requirements for good quality of care of patients and is relevant to all members of staff. Protection of staff from infection is now a major consideration and is backed by health and safety legislation. Hospitals should have an infection control organization which includes an infection control doctor, usually the medical microbiologist in the UK, and one or more infection control nurses, depending on the size of the hospital and the type of patient. These are members of the team who should meet daily or at least several times a week. The infection control committee is an expansion of the team and meets less frequently. It is important for approving policies and programmes, and for making recommendations which have a major financial implication to the Chief Executive. Collaboration with the community is also necessary and the Consultant in Communicable Disease Control (CCDC) should be a member of the infection control committee.

It is obviously necessary, in view of the problems described, for every hospital to have an infection control manual. To produce such a manual is a major task and it is time wasting for every hospital to produce it's own. This manual, originally produced by Dr. Damani and his colleagues for Craigavon hospital, covers all the main policies required in a hospital. It has been expanded to include basic information on the various topics and is now generally applicable to other hospitals in the UK and many other countries. It will be particularly useful in countries or hospitals which are setting up new infection control programmes. However, although national and hospital guidelines are important, individual departments differ and the final decisions should be made by local infection control staff.

This manual contains a wealth of practical advice, a number of useful tables, diagrams, definitions and essential references. The policies are detailed and provide sufficient instructions to carry out individual procedures. Infection control staff will find this manual useful for producing shorter manuals for individual wards. These should be introduced as part of an ongoing educational programme to ensure the manuals are not only read but are followed by nursing and medical staff and administrators. The manual should also be useful in preparing audit programmes. I congratulate Dr. Damani on producing a comprehensive and useful manual of procedures.

G. A. J. Ayliffe
1997

Preface to the Second Edition

A fundamental activity in health care establishments is to continually improve the quality of care and provide a safe working environment. Central to this activity is an effective infection control strategy, which prevents the acquisition of infection within the health care environment.

The second edition of this book has been thoroughly revised and rearranged. Four new chapters *Principles of infection control, Design and maintenance of health care facilities, Epidemiology and biostatistics*, and *Infection control information resources* have been added as I have found that these subjects are especially useful to infection control practitioners.

While revising the book I have made changes that are in keeping with current guidance and the recommendations made by various professional and statutory bodies with an overall intention to provide advice based on current evidence and the fundamental principles of infection control.

The scope of this book is intentionally broad and, whilst it does not attempt to cover all aspects of infection control in detail, it aims to serve as a practical manual on infection control procedures and provide essential information on the most important issues relating to infection control on a day-to-day basis.

Nizam N. Damani
November, 2002

Preface to the First Edition

...by forseeing in a distance, which is only done by men of talents, the evils which arise from them are soon cured; but when, from want of foresight, they are suffered to increase to such a height that they are perceptible to everyone, there is no remedy.

NICCOLÒ MACHIAVELLI

Prevention of infection acquired in the health care setting remains a major goal for all health care personnel because of increased morbidity and mortality for patients. In addition, it utilizes resources that could be used elsewhere in health care.

Studies in the UK, Europe and North America indicate that approximately 10% of patients develop infection whilst in hospital. Evidence in the US suggests that one third of hospital-acquired (nosocomial) infections could be prevented. Therefore financial benefit to the health care provider could be substantial by prevention of such infections.

Although in recent years there have been an increased allocation of resources directed to the problem on infection control services, the resources allocated have been constrained. This is because in the recent years the very nature of the hospital has changed. With the reduction in numbers of beds, the sickest patients have been concentrated in hospital and the throughput of patients has increased. Patients are often subjected to more aggressive diagnostic and therapeutic procedures and a greater number of health care workers (HCWs) are involved in the patient's management. In addition, newer varieties of the microorganisms are responsible for a wider spectrum of nosocomial infection, and bacterial isolates are becoming more resistant to the standard antibiotic therapies.

Although hospital-acquired infection has been worrying health care professionals for many years, more recently it is worrying patients and the public as well. This is due to emerging new pathogens coupled with heightened public awareness caused by AIDS, blood-borne hepatitis (B&C), methicillin-resistant *Staph. aureus* (MRSA), and more recently by *Clostridium difficile*, multidrug resistant tuberculosis (MDR-TB), vancomycin resistant enterococci (VRE) and *E. coli* 0157 making their control more problematic and challenging for infection control personnel world wide.

Until the 1960s, recommendations on the control of infection were subjective, based on personal observations and anecdotes. The art beginning to emerge but the science was lacking. It is only in the past two decades that infection control has been taken as a serious issue although there are still areas where practice is still ritualist and controversial. An attempt has been made in this book to provide practical advice to the HCW on the control of infection based on current scientific knowledge and recommendation from various bodies on prevention and control of infection in the health care setting.

Nizam N. Damani
1997

Acknowledgements

I would like to thank the following people who have made the production of this book possible:

- Dr. Christopher Armstrong, MRCPath, Consultant Microbiologist and Jemima Keyes, Infection Control Nurse, Craigavon Area Hospital for reading the manuscript and making helpful comments.

- Dr. Conall McCaughey, FRCPath, Consultant Virologist, The Royal Hospital Group, Belfast for reviewing Chapter 10 *Blood-borne hepatitis and HIV infections* and Chapter 11 *Protection for health care workers.*

- Dr. John Yarnell, MD, FFPHM, Senior Lecturer in Epidemiology and Public Health, Queen's University, Belfast for reviewing Chapter 5 *Epidemiology and Biostatistics.*

- Linda McAlister for secretarial assistance.

- Gavin Smith of Greenwich Medical Media for seeing the book through completion.

- Finally, I thank my wife Laila and my children Numair and Namiz for their understanding and willingness to accommodate their life to my chaotic schedules.

Contents

Foreword to the Second Edition vii

Foreword to the First Edition ix

Preface to the Second Edition.. xiii

Preface to the First Edition xv

Acknowledgements xvii

Abbreviations.. xxv

Glossary of Infection Control Terms xxvii

1. **Principles of Infection Control** 1
   Chain of Infection 1
   Body's Defense Mechanisms... 6
   Strategies to Control Health Care Associated Infection 7

2. **Administrative Arrangements** 9
   Infection Control Doctor.. 9
   Infection Control Nurse 10
   Infection Control Team 11
   Infection Control Committee 11
   Infection Control Link Nurse 12
   Policies and Procedures Manual 13
   Occupational Health and Safety 13
   Education and Training 13
   Risk Management in Infection Control 14

3. **Design and Maintenance of Health Care Facilities** 17
   Infection Control Risk Assessment 18
   The General Hospital Environment 18
   Patient's Accommodations 19
   Hand Washing Facilities 20
   Isolation Rooms 20
   Operating Theatres 22
   Ventilation and Air-Conditioning... 23

Cooling Towers and Water System 23
Construction, Renovation and Demolition 24

4. **Surveillance and Outbreak Control** 27
    Incidence of Various Nosocomial Infections 27
    Surveillance of Nosocomial Infection 28
    Methods of Surveillance 29
    Management of an Outbreak 30
    Look Back Investigations 35

5. **Epidemiology and Biostatistics** 39
    Cohort Studies 39
    Case-Control Studies 40
    Cross Sectional (Prevalence) Surveys 41
    Measures of Disease Frequency 42
    Measures of Association 43
    Bias and Confounders 44
    Confounders 45
    Biostatistics 46
    Measures of Central Tendency.. 46
    Measures of Dispersion 48
    Hypothesis Testing 49
    Error of Hypothesis Testing 49
    Test of Statistical Significance 49
    The *P* Value 50
    Confidence Intervals 50
    Sensitivity and Specificity 51

6. **Disinfection and Sterilization** 55
    Methods of Decontamination 55
    Risks of Infection from Equipment 57
    Chemical Disinfectants 58
    Chemical Disinfectants and Antiseptics 59
    Disinfection of Flexible Fibreoptic Endoscopes 69
    Environmental Cleaning 73
    Management of Infectious Spills.. 78
    Cleaning and Disinfection of Medical Equipment 78

7. **Isolation Precautions** 95
    Source Isolation 96
    Protective Isolation.. 98
    Practical Issues and Considerations 98
    Appendix I.. 114

8. **Prevention of Infections Caused by Multi-resistant Organisms** 119
    Methicillin Resistant *Staph. aureus* (MRSA)..................................... 121

Vancomycin Resistant Enterococci (VRE) 130

Multi-resistant Gram-negative Bacilli 134

9. **Prevention of Infection Caused by Specific Pathogens** 137

Tuberculosis (TB) 137

Clostridium difficile Infection 147

Legionnaires' Disease 151

Gastrointestinal Infections and Food Poisoning 155

Meningococcal Infections 160

Varicella zoster Virus (VZV) 165

Creutzfeldt-Jakob Disease (CJD) 169

Viral Haemorrhagic Fevers (VHFs) 175

Rabies 179

Infestations with Ectoparasites 180

10. **Blood-borne Hepatitis and Human Immunodeficiency Virus (HIV) Infections** 185

Viral Hepatitis 185

HIV Infection 188

Routes of Transmission 190

Occupational Risks to HCWs 192

Risks to Patients from HCWs 192

Responsibility of HCWs 193

Exposure-Prone Procedures 194

Surgical Procedure 194

Protection of the Newborn 198

Procedure after Death 199

11. **Protection for Health Care Workers** 203

Occupation Health Department 203

Measures to Protect HCWs 204

Management of Sharps Injury 205

Protection Against Tuberculosis 213

Pregnant HCWs 215

12. **Hand Hygiene and Personal Protective Equipment** 227

Personal Protective Equipment 235

13. **Prevention of Surgical Site Infections** 245

Surveillance 245

Microbiology 248

Pre-operative Patient Care 248

Operative Factors 252

Post-operative Factors 256

Other Factors 256

Environmental Cleaning of Operating Theatre 257

14.   **Prevention of Infection Associated with Intravenous Therapy** 261
      Sources of Infection 261
      Pathogenesis of Infection 262
      Education and Training 263
      Monitoring and Surveillance of Catheter-Related Infection 263
      Intravascular Catheters and Parenteral Solutions 264
      Selection of Catheter Type 264
      Selection of Insertion Site 265
      Aseptic Techniques 265
      Catheter Site Dressing Regimens 268
      In-line Filters 268
      Antimicrobial Prophylaxis 269
      Anticoagulant Flush Solutions 269
      Replacement of Intravascular Set, Tubings and
      Parenteral Fluids 269
      Replacement of Catheters 269
      Guidewire Exchange 270
      Catheter-Related Infections 270
      Device Reprocessing 270

15.   **Prevention of Infections Associated with Urinary
      Catheterization** 273
      Consideration Prior to Catheterization 273
      Maintenance of Catheter 274
      Removal of Catheter 278
      Use of Antimicrobial Agents 278
      Policy and Staff Training 279
      Re-use of Catheters 279

16.   **Prevention of Nosocomial Pneumonia** 283
      Pathogenesis 283
      Strategy for Prevention 285

17.   **Hospital Support Services** 291
      Food and Catering Service 291
      Staff Health/Hygiene 292
      Cook-chill Food Production Systems 292
      Texture Modified Products 293
      Food Trolleys 293
      Refrigerators 294
      Inspection 294
      Food Handlers 294
      Hospital Kitchen 294
      Ward Kitchens 295
      Ice Machines 295

Linen and Laundry Service 298

    General Principles to Prevent Infection 298

    Laundry Process 299

    Microbiological Sampling 300

    Staff Uniforms 300

    Mattresses and Pillows 301

    Air-fluidized Beds 301

Management of Clinical Waste 303

    Definition and Categorization of Clinical Waste 303

    Methods for Safe Handling of Clinical Waste........................... 304

    Methods for Safe Use, Handling and Disposal of Sharps 305

    Management and Disposal of Clinical Waste 308

Pest Control... 312

18. **Infection Control Information Resources** 315

    Internet Resources 315

    Books 317

    Computer Software... 321

Index 323

Abbreviations

AAFB	Acid and Alcohol Fast Bacilli		GRE	Glycopeptide resistant Enterococci
ACDP	Advisory Committee on Dangerous Pathogens		GISA	Glycopeptide resistant *Staphylococcus aureus*
A & E	Accident and Emergency Department		HAV	Hepatitis A Virus
AIDS	Acquired Immune Deficiency Syndrome		HBIG	Hepatitis B Immunoglobulin
			HBeAg	Hepatitis B e antigen
AZT	Azidothymidine (Zidovudine)		HBsAg	Hepatitis B surface antigen
			HBV	Hepatitis B Virus
BS	British Standard		HC	Health Circular
BBV	Blood-borne Viruses		HCV	Hepatitis C Virus
BSE	Bovine Spongiform Encephalopathies		HCW	Health Care Worker
CDC	Centers for Disease Control and Prevention		HEPA	High efficiency particulate air
CDSC	Communicable Disease Surveillance Centre		HEV	Hepatitis E Virus
			HIV	Human Immunodeficiency Virus
CFU	Colony forming units		HMSO	Her Majesty's Stationery Office
CI	Confidence Interval			
CJD	Creutzfeldt-Jakob Disease		HN	Health Notice
DHSS	Department of Health and Social Services		HSE	Health and Safety Executive
DoH	Department of Health		IV	Intravenous
EIA	Enzyme Immuno Assay		ICC	Infection Control Committee
ELISA	Enzyme Linked Immunosorbent Assay		ICD	Infection Control Doctor
ERCP	Endoscopic retrograde cholangiopancreatography		ICN	Infection Control Nurse
			ICT	Infection Control Team

ICU	Intensive Care Unit	RIBA	Recombinant immunoblot assay
MDA	Medical Device Agency		
MDR-TB	Multi-drug resistant Tuberculosis	SCBU	Special Care Baby Unit
		SSD	Sterile Supply Department
MRSA	Methicillin-resistant *Staphylococcus aureus*	SSI	Surgical Site Infection
		TB	Tuberculosis
NaDCC	Sodium Dichloroisocyanurate	UTI	Urinary Tract Infection
NNIS	National Nosocomial Surveillance System	vCJD	New variant Creutzfeldt-Jakob Disease
OPA	Orthophthaladehyde	VHFs	Viral Haemorrhagic Fevers
PCR	Polymerase Chain Reaction	VISA	Vancomycin resistant *Staphylococcus aureus*
PHLS	Public Health Laboratory Service		
		VRE	Vancomycin resistant Enterococci
ppm av Cl$_2$	Parts per million of available chlorine		
		VZIG	Varicella Zoster Immunoglobulin
QAC	Quaternary Ammonium Compound	WHO	World Health Organization

Glossary of Infection Control Terms

ANTISEPSIS

The destruction or inhibition of microorganisms on living tissues having the effect of limiting or preventing the harmful results of infection.

ANTISEPTIC

A chemical agent used in antisepsis.

CARRIER

A person (host) who harbours a microorganism (agent) in the absence of discernible clinical disease. Carriers may shed organisms into environment intermittently or continuously and therefore act as a potential source of infection.

CASE

A person with symptoms.

CHEMOPROPHYLAXIS

The administration of antimicrobial agents to prevent the development of an infection or the progression of an infection to active manifest disease.

COHORT

A group of patients infected or colonized with same microorganism, grouped together in a designated area of a unit or ward.

COLONIZATION

The presence of microorganisms at a body site(s) without presence of symptoms or clinical manifestations of illness or infection. Colonization may be a form of carriage and is a potential method of transmission.

COMMENSAL

A microorganism resident in or on a body site without causing clinical infection.

COMMUNICABLE PERIOD

The time in the natural history of an infection during which transmission may take place.

CONTACT — An exposed individual who might have been infected through transmission from another host or the environment.

CONTAMINATION — The presence of microorganisms on a surface or in a fluid or material.

DISINFECTANT — A chemical agent which under defined conditions is capable of disinfection.

ENDEMIC — The usual level or presence of an agent or disease in a defined population during a given period.

ENDOGENOUS INFECTION — Microorganisms originating from the patient's own body which cause harm in another body site.

EPIDEMIC — An unusual, higher than expected level of infection or disease by a common agent in a defined population in a given period.

EPIDEMIOLOGY — The study of the occurrence and cause of disease in populations.

EXOGENOUS INFECTION — Microorganisms originating from a source or reservoir which are transmitted by any mechanism to a person, i.e. contact, airborne routes etc.

FLORA — Microorganisms resident in an environmental or body site.

HOSPITAL-ACQUIRED INFECTION (*Nosocomial infection*) — Infection acquired during hospitalization; not present or incubating at the time of admission to hospital.

IMMUNITY — The resistance of a host to a specific infectious agent.

IMMUNOCOMPROMISED — A state of reduced resistance to infection that results from malignant disease, drugs, radiation illness or congenital defect.

INCIDENCE — The number of new cases of a disease (or event) occurring in a specified time.

INCIDENCE RATE — The ratio of the number of new infections or disease in a defined population in a given period to the number of individuals at risk in the population.

INCUBATION PERIOD	The time interval between initial exposure to the infectious agent and the appearance of the first sign or symptoms of the disease in a susceptible host.
INDEX CASE	The first case to be recognized in a series of transmissions of an agent in a host population.
INFECTION	The damaging of body tissue by microorganisms or by poisonous substances released by the microorganisms.
ISOLATION	The physical separation of an infected or colonized host from the remainder of the at risk population in an attempt to prevent transmission of the specific agent to other individuals and patients.
MICROBIOLOGICAL CLEARANCE	The reduction of the number of pathogenic microorganisms in a specimen below that detectable by conventional means.
MICROORGANISM	A microscopic entity capable of replication. It includes bacteria, viruses and the microscopic forms of algae, fungi and protozoa.
OUTBREAK	An outbreak may be defined as the occurrence of disease at a rate greater than that expected within a specific geographical area and over a defined period of time.
PATHOGEN	A microorganism capable of producing disease.
PATHOGENICITY	The ability of an infectious agent to cause disease in a susceptible host.
PREVALENCE RATE	The ratio of the total number of individuals who have a disease at a particular time to the population at risk of having the disease.
RESERVOIR	Any animate or inanimate focus in the environment in which an infectious agent may survive and multiply which may act as a potential source of infection.
SEROCONVERSION	The development of antibodies not previously present resulting from a primary infection.
SOURCE	Place where microorganisms are growing or have grown.

SPORADIC CASE	A single case which has not apparently been associated with other cases, excreters or carriers in the same period of time.
STERILE	Free from all living microorganisms.
STERILIZATION	A process which renders an item sterile.
STERILIZING AGENT (*Sterilant*)	An agent or combination of agents which under defined conditions leads to sterilization.
SURVEILLANCE	A systematic collection, analysis, and interpretation of data on specific events (infections) and disease, followed by dissemination of that information to those who can improve the outcomes.
SUSCEPTIBLE	A person presumably not possessing sufficient resistance (or immunity) against a pathogenic agent who contracts infection when exposed to the agent.
TRANSMISSION	The method by which any potentially infecting agent is spread to another host.
VIRULENCE	The intrinsic capabilities of a microorganism to infect host and produce disease.
ZOONOSIS	An infectious disease transmissible from vertebrate animals to humans.

Principles of
Infection Control

Hospitalized patients are more prone to develop infection as a result of surgery, invasive procedures and devices, immunosuppressive drugs, organ transplants etc. In addition, microorganisms flourish in health care setting and with breaks in infection control procedures and practices, along with patient's weakened defense mechanisms, help set the stage for nosocomial infections. Nosocomial infections lengthen patients' hospital stays and increase both morbidity and mortality. In addition, diagnosing and treating these infections puts intense pressure on the health services and health care budget.

Chain of infection

In order to control or prevent infection it is essential to understand that transmission of a pathogen resulting in colonization or infection requires the following six vital links (Fig. 1.1):

1. Causative agent
2. Infectious reservoir
3. Portal of exit from the reservoir
4. Mode of transmission
5. Portal of entry into the host
6. Susceptible host

Each link must be present for infection or colonization to proceed, and breaking any of the links can prevent the infection. The aim of isolation precautions is to interrupt these links.

1. Causative agent

The causative agent for infection is any microorganism capable of producing disease. Microorganisms responsible for infectious diseases include bacteria, viruses,

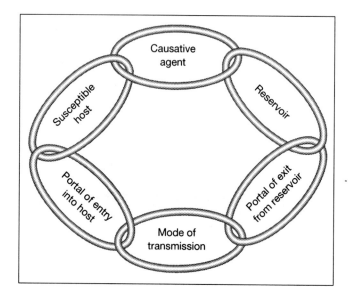

Figure 1.1 Figure showing chain of infection. An infection can occur only if the six components shown here are present. Removing any one link breaks the chain and prevents infection.

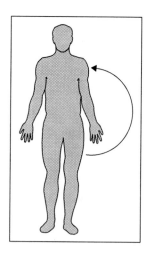

Figure 1.2 Endogenous or auto-infection where infection occurs from the patients' own colonizing microorganisms.

rickettsiae, fungi, and protozoa. Sometimes, microorganisms are part of patient's own body flora and can cause infection in the immunocompromised host. These infections are called *endogenous infections* (Fig. 1.2). Infections which are acquired from external sources are called *exogenous infections* (Fig. 1.3).

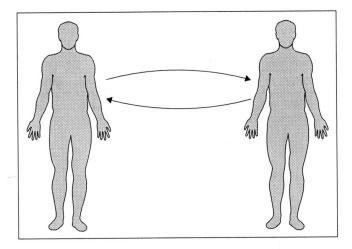

Figure 1.3 Exogenous or cross-infection where an infection occurs from an infected or colonized patient to other patients, health care workers and visitors or vice versa.

2. Reservoir of infection

The second link in the chain of infection is the reservoir, i.e. the environment or object in or on which a microorganism can survive and, in some cases, multiply. Inanimate objects, human beings, and animals can all serve as reservoirs, providing the essential requirements for a microorganism to survive at specific stages in its life cycle. *Pseudomonas* spp. survive and multiply in nebulizers and the hepatitis B virus (HBV) survives but does not multiply on the surface of haemodialysis machines.

Infectious reservoirs abound in health care settings, and may include everything from patients, visitors, and staff members to furniture, medical equipment, medications, food, water, and blood.

A human reservoir may be either a case or a carrier. A case is a patient with an acute clinical infection while a carrier is a person who is colonized with a specific pathogenic microorganism but shows no signs or symptoms of infection. A carrier may have a subclinical or asymptomatic infection, e.g. Hepatitis B virus.

Carriers fall into four categories: An *incubatory carrier* is one who has acquired the infection and has been incubating the illness but does not yet show symptoms. Incubation periods vary from one infectious disease to other (see page 114). A *convalescent carrier* is in the recovery stage of an illness but continues to shed the pathogenic microorganism for an indefinite period, e.g. a patient who has had a Salmonella infection commonly sheds the organism in his faeces even after symptoms disappear. An *intermittent carrier* occasionally sheds the pathogenic microorganism from time to time, e.g. some people are intermittent carriers of *Staphylococcus aureus*. A *chronic*

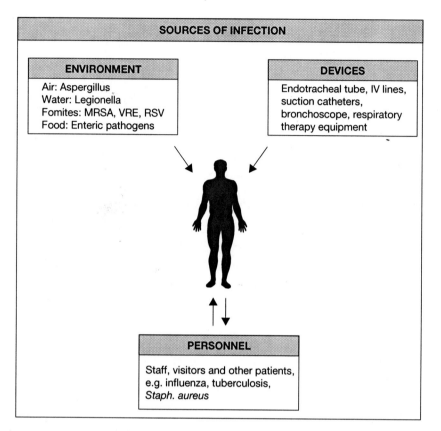

Figure 1.4 Summary of the modes by which various nosocomial infections are transmitted.

carrier always has the infectious organism in his system, e.g. chronic carriers of hepatitis B virus.

Carriers (especially when asymptomatic) may present a risk of transmission to susceptible patients in health care facilities because their illnesses go unrecognized and they and those around them are unlikely to take appropriate precautions against infection.

3. Portal of exit

The portal of exit is the path by which an infectious agent leaves its reservoir. Usually, this portal is the site where the microorganism grows. Common portals of exit associated with human reservoirs include the respiratory, genitourinary, and gastrointestinal tracts, the skin and mucous membranes and the placenta (transmission from mother to fetus).

4. Mode of transmission

The microorganism can be acquired by inhalation (through respiratory tract), ingestion (through gastrointestinal tract), inoculation (through accidental sharp injury or bites), contact (during sexual intercourse) and transplacental transmission (microbes may cross placenta from the mother to fetus). It is important to remember that *some microorganisms use more than one transmission route* to get from the reservoir to a new host.

Of the six links in the chain of infection, the mode of transmission is the easiest link to break and is key to control of cross-infection in hospitals.

Contact transmission: Contact is the most common mode of transmission of infection in the health care settings. Contact transmission may be subdivided into direct contact, indirect contact, and contact with droplets that enter the environment.

Direct contact: Direct contact refers to person-to-person spread of microorganisms through actual physical contact. Microorganisms with a direct mode of transmission can be transferred during such patient care activities as bathing, dressing changes, and insertion of invasive devices if the hands or gloves of health care worker (HCW) are contaminated. Diseases that spread by direct contact include scabies and herpes simplex (if direct contact with infected oral lesions or secretions occurs). *Handwashing is the most effective way to prevent transmission by the contact route.*

Indirect contact: Indirect contact occurs when a susceptible person comes in contact with a contaminated object. In health care settings, virtually any item could be contaminated with certain microorganisms, e.g. endoscopes, respiratory equipment, etc. Thorough cleaning, disinfection, and sterilization are essential in the health care setting to prevent nosocomial infection acquired from contaminated items and equipment.

Droplet transmission: Droplet transmission results from contact with contaminated respiratory secretions. A person with a droplet-spread infection coughs, sneezes, or talks, releasing infected secretions that spread through the air to the oral or nasal mucous membranes of a person nearby. Microbes in droplet nuclei (mucus droplets) can travel up to about 3 ft (1 m). Droplet transmission differs from airborne transmission in that the droplets don't remain suspended in the air but settle on surfaces. Examples of diseases spread by droplets include influenza, whooping cough, etc.

Airborne transmission: Airborne transmission occurs when fine microbial particles or dust particles containing pathogens remain suspended in the air for a prolonged period, and then are spread widely by air currents and inhaled. The tiny particles remain suspended in the air for several hours and may cause infection when a susceptible person inhales them. Examples of diseases spread by the airborne include pulmonary tuberculosis, varicella, and measles.

5. Portal of entry

The portal of entry is the path by which an infectious agent invades a susceptible host. Usually, this path is the same as the portal of exit. For example, the portal of entry for tuberculosis and diphtheria is through the respiratory tract, hepatitis B and Human Immunodeficiency Virus enter through the bloodstream or body fluids and Salmonella enters through the gastrointestinal tract. In addition, each invasive device, e.g. intravenous line, creates an additional portal of entry into a patient's body thus increasing the chance of developing an infection.

6. Susceptible host

The final link in the chain of infection is the susceptible host. The human body has many defense mechanisms for resisting the entry and multiplication of pathogens. When these mechanisms function normally, infection does not occur. However, in immunocompromised patients, where the body defenses are weakened, infectious agents are more likely to invade the body and cause an infectious disease. In addition, the very young and the very old are at higher risk for infection because in the very young the immune system does not fully develop until about age 6 months, while old age is associated with declining immune system function as well as with chronic diseases that weaken host defenses.

Body's defense mechanisms

The body's defense mechanisms fall into two general categories:

First line of defense: External and mechanical barriers such as the skin, other body organs, and secretions serve as the body's first line of defense. Intact skin, mucous membranes, certain chemical substances, specialized structures such as cilia, and normal flora can stop pathogens from establishing themselves in the body. The gag and cough reflexes and gastrointestinal tract peristalsis work to remove pathogens before they can establish a foothold. Chemical substances that help prevent infection or inhibit microbial growth include secretions such as saliva, perspiration, and gastrointestinal and vaginal secretions as well as interferon (a naturally occurring glycoprotein with antiviral properties). Normal microbial flora controls the growth of potential pathogens through a mechanism called microbial antagonism. In this mechanism, they use nutrients that pathogens need for growth, compete with pathogens for sites on tissue receptors and secrete naturally occurring antibiotics to kill the pathogens. When microbial antagonism is disturbed, such as by prolonged antibiotic therapy, an infection may develop; for example, antibiotic therapy may destroy the normal flora of the mouth, leading to overgrowth of *Candida albicans* and consequent thrush.

Second line of defense: If a microorganism gets past the first line of defense by entering the body through a break in the skin, white blood cells and the inflammatory response come into play. Because these components respond to any type of injury, their response is termed non-specific. The main function of the inflammatory response is to bring phagocytic cells (neutrophils and monocytes) to the inflamed area to destroy microorganisms.

If a pathogen gets past non-specific defenses, it confronts specific immune responses, cell-mediated immunity or humoral immunity. Cell-mediated immunity involves T cells. Some T cells synthesize and secrete lymphokines. Others become killer (cytotoxic) cells, setting out to track down infected body cells. Once the infection is under control, suppresser T cells bring the immune response to a close. Humoral immunity, mediated by antibodies, involves the action of B lymphocytes in conjunction with helper T cells. Antibodies produced in response to the infectious agent help fight the infection. In response to the effects of suppressor T cell activity antibody production then wanes. Impaired host defenses make patients more susceptible to infection. Conditions that may weaken a person's defenses include malnutrition, extremes of age, inherited and acquired immune deficiencies, chronic disease, immunosuppressive therapy, surgery and inadequate immunization.

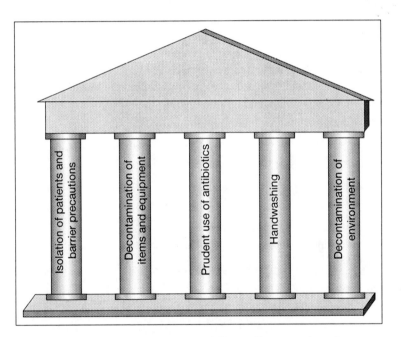

Figure 1.5 Five pillars of infection control. Surveillance and audit are essential tools to monitor the effectiveness of the programme.

Strategies to control health care associated infection

Strategies to control and prevent nosocomial infection fall into three main categories:

• Control *or* elimination of infectious agents

- Control of transmission
- Reservoir control

Control or elimination of the infectious agent: This is achieved by placing patients with suspected or proven infectious diseases under source isolation and applying barrier precautions. Infectious agents can be controlled or eliminated by effective disinfection and sterilization of items and equipments and thorough cleaning of the environment. This helps reduce the bioburden of microorganisms in health care facilities.

Control of transmission: This can be effectively achieved by handwashing, aseptic techniques and control of the health care environment. Proper handwashing has been shown to be effective in preventing the spread of infection. Basic aseptic technique must be practiced for sterile procedures e.g. insertion of intravenous lines and urinary catheters. Effective decontamination and control of the environment (e.g. mechanical ventilation) is essential to control transmission of microorganisms.

Reservoir control: Almost any piece of equipment used in health care facilities may harbour microorganisms and therefore act as a reservoir (e.g. respiratory therapy equipment and ventilator circuits, bedpans, urinals, bed linen etc). Interventions directed at controlling or destroying infectious reservoirs in health care facilities include using either disposable equipment or decontaminating equipment as soon as possible after use. In addition, both patients and health care workers may also act as reservoirs of infection. Identifying and treating these individuals will reduce the reservoirs and help prevent cross-infection.

References and further reading

Chin J. *Control of communicable disease manual*, 17th edn. Washington: American Public Health Association, 2000.

Garner J. The Hospital Infection Control Practice Advisory Committee. Guidelines for Isolation Precautions in Hospitals. *American Journal of Infection Control* 1996; **24**: 24–52.

Mims C, Nash A, Stephen J. *Mims' Pathogenesis of Infectious Disease*, 5th edn. London: Academic Press, 2000.

2

Administrative Arrangements

The provision of an effective infection control programme is a key to the quality and a reflection of the overall standard of care provided by that health care institution. Although the organization of an infection control programme varies from countries to countries depending on the available resources, in the majority of the countries the infection control programme is delivered through an Infection Control Team (ICT). The ICT is not only responsible for the day-to-day running of the infection control programme but is also responsible for setting priorities, applying evidence-based practice and advising hospital administrators on issues relating to infection control.

It is the responsibility of hospital administrator to ensure that adequate resources are given to infection control department. He/she should also managerially ensure that full support is afforded to the ICT so that agreed infection control programmes are implemented effectively.

Infection Control Doctor (ICD)

The ICD must be a registered medical practitioner. In the majority of countries, the role is performed either by a medical microbiologist or hospital epidemiologist. Hospital consultants in other disciplines (e.g. infectious diseases) may be appointed. Irrespective of their professional background, the ICD should have knowledge and experience in asepsis, hospital epidemiology, infectious disease, microbiology, sterilization and disinfection, and surveillance. It is recommended that one ICD is required for every 1,000 beds. The role and responsibilities of the ICD are summarized as follows:

- Serves as a specialist advisor and takes a leading role in the effective functioning of the ICT.

- Should be an active member of the hospital Infection Control Committee (ICC) and may act as its Chairman.

- Assists the hospital ICC in drawing up annual plans, policies and long-term programmes for the prevention of hospital infection.

- Advises the chief executive/hospital administrator directly on all aspects of infection control in the hospital and on the implementation of agreed policies.

- Participates in the preparation of tender documents for the support services and advises on infection control aspects.

- Is involved in setting quality standards, surveillance and audit with regard to hospital infection.

Infection Control Nurse (ICN)

An Infection Control Nurse or Practitioner is a registered nurse with an additional academic education and practical training which enables him or her to act as a specialist advisor in all matters relating to infection control. A recognized qualification in infection control should be held which will allow recognition of the ICN as a specialist practitioner.

The ICN is usually the only full-time practitioner in the ICT and therefore takes the key role in day-to-day infection control activities, with the ICD providing the lead role. It is recommended that one Infection Control Nurse is required for every 250 occupied beds. The role and responsibility of the ICN is summarized as follows:

- Serves as a specialist advisor and takes a leading role in the effective functioning of the ICT.

- Should be an active member of the hospital ICC.

- Assists the hospital ICC in drawing up annual plans and policies for infection control.

- Provides specialist nursing input in the identification, prevention, monitoring, and control of infection within the hospital.

- Participate in surveillance, investigation, and control of infection in the hospital.

- Identify, investigate and monitor infections, hazardous practice and procedures.

- Advice to the contracting departments, participating in the preparation of documents relating to service specifications and quality standards.

- Ongoing contribution to the development and implementation of infection control policy and procedure, participating in audit, and monitoring tools related to infection control and infectious diseases.

- Presentation of educational programmes and membership of relevant committees where infection control input is required.

It is essential that the ICN should have an expert knowledge of both general and specialist nursing practice and must also have an understanding not only of the functioning of clinical areas but also operational areas and services. He or she must also be able to communicate effectively with all grades of staff, negotiate and effect change, and influence practice.

Infection Control Team (ICT)

The ICT comprises the ICD and ICN. The ICT is responsible for the day-to-day running of infection control programmes. It is important that all acute hospitals should have an ICT, although smaller health care providers may not find this a viable option. In cases where the provision of an ICT is not practical, arrangements for the provision of and access to the infection control service should be arranged with nearby acute hospital.

The role of the ICT is to ensure that an effective infection control programme has been planned, co-ordinate its implementation, and evaluate the impact of such measures. Whilst they will actively participate in most of these areas, some aspects of the infection control programme may fall under the remit of others. In such cases the ICT will provide advice and direction, ultimately ensuring that all tasks reach completion. It is important to ensure that there is provision made for 24-hour access to the ICT for advice on infection prevention and control of infection, which would include both medical and nursing advice. The role of the ICT can be summarized as follows:

- Production of an annual infection control programme with clearly defined objectives.
- Production of written policies and procedures on infection control, including regular evaluation and update.
- Education of all grades of staff in infection control policy, practice and procedures relevant to their own area of practice.
- Surveillance of infection to detect outbreaks at the earliest opportunity and provide data that should be evaluated to allow for any change in practice or allocation of resource to prevent hospital-acquired infections.
- Provide advice to all grades of staff on all matters in relation to infection prevention and control on a day-to-day basis.
- Participate in the audit activity.

Infection Control Committee (ICC)

The hospital ICC is charged with the responsibility for the planning, evaluation of evidence-based practice and implementation, prioritization, and resource allocation of all matters relating to infection control.

The membership of the hospital ICCs should reflect the spectrum of clinical services and administrative arrangements of the health care establishment so that policy decisions take account of implementation issues. As a minimum, the committee should include:

- ICD or Hospital Epidemiologist who may act as a chairperson.

- Infection Control Nurse/Practitioner.

- Infectious Diseases Physician (if available).

- Chief executive or hospital administrator or his or her nominated representative.

- Director of Nursing or his/her representative.

- Occupational Health Physician or a representative.

- Representative from the major clinical specialties.

In addition in the UK, a Consultant in Communicable Disease Control should be included. Large institutions or those operating on multiple sites may need to enlarge this membership to ensure that all aspects of clinical service are adequately represented. Additionally, representatives of any other department may be invited as necessary. The ICC should meet regularly according to local need. A minimum of two planned meetings a year is recommended.

The function of local ICC is that of supporting the development of an effective infection control programme. The committee should discuss routine surveillance reports from the ICT, outbreaks of nosocomial infection, needle stick injury incidents, health care worker immunization and education, purchasing of equipment, etc. In addition, it is important that the members of the committee voice areas of concern including any problems relating to either infection control practice or policy, in particular highlighting areas which have not been addressed within their own sphere of responsibility.

Infection control link nurse

One effective way of developing infection control education and operational support can be through the development of a link system. It has been shown that competent infection control link nurses can motivate ward staff by enabling more effective practice. Sustained, consistent and senior management backing and interest are effective in supporting such link programmes and is essential in ensuring their success.

However, high staff turnover rates, adequate training time and recognition, the requirement for the ICT to monitor the link programmes are all resource pressures inherent in such schemes.

Policies and procedures manual

It is essential that each health care establishment should develop a manual of policies and procedures in infection control. The procedure manual should establish standards for performance in all aspects of infection control. The recommendations in the manual must be based on the relevant national guidelines. They should be practical, workable, necessary and sufficiently flexible to ensure their implementation. Policies and procedures should identify infection control indicators and desired outcomes. They should also include some basis for the risk assessment of each procedure.

A comprehensive procedures manual should include policy and procedures on:

- Cleaning and decontamination of surfaces and equipment.
- Procedures for isolation of patients.
- Management of spills or accidents with infectious substances.
- Hygiene and hand washing procedures.
- Use of protective clothing and equipment.
- Safe handling and transport of pathology specimens.
- Handling and cleaning of contaminated linen.
- Handling and disposal of clinical and related waste.
- Handling and disposal of sharps.
- Management of sharps injuries.

The infection control manual must be updated on regular basis. Staff should be informed of changes to current policy and procedures, as well as the introduction of new ones. New policies should be carefully monitored and should include HCWs feedback, with appropriate responses. The manual should be easily accessible and readily available to all HCWs.

Occupational health and safety

Employers have a responsibility to provide a safe work environment without risk to the health of their employees. In the health care setting, it is essential that *all* HCWs must be given adequate education and training on all issues relating to the control of infection. In addition, *employees also have a responsibility to comply with safety standards and procedures set by health care establishments*, and should ensure that their work practices do not jeopardize the health and safety of themselves or any other person.

Education and training

Managers of all health care establishments must ensure that all HCWs should be made aware of the importance and principles of infection control. They should also emphasize the importance of continuing education and training for all HCWs. New employees should be offered an orientation and induction programme to increase their awareness and to assist in their understanding of the institutional policies and programmes for infection control. Education and training programmes should be flexible enough to encourage participation.

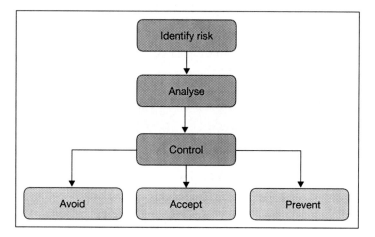

Figure 2.1 Principles of risk management.

Risk management in infection control

The purpose of risk management is to minimize exposure of health care workers, patient and visitors to sources of infection. The *primary aim of risk management is to be pro-active in the reduction of risks to the lowest level that is reasonably practicable.*

A practical approach to infection control risk management can be achieved by devising a structured care plan for each individual patient who is at risk from acquiring an infection and/or is a source of risk to others. This should be done using a formal cyclical process considering of the following:

Identification: Identification of activities and tasks that put patients and employees at risk of infection, the type of infectious agent involved, route of infection and the evidence that the disease can be spread this way.

Analysis: Analysis of the risk or problem e.g. evaluation of the infective dose of the infectious agent and the relationship between the dose received and the severity of the infection. In addition, analyse why they are happening – the possible causes could be inadequate knowledge, inadequate equipment, lack of motivation or lack of management reinforcement. Determine how often they are happening and do a cost benefit analysis.

Control: Think of the best possible solution and how the risk can be eliminated or minimized. If this is not possible can you accept the risk?

When the most suitable control method is implemented, it is essential that the corrective action should be evaluated and monitored by audit procedures. This approach can also be used for hazards or risks that arise from the environment or equipment, as well as patient-related risks.

References and further reading

Association of Medical Microbiologists, Hospital Infection Society, Infection Control Nurses Association and Public Health Laboratory Services. The Infection Control Standards Working Party. *Standards in Infection Control in Hospitals*. London: HMSO, 1993.

Astagneaue P, Brücker G. Organization of hospital-acquired infection control in France. *Journal of Hospital Infection* 2001; **47**: 84–87.

Barrett SP. Infection control in Britain. *Journal of Hospital Infection* 2002; **50**: 1106–1109.

Bassetti M, Topal J, Di Biagion A, Salvalaggio P, Basadonna GP, Bassetti D. The organization of infection control in Italy. *Journal of Hospital Infection* 2001; **48**: 83–85.

Daschner F. Cost-effectiveness in hospital infection control – lessons for the 1990s. *Journal of Hospital Infection* 1989; **3**: 325.

Department of Health and Public Health Laboratory Services. *Hospital Infection Control: Guidance on the control of infection in hospitals* (The Cooke Report). London: Department of Health, 1995.

Department of Health and Public Health Medicine Environmental Group. *Guidelines on the Control of Infection in Residential and Nursing Homes*. London: DoH, 1996.

Farrington M, Pascoe G. Risk management and infection control – time to get our priorities right in the United Kingdom. *Journal of Hospital Infection* 2001; **47**: 19–24.

Frank U, Gastmeier P, Rüden H, Daschner FD. The organization of infection control in Germany. *Journal of Hospital Infection* 2001; **49**: 9–13.

Hryniewicz W, Grzesiowski P, Ozoroowski T. Hospital infection control in Poland. *Journal of Hospital Infection* 2001; **49**: 94–98.

Huskins WC, Soule B. Infection control in countries with limited resources. *Current Opinion in Infectious Diseases* 1998; **11**: 449–455.

Jenner EA, Wilson JA. Educating the infection control team – past, present and future. A British perspective. *Journal of Hospital Infection* 2000; **46**: 96–105.

Jepsen OB. Infection control in Danish healthcare: organization and practice. *Journal of Hospital Infection* 2001; **47**: 262–265.

Leblebicioglu H, Unal S. The organization of hospital infection control in Turkey. *Journal of Hospital Infection* 2002; **51**: 1–6.

Lim VKE. Hospital infection control in Malaysia. *Journal of Hospital Infection* 2001; **48**: 177–179.

Melo-Cristino J, Marques-Lito L, Pina E. The control of hospital infection in Portugal. *Journal of Hospital Infection* 2002; **51**: 85–88.

Millward S, Barnett J, Thomlinson D. A clinical infection control audit programme: evaluation of an audit tool used by infection control nurses to monitor standards and assess effective staff training. *Journal of Hospital Infection* 1993; **24**: 219–232.

National Audit Office. *The management and control of hospital acquired infection in acute NHS Trusts in England.* London: The Stationary Office, 2000.

Plowman R, Graves N, Griffin N, *et al. Socioeconomic burden of hospital acquired infection.* London: Public Health Laboratories Services, 2000.

Ponce-de-Leon S. The needs of developing countries and the resources required. *Journal of Hospital Infection* 1991; **18** (Suppl. A): 376–381.

Reybrouck G, Vande Putte M, Zumofen M, Haxhe JJ. The organization of infection control in Belgium. *Journal of Hospital Infection* 2001; **47**: 32–35.

Rodriguez-Bano, Pascual A. Hospital infection control in Spain. *Journal of Hospital Infection* 2001; **48**: 258–260.

Scheckler WE, Brimhall D, Buck AS, *et al.* Requirements for infrastructure and essential activities of infection control and epidemiology in hospitals: A consensus panel report. *Infection Control Hospital Epidemiology.* 1998; **19**: 114–124.

Scottish Infection Manual. *Guidance on core standards for the control of infection in hospitals, health care premises and the community interface.* Published by the Scottish Executive, 1998.

Smith PW, Rusnak PG. Infection prevention and control in the long-term-care facility. *Infection Control Hospital Epidemiology* 1997; **18**: 831–849.

Sobayo EI. Nursing aspects of infection control in developing countries. *Journal of Hospital Infection* 1991; **18** (Suppl. A): 388–391.

Stone PW, Larson E, Kawar LN. A systematic audit of economic evidence linking nosocomial infections and infection control interventions. *American Journal of Infection Control* 2002; **30**: 145–152.

Teare EL, Peacock A. The development of infection control link nurse programme in a district general hospital. *Journal of Hospital Infection* 1996; **34**: 267–278.

UK Department of Health. *Risk Management in the NHS.* London: DoH, 1993.

Ward KA. Education and infection control audit. *Journal of Hospital Infection* 1995; **30** (Suppl.): 248.

Worssley MA. Nursing priorities and the contribution of the International Federation of Infection Control. *Journal of Hospital Infection* 1991; **18** (Suppl. A): 392–396.

Wright J, Stover BH, Wilkerson S, Bratcher D. Expanding the infection control team: development of the infection control liaison position for the neonatal intensive care unit. *American Journal of Infection Control* 2002; **30**: 174–178.

3

Design and Maintenance of Health Care Facilities

The provision of a safe environment within health care premises is a statutory obligation and must be part of the risk management strategy of hospital. The environment in which patients are nursed must be designed to reduce the risks of transmission of infection to a minimum.

Advances in medical treatment have changed the types of patients being admitted to hospital. Currently patients with impaired host defenses represent an increasing proportion of admissions to hospital and to reflect that, the design of health care facilities has undergone substantial changes. From an infection control perspective, the primary objective of hospital design should be to ensure that patients, especially immunocompromised ones, are at no greater risk of infection within the hospital than outside. Microbial flora of a health care facility can be influenced by its design and the Infection Control Team (ICT) plays a major role in this.

It is essential that the *ICT must be involved in the design, construction and commissioning of any new or upgraded building at an early stage.* Equally important is the engagement of the ICT when major decommissioning or demolition work is being planned as such situations can represent a threat to patient safety through the heavy release of microorganisms, particularly fungi, into the air. Therefore input from the ICT at the planning stage and through the entire life of the project is essential to ensure that the new health care premises meet with infection control requirements. Early involvement of the ICT in the process is essential to identify potential infection control issues early and provides an opportunity to design solutions prospectively. The ICT also play an important role in educating architects, engineers and construction workers about potential infection control risks and appropriate methods for reducing them, as they are the only personnel from a clinical background working on construction project. It is also important that the ICT should visit the construction site on a regular basis to ensure that agreed plans are been adequately implemented. It is the responsibility of the hospital administrator to ensure that the policies and procedures set forth by the ICT are incorporated into the contract.

Infection control risk assessment

The association between construction and the development of aspergillosis in immunocompromised patients and the association between hospitalization and legionellosis have been known for decades. Therefore it is essential that as part of the planning process for renovation and constructing of a health care facility, an infection control risk assessment should be conducted to determine the potential risk of transmission of microorganisms within the hospital. In general, the risks can be categorized as infections transmitted by air, water, or the environment.

The general hospital environment

Functional design of health care facilities should allow routine cleaning to be carried out efficiently. Surfaces, including walls, must be smooth, easy to clean and protected from damage. Unnecessary horizontal, textured and moisture-retaining surfaces, or inaccessible areas where moisture or soil will accumulate, should be avoided if possible. Where possible, all surfaces should be smooth and impervious.

To prevent dust accumulation, cupboards rather than shelves are recommended and cupboard doors should be easily washable. Consideration must be given to the design of radiators and other fixed or relatively immovable items, e.g. computer stations and their wiring, to ensure that all surfaces are accessible for cleaning. When furnishings and fittings are being selected, they must be assessed against their potential exposure to disinfectants, and finishes durable enough to withstand the appropriate cleaning of the hospital environment should be chosen. Items intended for domestic use are frequently inappropriate for the hospital setting. In equipment-processing areas, work surfaces should be nonporous, smooth and easily cleaned.

Walls and ceilings: Ideally, walls and ceilings should have a smooth, impervious surface that is easy to clean with minimal likelihood of dust accumulation. In general, pathogenic microorganisms do not readily adhere to walls or ceilings unless the surface becomes moist, sticky, or damaged. Little evidence exists that walls and ceilings are a major source for hospital-acquired infection. Wall coverings should be fluid resistant and easily cleaned, especially in areas where contact with blood or body fluids may occur, e.g. delivery suite, operating rooms, and laboratories. Finishing around plumbing fixtures should be smooth and water resistant. In addition, pipe penetrations and joints should be tightly sealed. Acoustical tiles should be avoided in high-risk areas because they may support microbial growth when wet. False ceilings may harbour dust and pests that may contaminate the environment if disturbed and should be avoided in high-risk areas unless adequately sealed.

Floor: Bacteria on hospital floors predominantly consist of skin organisms, e.g. coagulase negative staphylococci, *Bacillus* spp. and diptheroids; *S. aureus* and *Clostridium* spp. can also be cultured. However, the infection risk from contaminated floors is small. Gram-negative bacteria are rarely found on dry floors, but may be present after cleaning or a spill. Nevertheless, these microorganisms tend to disappear as the surface dries. All floors should have non-slip coverings. Where there is likely to be direct contact with patients, or with blood and body fluids, the surface of floors and walls should be made of smooth, impermeable, seamless materials, such as welded vinyl. Flooring should be able to be easily cleaned, in good repair and water resistant.

Carpet: Carpet harbours large numbers of microorganisms, e.g. coagulase negative staphylococci, *Bacillus* spp., fungi and vancomycin-resistant enterococci (VRE). These microorganisms can survive on carpets and may pose a greater risk of infection especially in high-risk areas after vacuuming. Therefore, their use in clinical areas should be avoided. In addition, carpets are expensive to clean and maintain, difficult to disinfect and become smelly with time.

If carpets are used in the health care facility, then they must be fitted with a moisture impermeable barrier. They should be well maintained to ensure that they are vacuumed daily and periodically steam cleaned. An appropriate choice of vacuum is important to minimize airborne dispersal of microorganisms.

Fixtures and fittings: All fixtures and fittings should be designed to allow easy cleaning and to discourage the accumulation of dust. When choosing material it is important to avoid porous *or* textured material. It must be durable, easy to clean, washable and able to withstand cleaning with abrasive disinfectant solutions.

Furniture: Various microorganisms have been recovered from furniture. Therefore, it is important that the furniture used by patients (beds, mattresses, chairs, tables etc.) must be durable and easily cleaned. Fabrics should be avoided, especially if soiling with blood and body fluids is possible. Upholstery and protective covers must be in good repair at all times and breaches in the material must be repaired or replaced immediately.

Curtains and blinds: Curtains must be easily washable and of a design that does not attract accumulated dust. Sufficient curtains must be purchased to enable single curtains to be replaced when soiled. There must also be a laundering programme in place, and the laundering process must not compromise the fire retardant finish. As there is no evidence to show that frequent changing produces any benefit; curtains need not be changed after discharge of every patient. Horizontal blinds carry a risk due to their high surface area with the potential for dust accumulation; vertical blinds are preferred.

Patient's accommodations

Outpatient accommodation: Patient waiting areas should have provision for separating patients who may be highly infectious. A triage system should be in place to identify such patients. Outpatients should have a separate room for patients with known or suspected infection. Every effort should be made to see these patients as quickly as possible.

Inpatient accommodation: To minimize the risk of cross-infection, hospitals should, wherever possible, restrict the number of beds per room/bay (ideally not more than four beds per room/bay); there should be at least 3.6 m between the centres of adjacent beds. Shared patient accommodation should include facilities such as toilets, baths and showers that are easy to clean and conveniently located to minimize unnecessary patient movement. Staff hand washbasins should also be located in patient areas.

Hand washing facilities

Hand washing is the single most important method of prevention of cross-infection in hospital. Health care facilities should have an adequate number of hand washbasins. Each patient room, examination room, and procedure room needs at least one sink. There must be a minimum of one sink per single room or one sink per 4–6 bedded cubicles. They should be located conveniently (i.e. preferably near the entrance) for easy access by the health care worker.

The hand washbasin should be large enough to prevent splashing. Too shallow a sink may cause contamination of hands by bacteria residing in the drain. They should be sealed to the wall or placed sufficiently far away from the wall to allow effective cleaning of all surfaces. Splash backs should be included to prevent wall damage. The surrounding area should be made of non-porous material to resist fungal growth. The tap outflow should not point directly into the sink outlets as gram-negative bacteria colonize 'U bends' causing splashing and dispersal of contaminated aerosols.

Taps should be fitted with an anti-splash device. Hand washbasins should be fitted with soap dispensers (i.e. operated by elbow, knee or foot) in order to further reduce possible cross-contamination. They should be supplied with both hot and cold water; preferably with a mixer tap to achieve correct temperature. The tap should be fitted with a hands-off control (e.g. elbow operated) to avoid contamination. Electronically operated systems may be an acceptable option in specialized areas such as theatres.

Isolation rooms

In an acute hospital, it is essential that adequate numbers of single rooms are available for the isolation of patients with suspected or confirmed infection. It is recommended that there is at least one single room for every 4–6 beds or there are four single rooms for each 24-bedded ward. Each side room should have a clinical hand basin at the port of exit, a patient's hand washbasin and an en-suite toilet and bathroom/shower. It should preferably have an ante-room.

Source isolation room

There should be at least one respiratory isolation room per 100 beds. Negative pressure ventilation is required only for conditions transmitted *via* the airborne route,

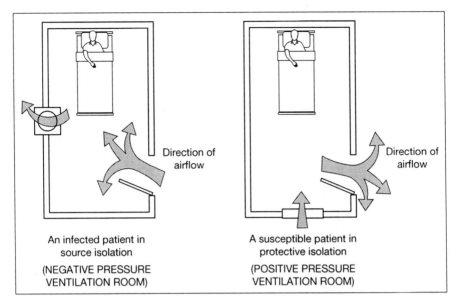

Figure 3.1 Isolation of patients.

e.g. tuberculosis, measles and chickenpox. Mechanically ventilated rooms should achieve 6–12 exchanges of air per hour and there should be adequate temperature and humidity regulation, such that windows need not be opened and doors can be kept closed when the rooms are in use. No recirculation of air should be permitted for respiratory isolation rooms. The exhaust air from isolation rooms should be vented to the exterior. *Where dual ventilation is present, there must be local safeguards to prevent accidental switching between positive and negative pressure.*

Regular maintenance and monitoring programmes must be established for ventilated rooms to ensure that the design criteria are met. Pressure and airflow must be monitored and filters must be replaced on a periodic planned basis according to written protocols. These rooms should be self-closing, and the walls, windows, ceiling, floor, and penetrations well sealed. Ideally, they should be located in areas where patients at high-risk will be cared for, e.g. emergency department, bronchoscopy suite, medical units etc. Isolation of patients with proven or suspected multiply drug-resistant *Mycobacterium tuberculosis* in a single room with negative pressure ventilation is essential.

Protective isolation room

Prevention of aspergillosis is particularly important in patients undergoing solid organ and bone marrow transplantation. In bone marrow transplant units, the air should be HEPA filtered with the air pressure in the room positive in relation to the corridor. In addition, rooms should be tightly sealed, especially around windows, and the air exchange rate should be high, i.e. ≥12 air exchanges per hour. It is important that air should be exhausted to the outside without recirculation.

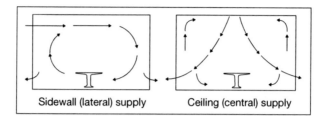

Sidewall (lateral) supply   Ceiling (central) supply

Figure 3.2 Airflow in conventionally ventilated operating theatre.

Operating theatres

To prevent contaminated air from reaching the operating theatre, mechanical ventilation is recommended. The air within the operating room should be at a positive pressure compared with other theatre suite rooms and with the external corridors. Theatre ventilation must be checked regularly and maintained by an appropriate engineer. The works and maintenance department must keep written records of all work on the ventilation system. Coarse and fine air filters must be replaced regularly according to the manufacturer's instructions or when the pressure differential across the filter indicates that a change is required.

Conventionally ventilated theatre

For a conventionally ventilated theatre, a minimum of 20 air changes per hour of filtered air should be delivered. The temperature of the room should be maintained at 18–25°C. The humidity should be maintained at 40–60% for staff comfort and to inhibit microbial growth. Additional ventilation units, such as mobile air cooling devices, must not be introduced into the theatre without consultation with the ICT.

The minimum standard for microbiological air counts for the operating room is 30 cfu m^{-3} (colony forming units per cubic metre of air) when the theatre is empty, and less than 180 cfu m^{-3} when in use. A conventionally ventilated theatre requires microbiological checks at commissioning, immediately after commissioning and at any major refurbishment, by the ICT. *Routine bacteriological testing of operating room air is not necessary* but may be useful when investigating an outbreak.

Ultra clean air theatre

It is now accepted that ultra clean air (<10 cfu m^{-3}) reduces the risk of infection in implant surgery. To achieve this, laminar flow systems (airflow 0.5 m s^{-1}) which deliver about 300 air changes per hour or special ventilation combined with bacteria impermeable clothing has to be used. The operating parameters for an ultra clean air theatre are different from those for a conventionally ventilated theatre, and depend upon the design of the system. In a fully walled enclosure, the airflow 1 m from the filter face should not fall below 0.3 m s^{-1}, but in a partially walled enclosure, because

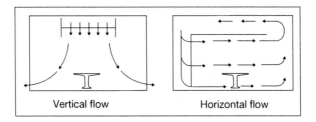

Vertical flow	Horizontal flow

Figure 3.3 Airflow in conventionally ultra clean operating theatre.

there is a greater diffusion of air, the airflow at 1 m from the floor (above the level of the operating table surface), should not be less than $0.2 \, \text{m s}^{-1}$. Bacterial counts at 1 m from the floor should be less than $1.0 \, \text{bcp m}^{-3}$ (bacteria carrying particles per cubic metre of air) of air in an empty enclosure and when tested during an operation there should be less than $10 \, \text{bcp m}^{-3}$ at the level of the operating table at the centre of the enclosure. Additionally, if the system is partially walled, then on each of the four sides at the periphery of the enclosure, the bacteriological count should not exceed $10 \, \text{bcp m}^{-3}$.

Ultra clean air theatres require assessment not only at commissioning, but at regular intervals as a part of the routine service to theatres, because factors other than simple ventilation parameters are important in determining the quality of the air. It is recommended that microbiological checks should be performed every 3 months because of the long incubation period for joint sepsis. Any system defect needs to be detected early and rectified quickly.

Ventilation and air-conditioning

A clear distinction must be made between ventilation provided as part of environmental patient comfort and that as part of the control of infection. Air-conditioning or ventilation systems in critical areas such as operating theatres, respiratory isolation rooms, bone marrow transplant units as well as in special treatment or procedural areas should maintain the inflow of fresh air and allows the temperature, humidity and purity (from dust, infectious agents, and gases) of the air to be maintained within prescribed limits. *Hospital air-conditioning systems must be monitored regularly and serviced* by the hospital estates department and/or other accredited service technicians. Maintenance schedules must be documented and carried out according to manufacturers' recommendations.

Cooling towers and water system

Respiratory tract infections from *Legionella* spp. are exclusively acquired from the environment, and hospital acquisition is well recognized. The highest concentrations of *Legionella* spp. are found in hot water storage tanks, cooling towers, and condensers. Therefore, cooling towers and water systems should be avoided where possible. If the construction of new cooling towers in the health care facilities is planned, it is important that they be sited and directed as far as practicable from patient and public areas. Drift must be directed away from the air-intake system and drift eliminators should be installed.

Adequate maintenance of wet cooling towers is essential and must be carried out in accordance with written policy, which must be based on national and international guidelines. A written record must be kept of detailed maintenance, including environmental test results. It is important that cooling towers should be drained when not in use. They should be mechanically cleaned to remove scale and sediment at regular intervals. Appropriate biocides should be used on a regular basis to prevent the growth of slime-forming organisms. Despite the potential presence of *Legionella* in the water supply, routine culturing of water in the absence of proven or suspected hospital transmission is not recommended.

Spa pools, heated swimming pools and other water systems are also potential sources of infection including *Pseudomonas* spp., *Legionella* spp. and *Cryptosporidium* spp. Each health care facility should develop guidelines based on relevant standards.

Construction, renovation and demolition

Environmental disturbances caused by construction, renovation and demolition activities in and around hospital markedly increase the airborne *Aspergillus* spp. spore counts in the indoor air, thereby increasing the risk of acquiring aspergillosis among immunocompromised patients. Although one case of healthcare-associated aspergillosis is often difficult to link to a specific environmental exposure, the occurrence of temporarily clustered cases increase the likelihood that an environmental source within the facility may be identified and corrected. Therefore it is essential that all the activities related to construction, renovation and demolition should be planned and coordinated by a multi-disciplinary team to minimize the risk of airborne infection both during projects and after their completion.

The ICT should carry out a risk assessment before initiating the project to identify potential exposures of susceptible patients to dust and moisture and determine the need for dust and moisture containment measures.

Microbiological sampling of air in health care facilities remains a controversial issue because of currently unresolved technical limitations and the need for substantial laboratory support.

References and further reading

American Institute of Architects: *Guidelines for Design and Construction of Hospital and Health Care Facilities*. Washington DC: The American Institute of Architects, 2001.

Anderson K, Morris G, Kennedy H, Croall J, Michie J, Richardson MD, Gibson B. Aspergillosis in immunocompromised paediatric patients: associations with building hygiene, design, and indoor air. *Thorax* 1996; **51**: 256–261.

Ayliffe GAJ, Collins BJ, Lowbury EJL, Babb JR, Lilly HA. Ward floors and other surfaces as reservoirs of hospital infection. *Journal of Hygiene* 1967; **65**: 515–536.

Ayliffe GAJ, Babb JR, Taylor LJ. The hospital environment. In: *Hospital-acquired infection: principles and prevention*. Oxford: Butterworth-Heinemann; 1999: 109–121.

Bartley J. (ed). *Construction and Renovation: APIC Infection control tool kit series.* Washington DC: Association for Professionals in Infection Control and Epidemiology, 2000.

Bartley JM. The role of infection control during construction in health care facilities. *American Journal of Infection Control* 2000; **28**: 156–169.

Carter CD, Barr BA. Infection control issues in construction and renovation. In: Herwaldt LA, Decker MD (eds). *A practical handbook for hospital epidemiologists.* Thorofare (NJ): Slack, Inc; 1997: 317–330.

Carter CD, Barr BA. Infection control issues in construction and renovation. *Infection Control Hospital Epidemiology* 1997; **18**: 587–596.

Centers for Disease Control and Prevention. Guidelines for preventing opportunistic infections among hematopoietic stem cell transplant recipients. *Morbidity and Mortality Weekly Report* 2000; **49**(RR-10): 1–125.

Centers for Disease Control and Prevention. Guidelines for preventing the transmission of *Mycobacterium tuberculosis* in health-care settings. *Morbidity and Mortality Weekly Report* 1994; **43**(RR-13): 1–132.

Cheng SM, Streifel AJ. Infection control considerations during construction activities: land excavation and demolition. *American Journal of Infection Control* 2001; **29**: 321–328.

Holton J, Ridgway GL. Commissioning operating theatres. *Journal of Hospital Infection* 1993; **23**: 153–160.

Kaatz GW, Gitlin SD, Schaberg DR, Wilson KH, Kauffman CA, Seo SM, *et al.* Acquisition of *Clostridium difficile* from the hospital environment. *American Journal of Epidemiology* 1988; **127**: 1289–1294.

Lai KK. A cluster of invasive aspergillosis in a bone marrow transplant unit related to construction and the utility of air sampling. *American Journal of Infection Control* 2001; **29**: 333–337.

Marshall JW, Vincent JH, Kuehn TH, Brosseau LM. Studies of ventilation efficiency in a protective isolation room by the use of a scale model. *Infection Control and Hospital Epidemiology* 1996; **17**: 5–10.

Noskin GA, Bednarz P, Reiner S, Suriano T, Peterson LR. Persistent contamination of fabric covered furniture by vancomycin resistant enterococci: implications for upholstery selection in hospitals. *American Journal of Infection Control* 2000; **160**: 2819–2822.

Neely AC, Maley MP. Survival of enterococci and staphylococci on hospital fabrics and plastic. *Journal of Clinical Microbiology* 2000; **38:** 724–726.

O'Connell NH, Humphreys H. Intensive care unit design and environmental factors in the acquisition of infection. *Journal of Hospital Infection* 2000; **45:** 255–262.

Pannuti CS. Hospital environment for high-risk patients. In: Wenzel RP (ed). *Prevention and control of nosocomial infections* 3rd edn. Baltimore: Williams and Wilkins; 1997: 463–489.

UK Department of Health. Technical memorandum 2025. *Ventilation in health care premises.* Part 1 Management Policy, Part 2 Design Considerations, Part 3 Validation and verification, Part 4 Operational management. London: HMSO, 1994.

UK Department of Health. Technical Memorandum 2040. *The control of legionella in healthcare premises – a code of practice.* Part 1 Management Policy, Part 2 Design Considerations, Part 3 Validation and verification, Part 4 Operational management. London: HMSO, 1994.

UK Department of Health. Health Building Note 26; *Operating Departments.* London: HMSO, 1991.

UK NHS Estates. *Infection Control in the built environment.* Norwich: The Stationary Office, 2002.

4

Surveillance and Outbreak Control

Approximately 10% of hospitalized patients develop infections every year. The rate of developing nosocomial or hospital-acquired infection in developing countries is as high as 25%. It has been estimated that up to one third of these infections are preventable.

An infection is classified as *nosocomial* if it was not present or incubating at the time the patient was admitted to the hospital. Infections should be considered nosocomial if they are related to procedures, treatments, or other events. Most nosocomial infections appear before the patient is discharged, although some are incubating at discharge and do not become apparent until later.

Thus, an infection is not considered nosocomial if it represents a complication or extension of an infectious process present on admission. In general, infections that occur more than 48–72 h after admission and within 10 days after hospital discharge are defined as *nosocomial* or *hospital-acquired*. The time frame is modified for infections that have incubation periods less than 48–72 h (e.g. gastroenteritis caused by Norwalk virus) or longer than 10 days (e.g. hepatitis A). Surgical site infections are considered nosocomial if the infection occurs within 30 days after the operative procedure or within 1 year if a device or foreign material is implanted.

Incidence of various nosocomial infections

Urinary tract infection (UTI): Most nosocomial UTIs develop after urinary tract manipulation. UTI arises in 20–25% of the hospitalized patients who have an indwelling urinary catheter. The risk of UTI increases if the patient has an indwelling urinary catheter for a longer duration.

Respiratory tract infections: Nosocomial pneumonia is the second most common hospital-acquired infection and has a mortality rate between 20–50%. Most respiratory nosocomial infections are linked to respiratory devices used to aid breathing or

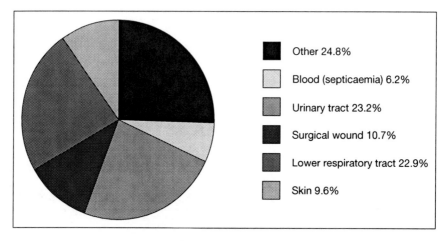

Legend:
- Other 24.8%
- Blood (septicaemia) 6.2%
- Urinary tract 23.2%
- Surgical wound 10.7%
- Lower respiratory tract 22.9%
- Skin 9.6%

Figure 4.1 Sites of the most common nosocomial infections: distribution according to the UK Prevalence Study (Emmerson AM, *et al*. 1996).

administer medications. Nosocomial pneumonia typically lengthens a patient's hospital stay by 4–9 days and is associated with very high morbidity and mortality.

Surgical site infections: Surgical site wound infections occur in up to 12% of surgical patients. Such infections lengthen hospital stays by about 6 days. Surgical site infections can occur in the incision as well as in the deep tissues of a wound.

Bloodstream infections: Nosocomial infections of the bloodstream account for approximately 6% of nosocomial infections. Although local infections outside the bloodstream are sometimes the source of infection, most bacteraemias are related to intravascular devices.

Surveillance of nosocomial infection

Surveillance of nosocomial infection is the foundation for organizing and maintaining an infection control programme. In addition, information obtained from surveillance data is a useful tool for the infection control team (ICT) and the infection control committee (ICC) in identifying areas of priority and allocating resources accordingly. Therefore it is essential that each health care establishment tailors its surveillance systems to maximize the use of all health care resources, given outcome priorities, population characteristics and institutional objectives.

The main objectives of surveillance are as follows:

- Reducing infection rates within health care facilities.
- Establishing endemic infection rates.

- Identifying outbreaks.
- Convincing medical personnel to adopt recommended preventive practices.
- Comparing infection rates between health care establishments.
- Evaluating control measures.

The process of surveillance must incorporate four key stages: data must be collected, recorded, analyzed and interpreted. The *most vital component of surveillance is ensuring that the information obtained is conveyed to those who may influence practice*, implement change or provide financial resources necessary to improve outcomes. It is a futile exercise to collect and record data without taking any further action.

Ideally surveillance should be carried out in all health care establishments to obtain baseline information on the frequency and type of nosocomial infections. Any increase in the rate of infection can then be quickly recognized and appropriate infection control action taken to minimize its transmission. A change in infection rates against a baseline rate can also be used to evaluate the effectiveness of new infection control policies and procedures.

Methods of surveillance

Different methods of surveillance exist and the findings are summarized in table 4.1 and table 4.2. The type of surveillance method depends on the local factors, i.e. the type and size of hospital, case mix and availability of resources. Continuous surveillance of an entire health care facility requires staff, IT resource and a well organized reporting system. *Targeted surveillance aimed at high risk areas is more effective and manageable* and is preferred in larger establishments. Irrespective of the methods used, *it is essential that data generated from the surveillance is appropriately risk-adjusted* for the generation of meaningful infection rates, especially when the information is released beyond the institution.

Surveillance methods should be flexible enough to accommodate technological changes within health care facilities, shortening lengths of stay and the necessity to provide post-discharge surveillance, including surveillance of procedures carried out in the community. Numerator and denominator data should be collected in all situations for the calculation of rates of infection. For surveillance purposes, the analysis of numerator data alone is meaningless.

A minimum data set for surveillance should include details of the infected individual, i.e. name or other unique identifier, date of birth, sex, hospital record number, ward or unit in the hospital, name of the consultant, unit involved, date of admission, date of onset of infection and date of discharge or death, site of infection or colonization, organism isolated with antibiotic sensitivities. This minimum data set should also include information on medical treatment/procedures at the time of infection and any other information relevant to why the infection may have occurred

Table 4.1 Various methods of surveillance used in infection control.

Methods	Sources of data	Comments
Continuing surveillance of all patients (CS)	Medical, nursing, laboratory records including temperature charts, X-ray and antibiotic treatment reports.	Time-consuming and not cost effective: infection rates are low in some specialties.
Ward liaison (WL)	Twice-weekly visits to wards. Discuss all patients with staff and review records.	Less comprehensive than CS, with similar disadvantages.
Laboratory-based (LB)	Laboratory records only.	Depends on samples taken and information on request forms.
Laboratory-based ward surveillance (LBWS)	Follow up of LB in wards.	Disadvantages of LB, but more accurate.
Laboratory-based ward surveillance and selected continuing surveillance (LBWS and CS)	As LBWS and reporting of outbreaks by ward staff and CS in special units. (e.g. ITU) or infections (e.g. wounds).	As LBWS, but early detection of outbreaks and incidence in studies in selected areas of infection.
Laboratory-based ward liaison (LBWL)	Combination of LB and LBWS.	Time-consuming but most sensitive after CS.

Adapted from Glenister HM, *et al.* An evaluation of surveillance methods for detecting infections in hospital inpatients. *Journal of Hospital Infection* 1993; **23:** 229–242.

including the patient's underlying medical risk factors, clinical outcome and an assessment of whether the incident was preventable.

Comparison of infection rates between establishments and the publication of such comparisons is a contentious issue and needs careful consideration and sensitive handling. This is mainly because the surveillance data may not be comparable, and the range of institutions involved will introduce confounding factors inherent in all surveillance systems. Problems of data interpretation can be overcome when surveillance systems are set up with clearly defined surveillance objectives included in the expected outputs of surveillance. Unfortunately, at this time, surveillance objectives rarely underpin surveillance methods.

Management of an outbreak

An outbreak may be defined *as the occurrence of disease at a rate greater than that expected within a specific geographical area and over a defined period of time* (Beck-Sague C, et al. 1997). Day-to-day surveillance is important to identify cases of nosocomial infections and other infectious diseases so that appropriate action is taken. Major outbreaks of transmissible infection in both the hospital and community require appropriate planning to ensure effective management of such episodes.

Table 4.2 Advantages and disadvantages of various surveillance strategies.

Strategy	Advantages	Disadvantages
Hospital-wide surveillance		
Incidence	Provides data on all infection sites, and units. Identifies clusters. Establishes baseline rates. Recognizes outbreaks early. Identifies risk factors.	Expensive. Labour-intensive and time-consuming. No defined management objectives. Large amounts of data collected and little time to analyse.
Prevalence	Inexpensive. Time efficient, can be done periodically.	Overestimates rates, important differences compared with incidence surveys.
Objective/ priority based	Adapts to hospitals with special interests and resources. Focuses on specific problems at the individual institution. Identifies risk factors. Can include post-discharge component.	No baseline infection rates. May miss clusters or outbreaks.
Targeted surveillance		
Site specific	Flexible, can be mixed with other strategies. Can include a post-discharge component.	No defined management objectives. No baseline rates in other units. May miss clusters.
Unit specific	Focuses on patients at greater risk. Requires fewer personnel. Simplifies surveillance effort.	Can miss clusters.
Rotating	Less expensive. Less time-consuming and labour-intensive. Includes all hospital areas.	
Outbreak	Valuable when used with all types of surveillance.	Thresholds are institution specific. No baseline rates provided.
Limited periodic surveillance	Decreases possibility of missing an outbreak. Liberates infection control nurse to perform other activities. Increase efficiency of surveillance.	May miss cluster.

Therefore it is important that the **health care facilities must draw up detailed outbreak control plans appropriate to local situations.** These plans should be discussed and endorsed by the hospital ICC and should include the criteria and method for convening the Outbreak Control Committee. The plan should also clearly address the areas of individual responsibilities, and action plans for all involved. Those who are or may be involved in the management of a major outbreak must be aware of such a policy and their individual role.

In an outbreak situation, communication to relevant staff is important. Effective outbreak investigation requires adequate laboratory support. It is particularly important to ensure that outbreak isolates are stored for further investigation. This is because many of the infectious agents that cause outbreaks in health care facilities are endemic organisms, and it may be necessary to use a typing system to evaluate which isolates are part of any putative outbreak. Although simple antimicrobial susceptibility testing may be enough to distinguish isolates, against a background of increasing resistance, other more sophisticated methods of typing may be necessary. These are usually available from a reference laboratory.

Recognition: The rapid recognition of outbreaks is one of the most important objectives of the routine surveillance of infection. Ideally, hospital surveillance systems should facilitate the early detection of outbreaks. In some instances, the occurrence of an outbreak may be obvious, such as in an episode of food poisoning that affects both health care workers (HCWs) and patients, while in other instances the onset may not be immediately apparent. Sometimes the outbreak may manifest itself clearly to the medical and nursing staff. However, some outbreaks may arise more insidiously and reach considerable proportions before they become apparent. These outbreaks are detected by the laboratory, but under some circumstances may be identified only through the vigilance of general nursing and medical staff.

Investigation: The principles for investigating outbreaks in hospitals are the same as for community-based outbreaks. There are three basic steps: i.e. (a) describing the outbreak, (b) developing a hypothesis and (c) testing the hypothesis with analytical epidemiology.

Once a possible outbreak has been recognized, the Infection Control Team should take immediate steps to collect information from the ward and the laboratory, determine whether an outbreak is occurring and establish a case definition. If the initial investigation confirms that an outbreak is occurring, it is important to establish its severity and initiate some immediate control measures. If, after the initial observation, it is established that no outbreak exists, then it is important that the person who has made the initial observation should be informed and the reason given. Ward staff may need reassurance and care should be taken not to discourage further reporting.

Outbreak control: Preliminary control measures should be introduced as soon as possible and be based on sound infection control practices such as patient isolation and/or hand washing. Heightened surveillance should be introduced to assess the

Summary for investigation of an outbreak

- Begin preliminary evaluation and determine a background rate of infection.

- Confirm the existence of an outbreak.

- Confirm the diagnosis using the microbiological methods.

- Create a case definition that may include laboratory and clinical data. Start with a broad case definition that can be redefined at a later date.

- Develop line listings by identifying and counting cases or exposures. Describe the data in terms of time, place and person. Remember that cases may have been discharged from the health care facilities.

- Construct an epidemic curve. This may indicate the source of the outbreak (see Figs 4.2 and 4.3).

- Develop and test the hypothesis. In larger outbreaks, a case-control method may be the most efficient way of testing a hypothesis: however, if a single hospital ward is affected, a retrospective cohort study is relatively easy.

- Take immediate control measures. Determine who is at risk of becoming ill. Look at changes that may have affected the rate of infection, e.g. new staff, new procedures, new laboratory tests, and health care worker:patient ratio, etc.

- Communicate information to relevant personnel.

- Screen personnel and environment as indicated.

- Write a coherent report (preliminary and final).

- Summarize investigation and recommendations to the appropriate authorities.

- Implement long term infection control measures for prevention of similar outbreaks.

impact of all control measures. As soon as possible, information about the outbreak, the investigation and the results should be conveyed to those at risk.

Outbreak control plan: Depending upon the nature of the infectious disease and number of cases involved, the Outbreak Control Committee should be convened. The membership of the committee varies depending upon the type of health care facilities.

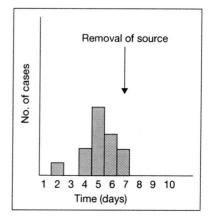

Figure 4.2 Epidemic curve of a ***point source outbreak***. Number of cases peaks and then disappears when a single source is identified and removed.

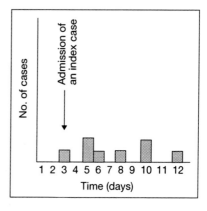

Figure 4.3 Epidemic curve of a ***common source outbreak***. Figure illustrates an index case and seven additional cases developing infection after exposure to the index case. The epidemic curve is relatively flat, spread over days and has breaks compared to figure 4.1.

The aim of the Outbreak Control Committee is to:

- Facilitate the investigation of the outbreak.
- Implement measures necessary to control the outbreak.
- Monitor the effectiveness of the control measures.
- Oversee communication to all relevant groups.
- Facilitate the medical care of patients.

Communication: The Outbreak Control Committee will inform the senior management of the hospital and other appropriate people on a regular basis. In an outbreak situation, it is good practice to have one designated person within the health care facility to respond to enquiries from the public, press and the media. That person should be kept informed of all the developments by the chairperson of the Outbreak Control Committee.

End of outbreak: At the end of an outbreak, the Outbreak Control Committee will prepare a final report. When the outbreak has been controlled, a final meeting of the Outbreak Control Committee should be held to:

- Review the experience of all participants involved in management of outbreak.

- Identify any shortfalls and particular difficulties that were encountered.

- Revise the outbreak control plan in accordance with the results.

- Recommend, if necessary, structural or procedural improvements which would reduce the chances of recurrence.

All outbreaks provide the opportunity to educate health care workers about infection control matters. *It is essential that all outbreaks, however minor, should be investigated thoroughly and the outcomes of such investigations documented.*

Look back investigations

Look back investigations refer to the process of identifying, tracing, recalling, counselling and testing patients or health care workers who may have been exposed to an infection. An example is the case of a health care worker who has undertaken exposure-prone procedures on surgical patients and is later found to be positive for a blood-borne virus, e.g. HIV, hepatitis B or C virus. A similar process may be needed if a breakdown in the normal processes of cleaning and disinfection or sterilization of instruments such as endoscopes is detected, allowing the potential for transfer of infection from one patient to another.

All types of look back investigation have the potential to cause a great deal of publicity. This can cause unnecessary anxiety in patients treated at the health care facility who have not been exposed to infection, as well as anger and distress among patients who were put at risk of infection. Look back investigations can take up a great deal of time and resources and should not be undertaken lightly.

The hospital and the local health authority should be involved at the outset and a planning team established with members who have expertise in infection control, infectious disease, microbiology, the discipline involved, public relations, representatives of the health authority; legal and indemnity issues should also be included. The procedures to be undertaken and how these are presented to at-risk patients and the public should be clearly worked out at the outset. These procedures should also clearly set out protocols for tracing, counselling and referral of at-risk patients in a timely manner. Test results should be available with minimal delay, and the planning team should ensure that the project is completed and a final report produced as soon as possible.

References and further reading

Association of Medical Microbiologists, Hospital Infection Society, Infection Control Nurses Association and Public Health Laboratory Services. The Infection Control Standards Working Party. *Standards in Infection Control in Hospitals.* London: HMSO, 1993.

Beck-Sague C, Jarvis W, Martone W. Outbreak investigations. *Infection Control Hospital Epidemiology* 1997; **18**: 138.

Coello R, Gastmeier P, de Boer AS. Surveillance of Hospital-Acquired Infection in England, Germany and the Netherlands: Will International Comparison of Rates Be Possible? *Infection Control and Hospital Epidemiology* 2001; **22**: 393–397.

Crowe MJ, Cooke EM. Review of case definitions for nosocomial infection – towards a consensus. *Journal of Hospital Infection* 1998; **39**: 3–11.

Emmerson AM, Ayliffe GAJ. Surveillance of Nosocomial Infections. *Clinical Infectious Diseases* 1996; **3**(2): 159–301.

Emmerson AM, Enstone JE, Griffin M, *et al.* The Second National Prevalence Survey of Infection in Hospitals – overview of the results. *Journal of Hospital Infection* 1996; **32**: 175–190.

Garner JS, Jarvis WM, Emori TG, Horan TC, Hughes JM. CDC definitions for nosocomial infections, 1988. *American Journal of Infection Control* 1988; **16**: 128–140.

Gaynes RP, Emoir TG. Surveillance of Nosocomial Infections. In: Abrutyn E (ed). *Saunders Infection Control Reference Service*, 2nd edn. Philadelphia: WB Saunders, 2001: 41–44.

Glenister HM, Taylor LJ, Cooke EM, Bartlett CLR. *A Study of Surveillance Methods for Detecting Hospital Infection.* London: Public Health Laboratory Services, 1992.

Glenister HM, Taylor LJ, Bartlett CLR, *et al.* An evaluation of surveillance methods for detecting infections in hospital inpatients. *Journal of Hospital Infection* 1993; **23**: 229–242.

Glynn A, Ward V, Wilson J, *et al. Hospital-Acquired Infection: Surveillance, Policies and Practice.* London: Public Health Laboratory Services, 1997.

Haley RW, Culver DH, White JW, *et al.* The efficacy of infection surveillance and control programs in preventing nosocomial infection in US hospitals (SENIC study). *American Journal of Epidemiology* 1985; **121**(2): 182–205.

Jarvis WR, Zara S. Investigation of Outbreaks. In: Mayhall CG (ed). *Hospital Epidemiology and Infection Control*, 2nd edn. Lippincott Williams & Wilkins 1999: 111–120.

Perl TM. Surveillance, reporting and the use of computers. In: Wenzel RP (ed). *Prevention and Control of Nosocomial Infections* 3rd edn. Baltimore: Williams & Wilkins, 1997: 127–161.

Public Health Laboratory Services: *Hospital Acquired Infection: Surveillance Policies and Practice.* London: PHLS, 1997.

Pottinger JM, Herwaldt LA, Perl TM. Basics of surveillance – an overview. *Infection Control and Hospital Epidemiology* 1997; **18:** 513–527.

Report from the National Nosocomial Infections Surveillance (NNIS) System. Nosocomial Infection Rates for Interhospital Comparison: Limitations and Possible Solutions. *Infection Control and Hospital Epidemiology* 1991; **12:** 609–621.

Report from the National Nosocomial Infections Surveillance (NNIS) System. National Nosocomial Infections Surveillance (NNIS) System Report, Data Summary from January 1992–June 2001. *American Journal of Infection Control* 2001; **29:** 404–421.

5

Epidemiology and Biostatistics

This chapter provides basic information about the epidemiological principles and statistical methods used in the practice of infection control surveillance, prevention and control. It is intended to be a brief introduction, since a thorough discussion of each of these concepts cannot be accomplished in one chapter. The reader who wishes to obtain more information on these topics should refer to the *References and further reading* list at the end of this chapter.

There are two major categories of epidemiological studies:

Experimental: In experimental studies, the investigator controls the exposures to specific factors and then follows the subjects to determine the effect of the exposure, e.g. a clinical trial of a new drug.

Observational: In observational studies, the group being compared is already defined and the investigator merely observes what happens. These observations are used to analyse outbreaks because the investigator is observing the outcomes to prior exposures over which the investigator has no control.

Case-control, cross-sectional and cohort are types of *observational* studies that typically consider features of the past, present and future respectively, to try to identify differences between the groups.

Cohort studies

Cohort studies are observational studies usually carried out over a number of years, and designed to investigate the aetiology of diseases or outcomes. The aim of such studies is to investigate the link between a hypothetical cause and a defined outcome. Prior to undertaking a cohort study, investigators should seek statistical advice regarding the number of subjects needed in each group.

Cohort studies originate with a hypothesis that the outcome (an infection or disease) is caused by exposure to an event (risk factor). Subjects exposed to the suspected risk factor (cases) and a similar group that have not been exposed (control) are identified. Often, a complete population sample (cohort) is followed prospectively over a period of time (usually a number of years) to identify the incidence of the outcome in both groups. These results are then analysed to determine if the group exposed to the risk factor has a higher incidence of disease than those not exposed. Cohort studies are usually prospective but they can be performed retrospectively if there is a clearly documented point of first exposure.

A cohort study with a case-control design is often called a nested case-control study.

Disadvantages of cohort studies

- Time-consuming and costly (unless the outcome has a high incidence and short latent period).

- Long studies inevitably increase the drop-out rates.

- Cohort studies are not useful investigations for rare diseases as large numbers of subjects are required.

Advantages of cohort studies

- The prospective design of the 'standard' cohort study provides an opportunity for accurate data collection that is not normally available from retrospective studies.

- The incidence, relative risk and attributable risk can be calculated from the results.

- An estimate of the time from exposure to disease development is possible.

- Occasionally, cohort studies can be performed retrospectively and can thus be cheaper and less time-consuming.

Case-control studies

Case-control studies are analytical epidemiological studies whose aim is to investigate the association between disease and suspected causes and are usually cross-sectional or retrospective in nature.

In case-control studies, people with an outcome (an infection or disease) are identified and their medical and social history examined retrospectively in an attempt to identify exposure to potential risk factors. A matched control group free from the disease or infection are also identified and data collected from them in an identical fashion. The two sets of data are compared to determine whether the disease group was exposed in significantly higher numbers to the suspected risk factors than the control group.

A case-control study must contain a sufficiently large number of study subjects in order to be able to detect an association, if one exists, between an exposure and a disease.

As the number of study subjects increases, the power to detect a statistically significant association increases.

When designing a case-control study it is important to tightly define what constitutes a 'case'. However, *in the initial stages of an outbreak, a case definition may be broad in order to identify all potential cases.* The case definition may be refined as the investigation progresses and potential risk factors are identified. If the number of cases is small, it is possible to include all of them in a case-control study. In a large outbreak, however, it may not be practical, or possible, to identify and include all of the cases. In this instance, cases are selected from those who are ill. Care must be taken to ensure that the cases selected are representative of the entire population with disease so that the study findings can be extrapolated to the whole population. Controls must come from the same environment where the cases' exposures occurred, i.e. they must be from the same population at risk for exposure and must be at the same risk of acquiring the disease. Controls should be similar to the cases in many respects except for the presence of the disease being studied. Ideally, controls should be randomly selected from the population at risk to avoid selection bias.

Disadvantages of case-control study

- It is not possible to calculate the true incidence and relative risk. The results should be expressed as odds ratios.

- The study design inevitably means that data are collected retrospectively and hence the information may not be available or may be of poor quality.

Advantages of case-control study

- These studies are relatively quick and cheap to perform.

- Case-control studies are useful for investigating rare diseases.

- Case-control studies can be used to evaluate interventions.

Case-control or cohort studies can be used in outbreak investigations to compare rates of infection in various populations in order to determine which exposures or risk factors are most likely responsible for the infection. A case-control study differs from a cohort study in that the subjects are enrolled into a case-control study based on whether or not they have a *disease*. In a cohort study, subjects are included in the study based on their *exposure* and are then followed for the development of disease. Case-control study is the method most commonly used to investigate outbreaks because it is relatively inexpensive to conduct, is usually of short duration and requires relatively few study subjects.

Cross-sectional (prevalence) surveys

Cross-sectional studies are descriptive studies in which a sample population's status is determined for the presence or absence of exposure and disease at the same time.

These surveys take a 'snapshot' of the population and thus detect the presence of disease at a point in time (prevalence) as opposed to the frequency of onset of the disease (incidence).

Measures of disease frequency

Rates

Rates describe the *frequency with which events occur*. In other words, a rate measures the occurrence of an event in a defined population over time. Rates are used to track trends, such as the occurrence of nosocomial infections over time. The rates most frequently used are incidence, prevalence, and attack rates. When an increase in a disease or other health-related event is suspected, rates can be calculated and used to determine if there is a change in the occurrence of disease from one period of time to the next.

Basic formula for all types of rates

$$\text{Rate} = \frac{\text{Numerator}}{\text{Denominator}} \times \text{Constant (k)}$$

where k = 100 for discharges and 1,000 for device-days (e.g. IV lines).

Incidence rates

Incidence rates are used to measure and compare the frequency of new cases or events in a population.

$$\text{Incidence rate} = \frac{\text{Number of new cases that occur in a defined period}}{\text{Population at risk during the same period}} \times k$$

where k = 100 for discharges and 1,000 for device-days (e.g. IV lines).

Prevalence rate

Prevalence is a measure of the number of active (new and old) cases in a specified population either during a given period of time (period prevalence) or at a given point in time (point prevalence). A prevalence rate is used to describe the current status of active disease at a particular time in a particular population. It is sometimes helpful to review the incidence and prevalence simultaneously.

$$\text{Prevalence rate} = \frac{\text{Number of all (new and existing) cases of a disease at specified period or point in time}}{\text{Population at risk during the same time period}} \times k$$

where k = 100 for discharges and 1,000 for device-days (e.g. IV lines).

Attack rate

Attack rate is another type of incidence rate that is expressed as cases per 100 population (or as a percentage). It is used to describe the new and recurrent cases of disease that have been observed in a particular group during a limited time period in special circumstances, such as during an epidemic.

$$\text{Attack rate} = \frac{\text{Number of new and recurrent cases that occur in a population in a specified time period}}{\text{Population at risk for same time period}} \times 100$$

Measures of association

Measures of association are used during outbreak investigations to evaluate the relationship between exposed and unexposed populations. These statistical measures can express the strength of association between a risk factor (exposure) and an outcome (disease).

Risks

Risk represents chance; usually the chance of an unwanted event. There are several ways to express risk, such as the relative risk, the odds ratio, the relative risk reduction or the absolute risk reduction. The measures of association used for outbreak investigations are the risk ratio (or relative risk) and the odds ratio.

Risk ratio

The *risk ratio* is the ratio of the attack rate (or risk of disease) in the exposed population to the attack rate (or risk of disease) in the unexposed population. If the value of the risk ratio (relative risk) is equal to 1, the risk is the same in the two groups and there is no evidence of association between the exposure and outcome. If the risk ratio is greater than 1, the risk is higher for the exposed group and exposure may be associated with the outcome. If the risk ratio is less than 1, the risk is lower for the exposed group and the exposure may possibly protect against the outcome.

Relative risk, absolute risk and individual risk

Relative risk provides an estimate of the chances of an exposed individual to develop an illness, complication or response to therapy in comparison with a non-exposed individual.

The *absolute risk* is the risk in the exposed and the non-exposed group as a whole and the individual risk computes the risk according to the levels of exposure. However one should remember that these chances have been calculated from observations of large groups of patients and the result of the group as a whole may not automatically apply to the patient that is presently sitting in front of you.

Table 5.1 The two-by-two contingency table.

	Disease	No disease	
Exposed	**a** number of individuals with *exposure and disease*	**b** number of individuals with *exposure* and *no disease*	a + b
Unexposed	**c** number of individuals with *no exposure* and *disease*	**d** number of individuals with *no exposure* and *no disease*	c + d
Total	a + c	b + d	N

a + b: total number with exposure
a + c: total number with disease
b + d: total number with no disease
c + d: total number with no exposure
N = a + b + c + d = total population in the study.

$$\text{Risk ratio (relative risk)} = \left(\frac{a/(a + b)}{a/(c + d)} \right) \quad \begin{array}{l}\text{(risk of disease in exposed compared}\\\text{to that in unexposed)}\end{array}$$

$$\text{Relative risk} = \frac{\text{Incidence rate among exposed}}{\text{Incidence rate among unexposed}}$$

Odds ratio

The *odds ratio* is similar to the risk ratio except that the odds, instead of the risk (attack rates), are used in the calculation. It is the ratio of the probability of having a risk factor if the disease is present to the probability of having the risk factor if the disease is absent. If the odds ratio is equal to 1, the odds of disease are the same if the exposure is present (i.e. there is no evidence of association between the exposure and disease). If the odds ratio is greater than 1, the odds of disease are higher for the exposed group and the exposure is probably associated with the disease.

$$\text{Odds ratio} = \frac{\begin{array}{c}\text{Number of diseased persons exposed } (a) \times \text{ number}\\\text{without disease and not exposed } (d)\end{array}}{\begin{array}{c}\text{Number of well persons exposed } (b) \times \text{ number}\\\text{with disease but not exposed } (c)\end{array}}$$

Bias and confounders

Bias

Bias refers to errors in study design and execution, and to interpretation and implementation of its results, which systematically influence the eventual outcome for the patient. Bias occurs in both quantitative and qualitative research and it can occur at any stage from conception of a study through to marketing and implementation of its results. Bias can be deliberate or unintentional.

The perfect study is one that is both accurate and precise without bias. An accurate study may be imprecise but not biased. A biased study can be precise but still be inaccurate.

The following are the most common and important biases occur in the study design:

Selection bias can occur when the cases selected for study do not represent the entire population at risk. This can occur if a non-random method is used to select study subjects (e.g. the selection is unconsciously or consciously influenced in some way) or if some of the study subjects are unavailable (e.g. they refuse to participate, their records are missing, their disease is mild and they do not seek medical care and are therefore not detected, and their disease is undiagnosed or misdiagnosed).

Information bias can occur if the information collected is incorrect because of inaccurate recall or because it is inconsistently collected (observer bias). Observer bias occurs when collection or interpretation of data about exposures is systematically different for persons who have the disease than those who do not or when data about outcomes are systematically different for persons who are exposed than for persons who are not exposed.

Bias can result from misuse of statistical tests. The most common types of bias are:

1. Using the wrong test for the data.
2. Inferring that there is no difference between treatments when the study is underpowered.
3. Multiple testing.

Confounders

Confounders are factors extraneous to the research question that are determinants of the outcome of the study. If they are unevenly distributed between the groups they can influence the outcome. A confounder need not be causal; it might be just a correlate of a causal factor. For example, age is associated with a host of disease processes but it is only a marker for underlying biological processes that are causally responsible for these diseases. Similarly, the water pump disconnected by John Snow in Limehouse was not the cause of the cholera, just the conduit that delivered the causal agent.

Procedures for dealing with confounders prior to a study include exclusion, stratified sampling, pairwise matching and randomization. After a study, corrections can be made by using standardization techniques, stratified analysis or multivariate analysis. Prior randomization, whenever possible, is the preferred method of eliminating the effect of confounders.

BIOSTATISTICS

It is important that those responsible for implementing infection control and quality management programmes are familiar with the statistical measures. Basic statistical methods can be used to organize, summarize and analyze data to determine if there are trends or associations in observations.

Numerous computer database and statistical programmes are available and these have virtually eliminated the need to calculate complicated mathematical formulas by hand or by using a hand held calculator. However, the investigator still needs to understand which statistical methods to use and when to use them. There are several computer software programmes that can be used to store, manage, and analyse epidemiological data. *Epi Info* is a software programme that was developed by the Centers for Disease Control and Prevention (CDC) to manage and analyse data collected during an epidemiological investigation and can be downloaded from the CDC web site www.cdc.gov free of cost.

Measures of central tendency

A set of data, which comprises a number of individual results for a particular single variable is said to make up a distribution in the group as a whole. Measures of central tendency describe the values around the middle of a set of data. The mean, median, and mode are the principal measures of central tendency.

Mean: Mean is an arithmetic *average of a group* of numbers. The value of the mean is affected by extreme values in the data set. When extreme values appear in a data set, the distribution of the data becomes skewed and the mean does not give a representative picture of the data.

Median: The median is *the middle number* or point in an ordered group of numbers – the value at which half of the measurements lie below the value and half above the value. The median is useful when there are extreme values in a data set, i.e. the data are skewed.

Mode: The mode is the *most frequently occurring value* in a set of observations. Mode is not often used as a measure of central tendency, particularly in small data sets.

In a normal (symmetric) distribution, the mean, median, and mode have the same values (Fig. 5.1). A curve of a histogram that is not symmetrical is referred to as skewed or asymmetrical. A curve that is said to be negatively skewed (Fig. 5.2) has a tail off to the left and most of the values are above the mean. The mean is less than the median, which is less than the mode. In contrast, a positively skewed (Fig. 5.3) curve value would depict a mirror image of this and the mean will be greater than the median, which will be greater than the mode.

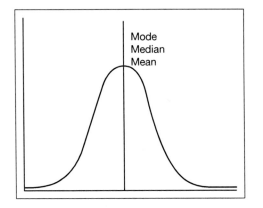

Figure 5.1 Symmetric distribution.

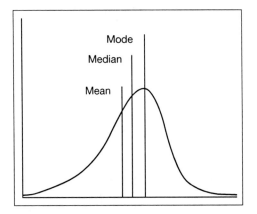

Figure 5.2 Negatively skewed distribution.

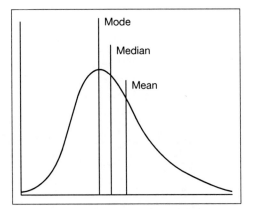

Figure 5.3 Positively skewed distribution.

Measures of dispersion

Measures of dispersion describe the distribution of values in a data set around the mean. The most commonly used measures of dispersion are range, deviation, variance and standard deviation.

The difference between the highest and lowest values in a data set is termed the *range*. The *deviation* is the difference between an individual measurement in a data set and the mean value for the set. A measurement may have no deviation (equal to the mean), or a positive deviation (greater than the mean). The *variance* measures the deviation around the mean of a distribution. The *standard deviation*, which may be represented as *s* or *SD*, is a measure of dispersion that reflects the distribution of values around the mean. A normal distribution represents the natural distribution of values around the mean with progressively fewer observations toward the extremes of the range of values. A normal distribution plotted on a graph shows a bell-shaped curve, in which 68.3% of the values fall within one standard deviation of the mean, 95.5% of the values fall within two standard deviation of the mean, and 99.7% of the values fall within three standard deviations of the mean (Fig. 5.4).

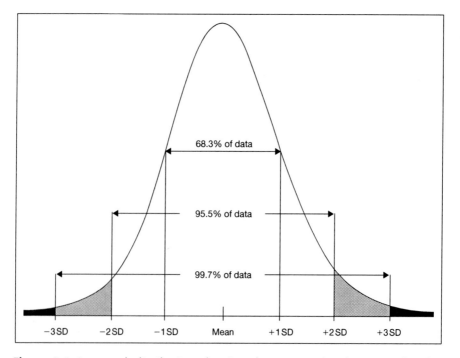

Figure 5.4 A normal distribution showing the area under the curve that lies between 1, 2 and 3 standard deviations on either side of mean.

Hypothesis testing

The traditional method of determining whether one set of data are different from another is hypothesis testing. By convention, the investigator will usually assume the null hypothesis, which predicts that the two sets of data are from the same population and therefore not different. The probability that the null hypothesis is correct is then determined. This probability is referred to as the *P* value. A *P* value of 0.10 tells us that there is a 0.10 probability or 10% chance that the null hypothesis (that there is no difference) is correct. An arbitrary cut-off of 0.05 or 5% has been chosen to indicate that the null hypothesis can be reasonably rejected. If the *P* value falls below this level, the observed difference is regarded as a true difference or a statistically significant difference. Of course there is a 5% chance that this inference is incorrect.

Error of hypothesis testing

An investigator's inference about an association can be wrong if the findings are due to bias or confounding in the study or to chance alone.

Type I (alpha) error: A type I (alpha) error occurs when an investigator states that there is an association when in fact there is no association, i.e. the investigator rejects a true null hypothesis.

Type II (beta) error: A type II (beta) error occurs when the investigator states that there is no association when in fact there is an association, i.e. the investigator fails to reject a null hypothesis that is actually false.

Although these errors are not always avoidable, the likelihood of making a type II error can be minimized by using a larger sample size. By choosing the statistical cut-off level, the investigator decides before beginning the study what probability of committing a type I error can be accepted (usually 5%).

Test of statistical significance

Z score

Z score is the simplest example of the statistical test which gives the deviation from the mean value expressed in standard deviation units. The Z score (or critical ratio) is the number of standard deviations that a value in a normally distributed population lies away from the mean. Thus, in a normally distributed population, 95% of the population lie within 1.96 Z scores of the mean.

Chi-square test

The chi-square test is commonly used in outbreak investigations to evaluate the probability that observed differences between two populations, such as cases and controls, could have occurred by chance alone if an exposure is not truly associated with disease. It is calculated by using two-by-two contingency tables (table 5.1). Because it takes a lot of patience to calculate chi-squares by hand, most investigators opt to use a computer with a statistical software package. The chi-square test can be used if the number of subjects in a study is approximately 30 or more. For smaller populations, or if the value of any of the cells in a two-by-two table is less than 5, the Fisher exact test should be used.

Fisher exact test

The Fisher exact test is used, for evaluating two-by-two contingency tables, is a variant of the chi-square test. The Fisher exact test is the preferred test for studies with few subjects. The formula for the Fisher exact test calculates the *P* value directly, so a table of chi-squares is not needed. However, in order to calculate the *P* value for the study, one must calculate the *P* value for the observations in the study and then add this *P* value to the *P* values of all possible combinations that have lower *P* values. This calculation should be done with the aid of a computer.

The *P* value

In the results of most research reports and scientific articles the *P* value seems to play a pivotal role. A *P* value less or greater than 0.05 conventionally indicates whether the findings are statistically, 'significant' or 'not significant' respectively.

This level of *P* value certainly means that there is statistical significance but does *not* necessarily mean that the results are clinically significant. Sometimes, a statistically significant difference may be clinically irrelevant.

Pitfalls of the *P* value

As has been mentioned earlier, the absence of a *P* value of 0.05 does not mean that there is no difference between the groups. The *P* value does not convey any information about the magnitude of differences between groups. Furthermore, the *P* value is equally influenced by the precision of the study results. Hence, a small (but consistent) difference may be highly statistically significant and a very large difference may lack statistical significance due to a variability of the test result. The *P* value can only be considered as an instrument to express the statistical certainty of a detected difference.

Alternatives to the use of the *P* value

Many researchers and biomedical journals prefer the use of 95% confidence intervals (CI) to the use of the *P* value. Briefly, a 95% CI reflects the range of differentiation that may be encountered in 95% of the cases if the experiment were repeated endlessly.

Confidence Intervals (CI)

Confidence intervals are estimates of where 'true' answers are most likely found. Whereas *P* values denote statistical significance, CI indicate clinical significance.

The CI (sometimes referred to as the margin of error) of a study with a stated probability (usually 95%) indicates that the true value of a variable, such as the mean, proportion, or rate, falls within the interval. In other words, a person using a 95% CI can be confident that if a study were repeated many times, the observed value would fall within the CI in 95 out of a 100 studies. Unlike the *P* value, which provides information on statistical significance only, the CI expresses the statistical precision of a point estimate and the strength of an association. The statistical precision is measured by the size (range) of the CI: the narrower the computed interval, the more precise the estimate. The strength of the association is measured by the magnitude of the difference in the measured outcomes between the two groups, e.g. the higher the numerical value of the risk ratio, the more likely the exposure is related to the outcome.

Confidence intervals provide an alternative to hypothesis testing when ratios of risk or rates are being compared. A 95% CI provides information on whether or not an observation is statistically significant with a *P* value less than or equal to 0.05. As noted previously, an odds (or risk) ratio of 1.0 means that the odds (or risk) of disease are the same between the comparison groups whether or not the exposure occurs. If the value of a risk ratio is greater than one, the risk of disease in the exposed population is greater than the risk of disease in the unexposed population. If a ratio of 95% CI does not include 1.0, then statistical significance is implied ($P \leq 0.05$). If the CI for an odds or risk ratio includes 1.0, then the findings are not statistically significant.

For example, if the odds ratio (the point estimate) for an exposure is said to be 8.1 with a 95% CI of 6.3–10.7, this means:

- persons with the disease were 8.1 times more likely to have been exposed to the risk factor than those without the disease, *and*

- one can be 95% confident (probability of 0.95) that the odds ratio in the population is between the confidence limits of 6.3 and 10.7 (i.e. it may be as low as 6.3 or as high as 10.7).

Although *P* values alone have traditionally been used to show the statistically significance between disease and risk factors in outbreaks, odds ratios/risk ratios and 95% CI are now frequently reported.

The calculation of CI depends on a representative sample from a normally distributed population. The width of the interval is determined by the degree of confidence desired (i.e. 90%, 95% or 99%), the variability of the data (standard error) and the number of observations (n). Larger numbers of observations result in narrower intervals.

Sensitivity and specificity

Sensitivity and specificity are terms that provide information about the accuracy of a diagnostic test. A diagnostic test is usually performed to establish the presence or absence of a disease. However, diagnostic tests are rarely 100% accurate and may give false-positive (i.e. the test indicates there is a disease, while this is in fact not true) or false-negative (i.e. the test falsely overlooks the presence of the disease) results.

The *sensitivity* of a test reflects the proportion of patients with the disease that have a positive test result, from the total number of patients with the disease. The *specificity* of a test reflects the proportion of healthy patients that have a negative test result, from the total number of patients that do not have the disease.

Test result	Disease present	Disease absent
Positive	True-positive (TP)	False-positive (FP)
Negative	False-negative (FN)	True-negative (TN)

Sensitivity = Percentage of cases with the disease who are detected by the test.

$$\frac{TP}{TP+FN} \times 100\%$$

Specificity = Percentage of people without the disease who were correctly labelled by the test as not diseased.

$$\frac{TN}{TN+FP} \times 100\%$$

Positive predictive value = Percentage of all test-positives who are truly positive (e.g. diseased).

$$\frac{TP}{TP+FP} \times 100\%$$

Negative predictive value = Percentage of all test-negatives who are truly negative (e.g. not diseased).

$$\frac{TN}{TN+FN} \times 100\%$$

References and further reading

Abramson JH. Making sense of data: *A self-instruction manual on the interpretation of epidemiology data*, 2nd edn. New York: Oxford University Press, 1994.

Birnbaum D, Sheps S. The merits of confidence intervals relative to hypothesis testing. *Infection Control and Hospital Epidemiology* 1992; 13: 553–555.

Centers for Disease Control and Prevention. *Principles of Epidemiology: An Introduction to Applied Epidemiology and Biostatistics*, 2nd edn. Atlanta, GA: US Dept of Health and Human Services, 1992.

Campbell MJ, Machin D. *Medical Statistics: A Common Sense Approach*. Chichester: John Wiley & Sons, 1990.

Edmiston CE, Josephson A, Pottinger J, *et al*. The numbers game: sample-size determination. *American Journal of Infection Control* 1993; 21: 151–154.

Freeman J, Hitchison GB. Prevalence, incidence and duration. *American Journal of Epidemiology* 1980; 112: 707–723.

Freeman J. Modern quantitative epidemiology in the hospital. In: Mayhall CG (ed.), *Hospital Epidemiology and Infection Control*, 2nd edn. Philadelphia: Lippincott Williams & Wilkins, 1999: 15–48.

Gaddis ML, Gaddis CM. Introduction to biostatistics: part 1, basic concepts. *Annals of Emergency Medicine* 1990; 19: 86–89.

Gaddis ML, Gaddis GM. Introduction to biostatistics: part 2, *Annals of Emergency Medicine* 1990; 19: 309–315.

Gaddis ML, Gaddis GM. Introduction to biostatistics: part 3, Sensitivity, specificity, predictive value, and hypothesis testing. *Annals of Emergency Medicine* 1990; 19: 591–596.

Gaddis ML, Gaddis GM. Introduction to biostatistics: part 4, statistical inference techniques in hypothesis testing. *Annals of Emergency Medicine* 1990; 19: 820–825.

Gaddis ML, Gaddis GM. Introduction to biostatistics: part 5, statistical inference techniques for hypothesis testing with nonparametric data. *Annals of Emergency Medicine* 1990; 19: 1054–1059.

Gaddis ML, Gaddis GM. Introduction to biostatistics: part 6, correlation and regression. *Annals of Emergency Medicine* 1990; 19: 1462–1468.

Gardner MJ, Aftman DG. Confidence intervals rather than *P* values: estimation rather than hypothesis testing. *British Medical Journal* 1986; 292: 746–750.

Giesecke J. *Modern Infectious Disease Epidemiology*, 2nd edn. London: Arnold, 2002.

Jackson MM, Tweeten SM. General principle of epidemiology. In: *APIC Infection Control and Applied Epidemiology: Principles and Practice*. St Louis: Mosby, 2000: 17.1–17.17.

Morris JA, Gardner MJ. Calculating confidence intervals for relative risks (odds ratios) and standardized ratios and rates. *British Medical Journal* 1988; 296: 1313–1316.

Mufloz A, Townsend T. Design and analytical issues in studies of infectious diseases. In: Wenzel RP, *Prevention and Control of Nosocomial Infections*. Baltimore: Williams & Wilkins, 1997: 215–230.

Ning L. Statistics in infection control studies. In: Wenzel RP. *Prevention and Control of Nosocomial Infections.* Baltimore: Williams & Wilkins, 1997: 231–240.

Phillips DY, Arias KM. Statistical methods used in outbreak investigation. In: Arias KM. *Quick reference to outbreak investigation and control in Health care facilities.* Gaithersbrug, Maryland: Aspen Publication; 2000: 191–209.

Riegelman RK, Hirsch RP. *Studying a Study and Testing a Test: How to Read the Health Science Literature,* 3rd edn. Philadelphia: Lippincott Raven, 1996.

Rowntree D. *Statistics without tears: A primer for non-mathematicians.* London: Penguin Books, 1981.

Tolly EA. Biostatistics for hospital epidemiology and infection control. In: Mayhall CG (ed.), *Hospital Epidemiology and Infection Control,* 2nd edn. Philadelphia: Lippincott Williams & Wilkins, 1999: 49–80.

Wacholder S, McLaughlin JK, Silverman DT, Mandel JS. Selection of controls in case-control studies. I. Principles. *American Journal of Epidemiology* 1992; **135:** 1019–1028.

Wacholder S, McLaughlin JK, Silverman DT, Mandel JS. Selection of controls in case-control studies. II. Types of controls. *American Journal of Epidemiology* 1992; **135:** 1029–1041.

Wacholder S, McLaughlin JK, Silverman DT, Mandel JS. Selection of controls in case-control studies. III. Design options. *American Journal of Epidemiology* 1992; **135:** 1042–1050.

6

Disinfection and Sterilization

Medical and surgical devices may serve as vehicles for the transmission of infectious diseases to susceptible hosts. Therefore it is important that all health care facilities should have a comprehensive disinfection policy. The aim of a disinfection policy is to make items and equipment safe for patients' use by effectively removing microorganisms by cleaning, disinfection and sterilization.

Methods of decontamination

The choice of method of disinfection or sterilization depends mainly on the type of material to be disinfected, the level of decontamination required for the procedure and the microorganisms involved. It is important to have a clear understanding of the terms and classification used in this context.

Cleaning: Cleaning of instruments before decontamination is an essential procedure. This allows the physical removal of microorganisms which prevents inactivation of the disinfectant by organic matter and allows complete surface contact during further decontamination procedures. Therefore *thorough cleaning of items is a prerequisite before disinfection and sterilization is commenced.*

Cleaning should be carried out by trained staff in the sterile supply department (SSD). Machine washing is the preferred option, however some instruments may require washing by hand. Staff performing these procedures must be trained in safe systems of work and wear appropriate protective equipments. During cleaning, care should be taken not to produce splashes, high pressure sprays or aerosols.

Disinfection by either heat or chemicals will destroy microorganisms but not bacterial spores. Chemical disinfection does not necessarily kill all microorganisms present but reduces them to a level not harmful to health. Chemical disinfection should only be used if heat treatment is impractical or may cause damage to the equipment. Chemical disinfectants are classified as chemical 'sterilant' which are used to disinfect heat-sensitive items if they can kill bacterial spores (which normally require prolonged exposure time); this process may be more accurately described as high-level disinfection.

The outcome of a disinfection procedure is affected by the presence of organic load (bioburden) on the item, type and level of microbial contaminant, prior cleaning of the object, disinfection concentration and exposure time, physical structure of the object and temperature and pH of the disinfection process.

Besides effective *cleaning* of items or equipments, the *concentration* and *contact time* are critical factors that determine the effectiveness of disinfection process.

Antiseptics: Chemicals used to kill microorganisms on skin or living tissue are known as antiseptics; disinfectants are used on inanimate objects only. Two factors must be evaluated in determining the effectiveness of antiseptics, i.e. the agents must have effective antimicrobial activity and must not be toxic to living tissues.

Sterilization is a process which achieves the complete destruction or removal of all microorganisms, including bacterial spores. Equipment and materials used in procedures involving a break in the skin or mucous membranes should be sterilized, e.g. surgical instruments and products intended for parenteral use or for instillation into sterile body cavities. In many procedures, high temperatures are used to achieve sterilization.

Dry heat sterilization: Dry heat sterilization requires higher temperatures for much longer exposure periods to kill all microorganisms. Exposure in an oven for 2 h at 170°C (328°F) is generally used for the dry heat sterilization of glassware and other items.

Moist heat sterilization: Moist heat is far more penetrating than dry heat and, hence, more effective for killing microorganisms. Steam under pressure is frequently used in sterilization procedures which can be achieved in an autoclave or sterilizer. A sterilizer is basically a chamber (see Fig. 6.1) that can withstand pressures of greater than two atmospheres. The materials to be sterilized are placed in a chamber, and the chamber is sealed. Steam is then transferred from a jacket into the chamber, forcing out all of the air to create a vacuum. The steam is held in the chamber for the necessary time and then vented from the chamber. Sterilizers have pressure gauges and thermometers that monitor the sterilization process. In addition to these, sterilizers are also monitored using chemical and biological indicators. The cycles most frequently used for sterilization are 134–138°C for 3 min, 121–124°C for 15 min or 115°C for 30 min.

If sterilization is not carried out in the hospital SSD then it is vital that sterilization procedures outside a central processing department promote the same level of safety and efficiency. Requirements include routine biological, mechanical and chemical monitoring to ensure that all parameters of sterilization are met before using the instrument on patients.

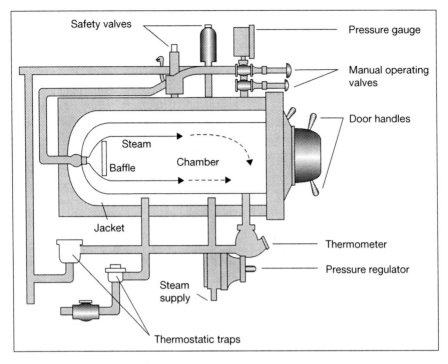

Figure 6.1 Diagram of a Sterilizer or an Autoclave showing basic features.
Reproduced from Atlas RM: *Microorganisms in our world*, St Louis Mosby, 1995.

Risks of infection from equipment

Spaulding outlined three categories of risks ('critical', 'semi-critical', and 'non-critical') from medical and surgical instruments based on the potential for the instrument to transmit infection if it is microbiologically contaminated before use. In 1991, Centers for Disease Control and Prevention (CDC) proposed an additional category designated 'environmental surfaces' to Spaulding's original classification. These are non-critical surfaces that generally do not come into direct contact with patients during care.

Critical or high risk items: Critical items are those that come into close contact with a break in the skin or mucous membrane or are introduced into a sterile body area. Items in this category should be sterilized by heat if possible. Heat-labile items may be treated with low-temperature steam and formaldehyde, ethylene oxide, or by irradiation. *Liquid chemical sterilant should be used only if other methods are unsuitable.*

Semi-critical or intermediate risk items: Semi-critical items are those that come into close contact with intact mucous membranes, or body fluids or are contaminated with particularly virulent or readily transmissible microorganisms or are to be used on highly susceptible patients or sites. In certain circumstances it may be preferable to transfer the items to the 'High Risk' category. *Disinfection by heat is preferred where this is possible.*

Non-critical or low risk items: Non-critical items are those that come into contact with normal and intact skin. Cleaning and drying of these items is usually adequate.

Minimal risk: Minimal risk items do not come into close contact with the patient or their immediate surroundings. Items in this category are either unlikely to be contaminated with significant numbers of potential pathogens, or transfer to a susceptible site on the patient is unlikely, e.g. bed-frames, lockers, flower vases, walls, floors, ceilings, sinks and drains. Cleaning and drying of these items is adequate.

Chemical disinfectants

Various chemical agents are used to disinfect items or equipment in a health care setting. Ideally, a disinfectant should have high germicidal activity. They should rapidly kill a wide range of microorganisms, including spores. The agent should be chemically stable and effective in the presence of organic compounds and metals. The ability to penetrate into crevices is desirable. It is essential that a disinfectant should not destroy the materials to which it is applied. Furthermore, it should be inexpensive and aesthetically acceptable.

Microorganisms vary in their sensitivity to particular antimicrobial agents. Generally, growing microorganisms are more sensitive than microorganisms in dormant stages, such as spores. Similarly, viruses are more resistant than other microorganisms to antimicrobial agents because they are metabolically dormant outside host cells.

Chemical disinfectants are hazardous substances and may cause damage on contact with skin, eyes or mucous membranes, by inhalation of vapours or by absorption through the skin. *Some individuals may be allergic to disinfectants,* or more sensitive to them than other people. This may take the form of skin rashes, contact dermatitis or, in rare cases, difficulty in breathing. Therefore it is important that *relevant safety precautions are observed when using chemical disinfectants.* Concentrated disinfectants should always be stored and handled with care and appropriate protective equipment must be worn. For certain chemical disinfectants (e.g. glutaraldehyde) proper ventilation is required.

The following points should be kept in mind when using chemical disinfectants:

- The efficacy of chemical disinfection is often uncertain and, wherever possible, disinfection by heat is preferable to chemical methods.

- All chemical disinfectants must be clearly labelled and used within the expiry date. They should be freshly prepared. They must be used at the correct concentration and stored in an appropriate container. Chemical disinfectant solutions must not be mixed or detergents added unless they are compatible.

- Disinfectant or detergent solutions must not be prepared and stored in multi-use containers for occasional use. Solutions prepared and stored in this manner may easily become contaminated with microorganisms; using such solutions will therefore readily contaminate a surface rather than clean it.

- Disinfectants can be corrosive and may damage fabrics, metals and plastics. Manufacturer's instructions must be consulted on compatibility of materials with the method of sterilization or disinfection.

Chemical disinfectants and antiseptics

Alcohol

Alcohol does not penetrate well into organic (especially protein-based) matter, and should therefore be used only on physically clean surfaces.

Uses: Alcohol impregnated wipes are used for disinfection of skin prior to injection. It can be used as a base for other antiseptics, e.g. chlorhexidine and iodine for pre-operative skin disinfection. Alcohol may be used for disinfecting physically clean equipment or hard surfaces as specified in the local disinfection policy.

Precautions: Alcohol should be stored in a cool place. *Alcohol-alcohol mixtures are flammable.* Do not allow contact with hot surfaces, flames, electrical equipment or other sources of ignition. *If an alcohol preparation is used to disinfect pre-operative skin, caution must be exercised whilst using diathermy as it may ignite, causing skin burns* if incorrectly used. Therefore all spirit-based skin cleaning and preparation fluids must have a cautionary statement, e.g. 'This preparation contains spirit. When use is to be followed by surgical diathermy, *do not allow pooling of the fluid to occur and ensure that the skin and surrounding areas are dry'.*

Do not leave bottles uncapped as alcohol vapours irritate mucous membranes, especially in an enclosed space. It may cause eye and skin irritation if used in a large quantity in an enclosed space, therefore its use should be avoided in a poorly ventilated area. If inhaled in large quantities, it may cause headache and drowsiness.

Chlorine-based disinfectants

Hypochlorites are the most widely used of the chlorine disinfectants. They are available as a liquid (sodium hypochlorite), or as a solid (calcium hypochlorite or sodium dichloroisocyanurate [NaDCC]). NaDCC tablets are stable and the antimicrobial activity of a solution prepared from NaDCC tablets may be greater than that of sodium hypochlorite solutions containing the same total available chlorine. Aqueous solutions of sodium hypochlorite are widely used as household bleach.

Table 6.1 Uses of hypochlorite and strengths of solution.

Uses	Dilutions	Available chlorine	
		(%)	(ppm)
Blood spills	1:10	1.0	10,000
Laboratory discard jars	1:40	0.25	2,500
General environmental disinfection	1:100	0.1	1,000
Disinfection of clean instruments	1:200	0.05	500
Infant feeding utensils, catering surfaces and equipment	1:800	0.0125	125

Reproduced with permission from Ayliffe GAJ, Coates D, Hoffman PN. *Chemical Disinfection in Hospitals*, 2nd edn. London: Public Health Laboratory Service, 1993.

Hypochlorites are fast acting, have a broad spectrum of antimicrobial activity, do not leave toxic residues and are not affected by water hardness. They are inactivated by organic matter, particularly if used in low concentrations. They are incompatible with cationic detergents. *Diluted solutions are unstable and should be freshly prepared daily.* In addition, decomposition is accelerated by light, heat and heavy metal. Chlorinated disinfectants are corrosive to metal, damaged plastic, rubber and similar components on prolonged contact, or if used at an incorrect concentration. They also *bleach fabrics, carpets or soft furnishings*.

Uses: Hypochlorite is very active against viruses and is the disinfectant of choice for environmental decontamination following blood spillage from a patient with known or suspected blood-borne viral infection. It is also incorporated into some non-abrasive cleansing agents which may be used for environmental disinfection on hard surfaces such as baths or sinks. It is used in water treatment and in food preparation areas and milk kitchen. Other uses in hospital and the recommended in-use concentrations are shown in Table 6.1.

Precautions: Chlorinated disinfectants can cause irritation of the skin, eyes and lungs if used frequently in a poorly ventilated area. They *should not be used in the presence of formaldehyde as some of the reaction products are carcinogenic.* Appropriate protective equipment must be worn when hypochlorite is handled, whether in liquid or powdered/granulated form. Skin and eyes should be protected when using undiluted hypochlorite solutions. *Sodium hypochlorite should not be mixed with ammonia or acid or acidic body fluids (e.g. urine), as toxic chlorine gas will be released.*

Phenolics

Phenol (carbolic acid) is probably the oldest recognized disinfectant. Its use as a germicide in operating rooms was introduced by Joseph Lister in 1867. Phenol and its chemical derivatives (phenolics) disrupt plasma membranes, inactive enzymes, and denature proteins, thereby exerting antimicrobial activities. They are usually

MICROORGANISMS		EXAMPLES	LEVEL OF DISINFECTION
PRIONS		Agents for Creutzfeld-Jakob disease.	PRION REPROCESSING
BACTERIAL SPORES		*Bacillus subtilis, Clostridium sporogenes, Clostridium difficile*, etc.	STERILIZATION
COCCIDIA		*Cryptosporidium*	
MYCOBACTERIA		*Mycobacterium tuberculosis*	HIGH LEVEL DISINFECTION
NONLIPID OR SMALL VIRUSES		Poliovirus, Coxsackie virus, Rhinovirus, etc.	INTERMEDIATE LEVEL DISINFECTION
FUNGI		*Trichophyton* spp., *Cryptococcus* spp., *Candida* spp., etc.	
VEGETATIVE BACTERIA		*Pseudomonas aeruginosa, E. coli, Staph. aureus, Salmonella* spp., *Neisseria meningitidis, Enterococci*, etc.	LOW LEVEL DISINFECTION
LIPID OR MEDIUM-SIZED VIRUSES		Herpes simplex, Cytomegalovirus, Respiratory syncytial, Hepatitis B, Human Immunodeficiency Virus (HIV), etc.	

Figure 6.2 Descending order of resistance to germicidal activity of chemical disinfectants against various microorganisms.

Reproduced with modification from Block SS: *Disinfection, Sterilization and Preservation*, 4th edn. Philadelphia, Lea & Febiger, 1991.

supplied in combination with a detergent to aid the cleaning process. They also retain their activity in the presence of organic material. They are incompatible with cationic detergents and absorbed by rubber and plastics. Cresols, which are phenolic derivatives of coal tars, are good disinfectants. The active ingredient in Lysol, a commonly used household disinfectant, is the cresol *o*-phenylphenol. The distinctive aroma of these phenolics gives many hospitals their characteristic smell.

Uses: Phenols are used for environmental disinfection. Routine-use dilution for the commonly used clear soluble phenolics is 1% v/v for 'clean' (low organic soiling) and 2% v/v for 'dirty' (high organic soiling) conditions. They are the agents of choice for mycobacteria including *M. tuberculosis* in the environment. Clear soluble (2%) phenolics can be used in laboratory discard jars in bacteriology.

Table 6.2 Antimicrobial activity of antiseptic agents.

Group	Gram-positive bacteria	Gram-negative bacteria	Mycobacteria	Fungi	Viruses	Speed of action
Alcohols	+++	+++	+++	+++	+++	Fast
Chlorhexidine (2% and 4% aqueous)	+++	+++	+	+	+++	Intermediate
Hexachlorophane (3% aqueous)	+++	++	+	+	+	Intermediate
Iodine compounds	+++	+++	+++	++	+++	Intermediate
Iodophors	+++	+++	+	++	++	Intermediate
Phenol derivatives	+++	+	+	+	+	Intermediate
Triclosan	+++	++	+	−	+++	Intermediate
Quaternary ammonium compounds	+	++	−	−	+	Slow

Activity: +++: Good; ++: Moderate; +: Poor; −: no activity or not sufficient.

Table 6.3 Antimicrobial activity and summary of properties of disinfectants.

Disinfectant	Antimicrobial activity					Other properties			
	Bacteria	Mycobacteria	Spores	Viruses		Stability	Inactivation by organic matter	Corrosive/ damaging	Irritant/ sensitizing
				Enveloped	Non enveloped				
Alcohol 60–70% (ethanol or isopropanol)	+++	+++	−	++	++	Yes (in closed container)	Yes (fixative)	Slight (lens cements)	No
Chlorine releasing agents (0.5–1% available chlorine)	+++	+++	+++	+++	+++	No (<1 day)	Yes	Yes	Yes
Clear soluble phenolics (1–2%)	+++	++	−	++	+	Yes	No	Slight	Yes
Glutaraldehyde (2%)	+++	+++	+++	+++	+++	Moderately (14–28 days)	No (fixative)	No	Yes
Peracetic acid (0.2–0.35%)	+++	+++	+++	+++	+++	No (<1 day)	No	Slight	Slight
Peroxygen compounds* (3–6%)	+++	±	±	+++	±	Moderately (7 days)	Yes	Slight	No

Good = +++, Moderate = ++, Poor = +, Variable = ±, None = −.
*Activity varies with concentration.

Precautions: Respiratory irritation may occur if used at concentrations above those listed in the disinfection policy. Appropriate protective clothing must be worn when handling phenolic disinfectants. Skin and eyes must be protected while 'making up' or discarding a phenolic solution. Phenolic disinfectants can be absorbed through the skin, therefore skin must be protected during its use. Use latex gloves for intermittent use; medium weight washing up gloves are appropriate for more prolonged contact.

Phenolic disinfectants should not be used to clean infant bassinets and incubators because of the occurrence of hyperbilirubinaemia in infants. If phenolics are used to clean nursery floors, they must be diluted according to the manufacturer's recommendation. *Phenol must not be used on items and equipments that may come into contact with skin or mucous membranes.* Phenolic disinfectants may taint food and should not be used on food preparation surfaces.

Chlorhexidine

Chlorhexidine is inactivated by soap, organic matter and anionic detergents. It also stains fabrics brown in the presence of chlorine-based disinfectants.

Uses: Used exclusively as an antiseptic where contact with skin and mucous membranes is involved. Chlorhexidine solutions are usually combined with detergent which is used for hand disinfection or with alcohol which is useful if rapid disinfection is required for physically clean hands. It is combined with alcohol for pre-operative skin disinfection and with other antiseptics for cleaning dirty wounds.

Precautions: Chlorhexidine is relatively non-toxic. *It must not be allowed to come into contact with the brain, meninges, eye or middle ear.*

Iodine and iodophors

This group includes aqueous iodine and tincture of iodine. It is inactivated by organic matter and may corrode metals. Iodophors do not stain skin and are non-irritant.

Uses: Alcoholic preparations containing iodine and iodophors are suitable for pre-operative skin preparation. Povidone iodine detergent preparations are used for surgical hand-disinfection.

Precautions: Use gloves for prolonged handling of iodine/iodophors preparation. An alcoholic iodophor is less irritant than an alcohol/iodine mixture. Tincture of iodine and aqueous iodine solutions can cause skin reactions in some individuals; therefore iodophor solution is usually preferred.

Quaternary ammonium compounds (QAC)

The most widely used cationic detergents are QAC. Several quaternary ammonium cationic detergents are used as antiseptic agents. These compounds are relatively non-irritating to human tissues at concentrations that are inhibitory to micro-organisms. However, they act slowly and are inactivated by soaps, anionic detergents and organic matter. Their antimicrobial activity is lowered if they are absorbed by porous or fibrous materials such as gauze bandages. Hard water containing calcium or magnesium ions interferes with their action. They can also cause metal objects to rust.

Uses: QAC may be used as antiseptics for cleaning dirty wounds. They should not be used in operating theatres because of the danger that they will permit growth of *Pseudomonas* spp. which can cause infection in surgical wounds (see below). Their use as an environmental disinfectant is usually not recommended.

Precautions: QAC inhibit the growth of bacteria (bacteriostatic) but do not kill them. *Gram-negative bacilli (e.g. Pseudomonas spp.) may cause contamination and grow in diluted solution.* Therefore, any unused solutions should be discarded immediately after use. *Decanting from one container and topping-up should be avoided.* This can result in contamination and promote growth of Gram-negative bacilli which may then colonize the wound. The correct strength of solution should be obtained from the pharmacy. Single-use sachets should be used, if possible. Liquid should be stored in closed bottles until immediately before use. Benzalkonium chloride is one of the leading allergens amongst health care personnel.

Hexachlorophane

Hexachlorophane is a chlorinated bisphenol and one of the most useful of the phenol derivatives. Unlike most phenolic compounds, hexachlorophane has no irritating odour and has a high residual action. Hexachlorophane is not fast acting and its rate of killing is classified as slow to intermediate. The major advantage of hexachlorophane is its persistence. Soaps and other organic materials have little effect. Hexachlorophane is more effective against Gram-positive than against Gram-negative bacilli.

Uses: Hexachlorophane (0.33%) powder has good residual effect on the skin and can be used as an anti-staphylococcal agent. *Use of hexachlorophane on broken skin or mucous membranes or for routine total body bathing is contraindicated. Hexachlorophane should not be applied on neonates* because it can cause neurological damage.

Triclosan

Triclosan phenol or Irgasan is a diphenyl ether. It can be absorbed through intact skin but appears to be non-allergenic and non-mutagenic with short term use. Its speed of killing is intermediate but it has excellent persistent activity on skin. Its activity is only minimally affected by organic matter. It is commonly used in deodorant soaps and health care hand washes. It has a similar range of antimicrobial activity as hexachlorophane but exhibits no documented toxicity in neonates.

Aldehydes

Glutaraldehyde

Most preparations of glutaraldehyde are non-corrosive to metals and other materials and inactivation by organic matter is very low. Alkaline solutions require activation; once activated they remain active for 2–4 weeks depending on the brand or preparation used and the frequency of use. Acidic solutions are stable and do not require activation, but slower in activity than alkaline buffered solutions.

Uses: 2% glutaraldehyde is used to disinfect heat-sensitive items such as endoscopes.

Precautions: Glutaraldehyde may be irritant to the eyes and nasal pathway and may cause respiratory illness (asthma) and allergic dermatitis. Glutaraldehyde should not be used in an area with little or no ventilation, as exposure is likely to be at or above the current Occupational Exposure Standards (OES: 0.2 ppm/0.7 mg m^{-3}, 10 min only). *Eye protection, a plastic apron and gloves must be worn when glutaraldehyde liquid is made up, disposed of, or when immersing instruments.* Latex gloves may be worn and discarded after use if the duration of contact with glutaraldehyde is brief, i.e. less than 5 min. For longer duration, nitrile gloves must be worn. It should be stored away from heat sources and in containers with close-fitting lids.

Formaldehyde

Uses: Formaldehyde is used mainly as a gaseous fumigant to disinfect safety cabinets in the laboratory and to fumigate the rooms of patients with highly dangerous pathogens. These uses may only be carried out by fully trained persons.

Precautions: Formaldehyde is a potent eye and nasal irritant and may cause respiratory distress and allergic dermatitis. Gloves, goggles and aprons should be worn when preparing and disposing of formaldehyde solutions. Monitoring may be required if formalin is used regularly as a disinfectant.

Peracetic acid

Peracetic acid is characterized by a very rapid action against all microorganisms. A special advantage of peracetic acid is that it has no harmful decomposition products and leaves no residue. It remains effective in the presence of organic matter and is sporicidal even at low temperatures. Peracetic acid can corrode copper, brass, bronze, plain steel, and galvanized iron but these effects can be reduced by additives and pH modifications. It is considered unstable, particularly when diluted. The advantages, disadvantages, and characteristics of peracetic acid are listed in Table 6.4.

An automated machine using peracetic acid chemically sterilizes medical, surgical and dental instruments including endoscopes and arthroscopes. It is more effective than glutaraldehyde at penetrating organic matter such as biofilms. It is used as a cold 'sterilant' to disinfect endoscopes. The solution is activated to provide the appropriate in-use strength. Once prepared, the current manufacturer's recommendation is that it should be used within 24 h.

Table 6.4 Summary of advantages and disadvantages for liquid chemical sterilants used primarily as high-level disinfectants.

Sterilization method	Advantages	Disadvantages
Peracetic acid	• No activation required. • Odour of irritation not significant.	• Materials compatibility concerns (lead, brass, copper, zinc) both cosmetic and functional. • Limited clinical use.
Glutaraldehyde	• Numerous use studies published. • Relatively inexpensive. • Excellent materials compatibility.	• Respiratory irritation from glutaraldehyde vapour. • Pungent and irritating odour. • Relatively slow mycobactericidal activity. • Coagulates blood and fixes tissue to surfaces.
Hydrogen peroxide	• No activation required. • May enhance removal of organisms. • No disposal issues. • No odour or irritation issues. • Compatible with metals, plastics and elastomers. • Does not coagulate blood or fix tissues to surfaces. • Inactivates *Cryptosporidium*.	• Material compatibility concerns for brass, zinc, copper, and nickel/silver plating (cosmetic only). • Serious eye damage if contacted.
Ortho-phthaladehyde	• Fast acting high-level disinfectant. • No activation required. • Odour not significant. • Excellent materials compatibility. • Does not coagulate blood or fix tissues to surfaces.	• Stains skin, clothing and environmental surfaces. • Limited clinical use.
Peracetic acid (Steris System 1)	• Rapid sterilization cycle time (30–45 min). • Low-temperature (50–55°C) liquid immersion sterilization. • Environmental friendly by–products (acetic acid, O_2, H_2O). • Fully automated. • No adverse health effects to operators. • Compatible with wide variety of materials and instruments.	• Potential material incompatibility (e.g. aluminium anodized coating becomes dull). • Used for immersible instruments only. • Biological indicator may not be suitable for routine monitoring. • One scope or a small number of instruments can be processed in a cycle. • More expensive (endoscope repairs,

Table 6.4 *Continued*

Sterilization method	Advantages	Disadvantages
	• Does not coagulate blood or fix tissues to surfaces. • Rapidly sporicidal. • Provides procedure standardization (constant dilution, perfusion of channel, temperatures, exposure).	operating costs, purchase costs) than high-level disinfection. • Serious eye and skin damage (concentrated solution). • Point-of-use system, no long-term sterile storage.

Adapted and modified from Rutala WA, Weber DJ. Disinfection of endoscopes: Review of chemical sterilants used as high-level disinfectants. *Infection Control and Hospital Epidemiology* 1999; **20:** 69–76.

Hydrogen peroxide

Hydrogen peroxide works by the production of destructive hydroxyl free radicals that can attack membrane lipids, DNA, and other essential cell components. Hydrogen peroxide is active against a wide range of microorganisms. Under normal conditions hydrogen peroxide is extremely stable when properly stored (e.g. in dark containers). Hydrogen peroxide and peroxygen compounds have low toxicity and irritancy.

Uses: Commercially available 3% hydrogen peroxide is a stable and effective disinfectant when used on inanimate surfaces. It has been used in concentrations from 3 to 6% for the disinfection of soft contact lenses, tonometer, biprisms, ventilators and endoscopes.

Precautions: A chemical irritation resembling pseudomembranous colitis has been reported in a gastrointestinal endoscopy unit with use of 3% hydrogen peroxide. As with other chemical sterilants, dilution of hydrogen peroxide must be monitored by regularly testing the minimum effective concentration (i.e. 7.5–6.0%). Hydrogen peroxide has not been widely used for endoscope disinfection because of concerns that its oxidizing properties may be harmful to some components of the endoscope. Manufacturer's approval should be obtained before using on equipment where corrosion may present problems, such as endoscopes or centrifuges.

Ortho-phthaladehyde (OPA)

OPA has an excellent antimicrobial activity. The product currently marketed as a sterilant is a premixed, ready-to-use chemical that contains 7.5% hydrogen peroxide and 0.85% phosphoric acid (to maintain a low pH).

OPA has several potential advantages compared to glutaraldehyde. It has excellent stability over a wide pH range (pH 3–9), is not a known irritant to the eyes and nasal passages, does not require exposure monitoring, has a barely perceptible odour, and requires no activation. OPA, like glutaraldehyde, has excellent material compatibility. A potential disadvantage of OPA is that it stains proteins grey (including unprotected skin) and thus must be handled with caution. However, skin staining would indicate improper handling that requires additional training and use of personal protective equipment, e.g. gloves, eye and mouth protection, fluid-resistant gowns. In addition, equipment must be thoroughly rinsed to prevent discoloration of a patient's skin or mucous membrane. Since OPA was only recently cleared for use as a high-level disinfectant, only limited clinical studies are available. Disposal must be undertaken in accordance with local regulations; OPA solution may require neutralization before disposal to the sanitary sewer system.

Ethylene oxide

Ethylene oxide has several applications as a sterilizing agent. The ethylene portion of the molecule reacts with proteins and nucleic acids. Ethylene oxide kills all microorganisms and endospores. It is toxic and explosive in its pure form, so it is usually mixed with a non-flammable gas such as carbon dioxide or nitrogen. A special autoclave-type sterilizer is used for ethylene oxide sterilization. Because of their ability to sterilize without heat, gases like ethylene oxide are also widely used on medical supplies and equipment that cannot withstand steam sterilization. Examples include disposable sterile plastic-ware such as syringes and Petri plates, linens, sutures, lensed instruments, artificial heart valves, heart-lung machines and mattresses.

Disinfection of flexible fibreoptic endoscopes

The number of endoscopic procedures used on patients for diagnostic and thera-peutic reasons is increasing each year. Although the overall incidence of infection following endoscopy is very low, it can only be avoided by maintaining the highest standards of decontamination after each use.

Rigid endoscopes (e.g. arthroscopes) are relatively easy to clean while flexible endo-scopes (e.g. bronchoscopes and gastrointestinal endoscopes) are complex and difficult to clean, disinfect and sterilize.

Endoscopes (e.g. arthroscopes, cystoscopes, laparoscopes) that pass through normally sterile tissues must be subjected to a sterilization procedure before each use; if this is not feasible due to damage caused by exposure to high sterilizing temperatures, they should receive high-level disinfection using liquid chemicals.

The *endoscope must be disinfected according to the written protocol based on the manufacturer's recommendations.* Effective decontamination of endoscopes requires input from:

- The user of the instrument who is familiar with the risks associated with the procedure.
- Infection control personnel who are responsible for advising on the selection and use of a suitable decontamination process.

- Endoscopy nurse, sterile services personnel or other persons responsible for processing.

- Instrument manufacturer or supplier who is familiar with the design and function of the item and its compatibility with heat and chemical disinfectants.

Cleaning and high-level disinfection or sterilization should be undertaken before the endoscopy list, between each patient, at the end of the list and prior to inspection, service or repair. This should be carried out by fully trained staff using appropriate protective equipment.

A log should be maintained indicating, for each procedure, the patient's name and medical record number (if available), the procedure, the endoscopist, and the serial number or identifier of the endoscope used.

Endoscopic unit

Facilities where endoscopes are used and disinfected should be designed to provide a safe environment for health care workers (HCWs) and patients. Air-exchange equipment (e.g. ventilation system, exhaust hoods) should be used to minimize the exposure of all persons to potentially toxic vapours (e.g. glutaraldehyde). The vapour concentration of the chemical sterilant used should not exceed allowable limits.

Personnel responsible for the reprocessing of endoscopes must receive training in the reprocessing of equipment to ensure proper cleaning and high-level disinfection or sterilization is carried out. Competency testing of personnel should be done on commencement of employment and then on an annual basis. All personnel working in an endoscopy unit must be educated about the biological, chemical, and environmental hazards. Personal protective equipment (e.g. gloves, eyewear, and respiratory protection) should be readily available and should be used as appropriate. *Staff should also be immunized against hepatitis B virus.*

Chemical disinfectants

The problems associated with the use of the most commonly used disinfectant, glutaraldehyde, have prompted the development of non-aldehyde alternatives (see Table 6.4). It is essential that advice is sought from the endoscope manufacturer on compatibility with any new disinfectant or process.

Formulations containing glutaraldehyde, OPA, hydrogen peroxide, chlorine, peracetic acid, and both hydrogen peroxide and peracetic acid can achieve high-level disinfection if the objects are properly cleaned and exposed to disinfectant solution at recommended concentrations and for recommended exposure times. *The selection and use of new disinfectants in the health care facilities should be approved by the persons or committees responsible for selecting disinfectants* and should be guided by information in the scientific literature.

It is essential that exposure time beyond the minimum effective time should not be used because of risk of damage to delicate instruments. Avoid the use of high-level disinfectants on an endoscope if the endoscope manufacturer warns against use because of functional damage (with or without cosmetic damage).

Routine testing of the disinfectant solution should be performed to ensure minimal effective concentration of the active ingredient. Check the solution each day of use (or more frequently) and document the results. If the chemical indicator indicates that the concentration is less than the minimum effective concentration, discard the solution.

Cleaning and disinfection of the endoscope

Thorough manual cleaning of the instrument and its internal channels with detergent is the most important part of the disinfection procedure. Without this, dry residual organic material such as blood or mucous may prevent penetration of the disinfectant. It also ensures better contact between the disinfectant or sterilant and removal of any remaining microorganisms in subsequent stages of decontamination. Cleaning with warm water and a neutral or enzymatic detergent is recommended, though advice on suitable cleaning agents should be sought from the endoscope's manufacturer. The detergent should be changed frequently to prevent its contamination with organic matter. It is important that the instrument is in full working order and that a 'Leak Test' has been performed to ensure that it is watertight prior to any cleaning procedure.

There are many automatic endoscope reprocessors available that are capable of cleaning as well as disinfecting endoscopes. However, *it is essential that initial manual cleaning at the point of use is performed* to ensure the effectiveness of subsequent processing and prevent the machine and the disinfectant becoming contaminated with excess organic matter or body fluids.

Ultrasonic washers may be used for most rigid endoscope components and accessories with the exception of the telescope. All lumens should be irrigated after ultrasonic cleansing to remove dislodged organic matter. Irrigation pumps are available for flushing instrument lumens and components.

- *All accessories should be disconnected and disassembled as far as possible and completely immersed in the enzymatic detergent.*

- All of the channels should be flushed and brushed, if accessible, to remove all organic materials (e.g. blood, tissue) and other residue.

- Reusable accessories (e.g. biopsy forceps or other cutting instruments) that break the mucosal barrier should be cleaned and then sterilized between each patient.

- External surfaces and accessories of the devices should be cleaned using a soft cloth, sponge, or appropriate brushes.

- The *instrument must be completely immersed in the high-level disinfectant,* ensuring that all channels are perfused.

- Detergents should be discarded after each use, as these products are not microbicidal and may allow microbial growth.

- The instrument and its channels should be thoroughly forced-air dried. A final drying step that includes flushing all channels with alcohol followed by purging the channels with air greatly reduces the possibility of recontamination of the endoscope by waterborne microorganisms.

- Endoscopes should be hung in a vertical position to facilitate drying. *Endoscopes should be stored in a manner that will protect them from contamination.*

- After high-level disinfection, endoscopes (including channels) must be rinsed with sterile water, filtered water, or tap water, followed by a rinse with 70–90% ethyl or isopropyl alcohol.

- The water bottle, used to provide intra-procedural flush solution, and its connecting tube should be sterilized or receive high-level disinfection at least daily. Sterile water should be used to fill the water bottle.

- After decontamination, *final rinsing of endoscopes and accessories with sterile water is important* as many of the agents used for this process deposit toxic residues which must be adequately rinsed off before the endoscope can be used.

Automatic endoscope reprocessor

If an automatic endoscope reprocessor is used, the endoscope should be placed in the reprocessor and the air channel connectors attached according to the manufacturer's instructions to ensure exposure of all internal surfaces with the high-level disinfectant/chemical sterilant. Since design flaws have compromised the effectiveness of the automatic endoscope reprocessor, the infection control staff should routinely review the scientific literature to ensure that all components of the endoscope are effectively reprocessed.

Problems due to inadequate decontamination

Major problems leading to inadequate decontamination include inadequate cleaning which may lead to failure to remove deposits of blood, faeces, tissue, mucous, microorganisms, film or slime. These may result in infection, misdiagnosis or instrument malfunction.

A number of factors have been associated with contamination of machines:

- Inadequate cleaning and maintenance of the machine.
- The use of static water, i.e. within pipework or tank.

- The use of water of poor microbiological quality.

- The use of hard water.

- Inadequate cleaning of the endoscope.

- The formation of biofilm within the machine.

All tank and fluid pathways in endoscope washer/disinfectors should be regularly drained, cleaned and disinfected to prevent colonization of the fluid pathway which could be responsible for misdiagnosis of a patient's infection. Disinfection should be performed at the start of each session prior to using the endoscope reprocessor. *Water used to rinse endoscopes following disinfection must be of a suitable quality* with respect to hardness and freedom from microbiological contamination.

A record must be kept of the number of washing cycles to ensure that the disinfectant is not unreasonably diluted or neutralized by organic matter. Appropriate records on disinfection of the equipment must be maintained by the department.

Microbiological quality of water or other fluids

Hardness of water results in the build-up of lime scale on the internal pipework of the washer/disinfector and poor microbiological quality of water may result in microbial contamination. Use pre-sterilized bottled water for stand alone machines and pre-treated water for machines connected to the main water supply. *Tap water may contain microbes including* Pseudomonas *spp. and* Mycobacterium *spp.* and there are many reports of procedure-acquired infection with these organisms. *Misdiagnosis of tuberculosis has been reported due to contamination of the instruments with environmental mycobacteria* (e.g. *M. chelonae*) from the rinse water which subsequently contaminated bronchial washings sent for culture. Therefore, sterile water is recommended for the final rinsing of all types of endoscope to be used for all invasive procedures.

Renewal of disinfectant

Serial processing of endoscopes in automated systems may reduce disinfectant potency due to constant dilution of the disinfectant by wet instruments. Therefore, disinfectant should be changed frequently; at least weekly, depending on usage and its contamination with organic matter. The concentration of glutaraldehyde in the solution should not be allowed to fall below 1.5% and solutions must not be used beyond the manufacturer's recommended post-activation life. Test kits are available which indicate glutaraldehyde concentration. The rinse water should also be changed regularly to avoid build-up of glutaraldehyde on the instrument and eyepiece assembly, as residues may cause skin and eye irritation.

Environmental cleaning

Effective environmental cleaning is essential because microbiologically contaminated surfaces may act as a reservoir of potential pathogens. *The transfer of microorganisms*

from environmental surfaces to patients is largely via hand contact with the contaminated surface. While handwashing is important to minimize the impact of this transfer,
cleaning is a form of decontamination that renders the environmental surface safe by
reducing the number of microorganisms and helps prevent cross-infection.

Housekeeping surfaces requires regular cleaning and removal of soil and dust. Dry
conditions favour the persistence of Gram-positive cocci (e.g. coagulase-negative
staphylococci) in dust and on surfaces, whereas *moist, soiled environments favour the
growth and persistence of Gram-negative bacilli.* Fungi are also present on dust and
proliferate in moist, fibrous material. *Hot water and detergent are sufficient
for most purposes.* Thorough cleaning and adequate disinfection is particularly
indicated for pathogens that can survive in the general environment for prolonged
periods, e.g. the spores of *Clostridium difficile,* vancomycin resistant enterococci
(VRE) and MRSA. *Routine environmental swabbing to monitor the effectiveness of
cleaning process should not be done.*

Cleaning removes organic matter, salts, and visible soils, all of which interfere with
microbial inactivation. The physical action of scrubbing with detergents and surfac-
tants and rinsing with water during environmental cleaning effectively removes
microorganisms. *Adding detergent aids cleaning* because one end of the detergent
molecule is hydrophilic and mixes well with water. The other end is hydrophobic and
is attracted to non-polar organic molecules. If the detergents are electrically charged,
they are ionic. Anionic (negatively charged) detergents are only mildly bactericidal.
Anionic detergents are used as laundry detergents to remove soil and debris. They
also reduce the number of microorganisms associated with the item being washed.
Cationic (positively charged) detergents are highly bactericidal.

Cleaning of environmental surfaces

Strategies for cleaning and disinfecting surfaces in patient care areas take into
account:

- Potential for direct patient contact.
- Degree and frequency of hand contact.
- Potential contamination of the surface with body substances or environ-
  mental sources of microorganisms (e.g. soil, dust, or water).

The number and types of microorganisms present on environmental surfaces are
influenced by several factors:

- Number of people in the environment.
- Amount of activity.
- Amount of moisture.
- Presence of material capable of supporting microbial growth.

Procedure for terminal cleaning of a room

Terminal cleaning of a room should be done when a patient who has been under source isolation is discharged. *Fumigation of the room is not necessary*. The following procedure should be followed:

- Domestic staff should wear appropriate personal protective equipment, e.g. household-type gloves, disposable plastic apron.

- Discard all disposable items or equipment as appropriate. Seal clinical waste bags before leaving the room and dispose off according to local policy.

- Remove any items or equipment to the dirty utility area for cleaning and disinfection. Send appropriate items to SSD for sterilization.

- Gently place all linen into the appropriate laundry bags. Bags must be sealed before leaving the room or the area.

- Dust the high ledges, window frames and curtain tracks.

- Wet clean all ledges, fixtures and fittings, including taps and door handles.

- Vacuum clean fixtures, fittings and floor. Only use a suitable vacuum cleaner with a high filter mechanism.

- The bed mattresses should be wiped with warm water and detergent and dried thoroughly. If disinfection is required use appropriate disinfectant, e.g. freshly prepared hypochlorite (1:100 dilution) solution.

- Wash sink with warm water and detergent. Rinse and dry thoroughly. Hypochlorite/detergent cleanser may be used, if indicated.

- Wash floor and spot clean walls with detergent solution. Rinse and dry thoroughly.

- Open windows, if required, to facilitate thorough drying of all surfaces.

- The room may be re-used again by the next patient when all surfaces are dry.

NOTE: Routine environmental swabbing to monitor the effectiveness of cleaning process should not be done.

- Rate at which organisms suspended in the air are removed.
- Type of surface and orientation, e.g. horizontal or vertical.

Housekeeping surfaces can be divided into two groups: those with minimal hand contact (e.g. floors, wall, window sills and ceilings) and those with frequent hand contact. Horizontal surfaces with minimal hand contact in routine patient-care areas require cleaning on a regular basis, when soiling or spills occur, and when a patient is discharged. Cleaning of walls, blinds, and window curtains is recommended when they are visibly soiled. *Areas of frequent hand contact should be cleaned more frequently than surfaces with minimal hand contact.* The methods and frequency for these processes, and the products used, are a matter for local policy.

Cleaning special-care areas

Since immunosuppressed patients are more susceptible to infection, it is essential that the following points should be taken into consideration when cleaning is undertaken in such an area:

- Wet dusting of horizontal surfaces should be done daily with cleaning cloths pre-moistened with a water and detergent. It is important that care should be taken to avoid patient contact with the detergent/disinfectants.

- Since dispersal of microorganisms in the air from dust or aerosols can be problematic for these patients, the cleaning equipment that produces mists or aerosols should be avoided. There is the potential for vacuum cleaners to serve as dust disseminators if they are not operating properly. Therefore it is essential that the vacuum cleaner should be equipped with high efficiency particulate air (HEPA) filters, especially for the exhaust. They should be used in any patient care area where immunosuppressed patients are present. Doors to patients' rooms should be closed when vacuuming areas where immunosuppressed patients are located. Bacterial and fungal contamination of filters in cleaning equipment is inevitable, and these filters should be cleaned regularly or replaced as per equipment manufacturer recommendation.

Cleaning method and equipment

It is essential that the *methods of cleaning produce minimal mists and aerosols or dispersion of dust in patient care areas.* Bucket solutions become contaminated almost immediately during cleaning, and continued use of the solution transfers increasing numbers of microorganisms to each subsequent surface to be cleaned. Therefore, cleaning solutions should be replaced frequently. Another reservoir for microorganisms in the cleaning process may be diluted solutions of the detergents or disinfectants (e.g. phenolics). Therefore it is essential that *fresh cleaning solution should be made daily and any remaining solution discarded after use.*

Management of blood spills

Splashes and drips

Procedure

• Wear non-sterile gloves for this procedure.

• Wipe the area immediately with paper towel soaked in hypochlorite (household bleach) solution 1:100 dilution; alternatively a disposable alcohol wipe can be used.

• Rinse treat surface with clean water as hypochlorite solution may be corrosive.

• Clean the area with water and detergent.

• Dry the surface with disposable paper towels.

• Discard gloves and paper towels as clinical waste according to local policy.

• Wash and dry hands immediately.

Larger spills

Procedure

• Sprinkle the spill with NaDCC granules until the fluid is absorbed if the quantity is small (≤30 ml). For larger spills, cover the spillage with paper towels to absorb all liquid and carefully pour a freshly prepared hypochlorite (household bleach) solution 1:10 dilution.

• Leave the spill for a contact period of about 3 minutes to allow for disinfection.

• Depending on the method used, either scoop up the absorbed granules or lift the soiled paper towels and discard into a yellow plastic waste bag as clinical waste.

• Wipe the surface area with fresh hypochlorite (1:100 dilution) solution and rinse with clean water as the hypochlorite solution may be corrosive.

• Dry the surface with disposable paper towels.

• Remove gloves and plastic apron and discard as clinical waste according to local policy.

• Wash hands and dry immediately.

Another source of contamination in the cleaning process is the cleaning cloth or mop head, especially if left soaking in dirty cleaning solutions. Laundering of cloths and mop heads after use, and allowing them to dry before reuse, can help to minimize the degree of contamination. A simplified approach to cleaning involves replacing soiled cloths and mop heads with clean items each time a bucket of detergent is emptied and replaced with fresh, clean solution. *Buckets should be emptied after use, washed with detergent and warm water and stored dry. Mops should be cleaned in detergent and warm water, then stored dry.* Disposable cleaning cloths and mop heads are an alternative option, if costs permit.

Brooms disperse dust and bacteria into the air and should not be used in patient areas. Dust-retaining materials, which are specially treated or manufactured to attract and retain dust particles, should be used as they remove more dust from surfaces.

Management of infectious spills

There is no documented evidence that any blood-borne virus (HIV, Hepatitis B or C) has been transmitted from an environmental surface. Nonetheless prompt removal and surface disinfection of an area contaminated by either blood or body fluids is necessary as a part of good infection control practice. Health care facilities should have management systems in place for dealing with blood and body substance spills. Protocols for spills management should be included in procedural manuals and emphasized in ongoing education and training programmes.

Management of a spill depends on a number of factors, including:

- The nature of the spill (e.g. sputum, vomit, faeces, urine, blood or laboratory culture).
- The pathogens most likely to be involved in these different types of spills (e.g. *Mycobacterium tuberculosis* in sputum).
- The size of the spill (e.g. spot, small or large spill).
- The type of surface (e.g. carpet or impervious flooring).

It is not necessary to use bleach for managing all spills but it may be used if the circumstances indicate that it is necessary. Spills of blood and high risk body fluids should be removed as soon as possible and the area washed with detergent/disinfectant and dried as outlined on page 77.

Cleaning and disinfection of medical equipment

Manufacturers of medical equipment should provide care and maintenance instructions specific to their equipment. These instructions should include information about materials compatibility with chemical disinfectants, whether or not the equipment can be safely immersed for cleaning, and how the equipment should be decontaminated if servicing is required. In the absence of manufactures' instructions, a member of the Infection Control Team should be consulted.

Decontamination of equipment prior to inspection, service or repair

Equipment and items which have been contaminated by contact with blood and high risk body fluids, pathological specimens, or exposure to patients in isolation will require decontamination prior to examination by third parties who perform inspection, service or repair. It is the responsibility of the individual heads of departments to ensure the policy is implemented. It is important that all decontamination procedures should be undertaken by suitably qualified and trained staff. The method of decontamination to be used should be one that does not damage the article or any of its components and could include steam sterilization, dry heat, or chemical methods. In cases of doubt about the appropriate method, advice should be sought from:

- The manufacturer or agent.

- Hospital engineering staff.

- The sterile services manager.

- A member of the Infection Control Team.

A record of the procedures used should be kept in the equipment log book. *A written declaration of decontamination status should be provided.* If the equipment is to leave the premises, the certificate/statement should be enclosed in an envelope affixed to the outside of the package.

In certain situations, equipment may not be decontaminated before inspection, service or repair, either because the equipment is subject to investigation as the result of a complaint or it may not be adequately decontaminated without engineering assistance. In such cases, the advice of the investigating body or engineering department should be sought. If such an item is to leave the premises, the following precautions must be taken:

- A prior warning should be given to the intended recipient.

- The condition of the item should be clearly labelled on the outer packaging.

- The packaging should be suitably robust to ensure that the inner pack cannot contaminate the outer pack or become damaged in transport.

- The agreement of any transporters may be required.

Decontamination of suction equipment

Suction systems can either be: (i) fixed unit, which can be used with a reusable (suction jar) or disposable (liner) reservoir or (ii) portable unit which is usually used with re-usable suction jar. Suction tubing, handles and catheters are all disposable. Suction containers or reservoir can either be disposable or non-disposable. When emptying non-disposable suction jar the following precautions should be taken:

- A plastic apron and household gloves should be worn. In addition, eye protection should be worn if the patient belongs to a *high risk* group. High filtration mask should be worn for a patient with pulmonary tuberculosis.

- The jar must be disconnected from the vacuum system, carried carefully to the dirty utility room and poured gently into the sluice hopper. The contents should be flushed with copious amounts of running water.

- The jar should be rinsed and then washed with a neutral pH detergent and hot water solution. It should be rinsed again in fresh water and dried with disposable wipes.

- A weak solution of sodium bicarbonate (mucolytic agent) may be used to help remove mucous material. Alternatively the suction jar may be machine washed in a washer/disinfector unit.

- The bottle should be emptied when full and cleaned at least daily irrespective of the amount of fluid aspirate. Fresh tubing should be attached just prior to use.

- The routine use of a disinfectant is not necessary for cleaning suction jars as the organic matter in the contents readily inactivates disinfectants. The only exception to this is when the patient has pulmonary tuberculosis or other infectious diseases. In such cases send the equipment to SSD for decontamination.

- A fresh single-use disposable suction catheter must be used each time a patient undergoes tracheo-bronchial aspiration. Yankaeur suction catheters or handles can be re-used on the same patient provided they are flushed after use by drawing a sodium bicarbonate solution through the tip followed by aspirating the air for 20 s, drying with a disposable tissue and storing in a protective cover. Approximately 10 ml of an anti-foaming agent may be added just prior to use to prevent excessive foaming of the bottle contents, which may wet the filter and enter the pump mechanism. The filter should be changed between patients or if it becomes moist or discoloured or used by an infected patient.

Table 6.5 Disinfection procedures for individual items and equipment.

Equipment or site	Suggested method(s)	Acceptable alternative or additional recommendations
Airways and endotracheal tubes	Single-use disposable or heat sterilize in the SSD.	Use single-use disposable item or heat sterilize for patients with known infections, e.g. tuberculosis, AIDS, etc.
Ampoules	Wipe neck with a 70% isopropyl alcohol impregnated swab and allow to dry before opening or piercing.	When a sterile ampoule exterior is required it will be processed by the SSD, by agreement with medical and pharmaceutical staff. Do not immerse an ampoule in a disinfectant solution.
Apnoea and enuresis monitors	Clean and dry regularly as part of a routine. If contaminated disinfect and then rinse and dry.	
Arm splint	Wash with detergent, rinse and dry.	
Auroscope tip	Use single-use tips and discard after single-use. If reusable tip then wash and disinfect between patient use.	
Babies feeding bottles and teats	Use pre-sterilized or heat-treated feeds. *Non-disposable bottles:* Wash thoroughly, rinse and place in fresh hypochlorite (125 ppm av Cl_2) solution for 30 min.	Chemical disinfectant should be used only when other methods are unavailable. Non-disposable bottles which originate from a milk kitchen must be returned for disinfection.
Baths	*Non-infected patients:* Clean with detergent or use a non-abrasive cream cleanser to remove stain or scum if necessary. Rinse and dry after cleaning, before and after use.	*Infected patients:* Disinfect by cleaning with a chlorine-based agent or non-abrasive chlorine releasing powder. *Patients with open wounds:* For patients with unhealed wounds and those who are immunocompromised, disinfect before use with a non-abrasive hypochlorite powder. Apply powder to a wet surface, rinse thoroughly and dry.
Bath water	Do not add an antiseptic bath additive routinely.	For staphylococcal dispensers seek advice from a member of the ICT.

Table 6.5 *Continued*

Equipment or site	Suggested method(s)	Acceptable alternative or additional recommendations
Beds and cots	Wash with detergent and dry.	*Infected patients:* Use hypochlorite (1,000 ppm av Cl$_2$) solution for disinfection. Do not use phenolic disinfectants on infant cots, prams or incubators as residual fumes may cause respiratory irritation.
Bed-frames	For normal cleaning use detergent and hot water. Perform cleaning after discharge of each patient and regularly in the case of long stay patients.	*Infected patients:* Wipe with disinfectant, wash with detergent, rinse and dry.
Bedpans and urinals	Dispose after single-use. If reusable heat disinfect in a washer/disinfector (80°C for 1 min). Store dry.	*Infected patients:* Gloves and plastic aprons must be worn when handling contaminated items from infected patients. Alternatively, single-use disposable items may be used. These should always be disposed of into a macerator unit.
Birthing pools	Use disposable pool liner. Clean and disinfect paying particular attention to the outlet.	
Bowls (washing)	Individual wash bowls should be available for each patient. After each use, wash with detergent, rinse, dry and store inverted and tilted forward to avoid trapping of water which may harbour microorganisms.	*Infected patients:* After thorough cleaning, disinfect by wiping with a disinfectant solution.
Bowls (surgical, sterile)	Return to SSD for autoclaving.	
Bowls (vomit)	Empty and rinse. Wash with detergent and hot water, rinse and dry.	For infected patients [*see above under Bowls (washing)*].
Breast pumps	For single patient use only. Wash with detergent and water and then rinse.	

Table 6.5 *Continued*

Equipment or site	Suggested method(s)	Acceptable alternative or additional recommendations
	Immerse in hypochlorite (125ppm av Cl$_2$) solution for 30min. Before use by subsequent patients clean, disinfect and autoclave.	
Cardiac monitors, defibrillators and ECG equipment	If patient contact, then surface clean and disinfect unless disposal is necessary (if single-use item).	
Carpets	Suction clean daily with a vacuum cleaner with an effective filter. Shampoo periodically by hot water extraction or when soiled.	For known contaminated spills, disinfect with an agent that does not damage carpet and then clean with a detergent. Seek advice from the Infection Control Nurse.
Cheatle forceps	Do not use.	If used in an exceptional circumstance, autoclave daily and store in a fresh 1% clear soluble phenolic disinfectant which must be changed daily.
Cleaning equipment	*Mops:* The detachable heads of used mops must be machine laundered, thermally disinfected and dried daily. *Mop bucket:* Wash with detergent. Rinse, dry and store inverted. *Scrubbing machine:* Drain reservoir after use and store dry.	Colour coded cleaning equipment should be used for each area, i.e. clinical, non-clinical, kitchen and sanitary area according to the local policy.
Commodes	For single patient use only, wash with detergent and rinse. Between use clean and disinfect.	If faecal contamination has occurred, remove soil with tissue. Wash with detergent and hot water. Wipe with disinfectant, wash, rinse and dry.
Crockery and cutlery	Machine wash with rinse temperature above 80°C and dry or hand wash in detergent and hot water (approx. 60°C), rinse and allow to dry thoroughly. Rubber gloves will be required at this temperature.	*Infected patients:* For patients with enteric infections or open pulmonary tuberculosis, heat disinfect in a dishwasher.

Table 6.5 *Continued*

Equipment or site	Suggested method(s)	Acceptable alternative or additional recommendations
Drains	Clean regularly as outlined in the maintenance programme. Chemical disinfection is not required.	When blockage occurs, contact Works and Maintenance Department.
Drip stands	Clean after each use.	
Duvets	Launder to thermal disinfection temperatures.	Launder after each patient use, weekly or if visibly soiled.
Endoscopes	*Flexible fibreoptic endoscopes:* (See page 69). *Arthroscopes and laparoscopes:* Clean and wash thoroughly. Rinse, dry and send to SSD for sterilization.	
	If this is not possible a 10 min exposure to alkaline glutaraldehyde is used. The instrument must be dismantled before disinfection and rinsed in sterile water afterwards.	If used on a patient where tuberculosis is suspected, then the contact time with 2% alkaline glutaraldehyde must be extended to 60 min.
	Procto/sigmoidoscope: Clean and wash thoroughly. Rinse and dry and send it to SSD for sterilization or use disposable if available.	
	If this is not possible a 10 min exposure to 2% alkaline glutaraldehyde must be dismantled and thoroughly cleaned before disinfection and rinsed in sterile water afterwards.	If used on a patient where tuberculosis is suspected, then the contact time with 2% alkaline glutaraldehyde must be extended to 60 min.
Enteral feeding lines	Single-use disposable.	
Floors (dry cleaning)	Vacuum clean or use a dust-attracting dry mop.	Never use brooms in patient areas.
Floors (wet cleaning)	Wash with a detergent solution. Disinfection is not routinely required.	If contaminated, disinfect and clean.
Fixtures and fittings	In clinical areas damp dust daily with detergent solution.	In known contaminated and special areas, damp dust with a disinfectant solution.

Table 6.5 *Continued*

Equipment or site	Suggested method(s)	Acceptable alternative or additional recommendations
Furniture and ledges	In clinical areas damp dust daily with warm water and detergent.	
Haemodialysis machines	Clean and disinfect, paying particular attention to the microbial quality of water and the fluid pathway. Regular microbiological monitoring is essential to validate effective disinfection.	
Hoist (patient)	Sling to be washed with detergent, rinse and dry between patients. Examine material and clips for wear or damage before each use. Surface clean the hoist.	
Humidifiers	Clean and sterilize device between patients and fill with sterile water which must be changed every 24 h or sooner if necessary. Single-use disposables are available.	Seek advice from the ICT.
Hydrotherapy pools	Filter, drain and clean regularly as part of a routine. Maintain disinfectant levels within water. Microbiological monitoring is recommended.	
Infant incubators	After use, wash all removable parts and clean with detergent. Clean and dry regularly as part of a routine. If contaminated disinfect and then rinse and dry.	*Infected patients:* After cleaning, wipe with 70% isopropyl alcohol impregnated wipe or with hypochlorite (125 ppm av Cl_2) solution before re-use. *Do not* use phenolic disinfectant. Alcohol may damage the plastic surfaces. Please refer to the manufacturer's instructions.
Instruments (surgical, sterile)	Return to SSD for machine washing and sterilization. Transport safely in a closed rigid container.	Contaminated instruments should be cleaned by trained staff in SSD before sterilization.

Table 6.5 *Continued*

Equipment or site	Suggested method(s)	Acceptable alternative or additional recommendations
Laryngoscope blade	Wash with detergent, rinse, dry and wipe with an alcohol impregnated wipe.	Contaminated instruments should be sterilized in SSD.
Linen	Refer to the local policy.	
Locker tops	Treat as 'Fixtures and Fittings'.	
Mattresses and pillows	Clean and disinfect the cover regularly as part of a routine. Rinse thoroughly and dry. Mattresses should be enclosed in a waterproof cover and routinely inspected for damage.	Should be protected by a waterproof cover. *Infected patients:* Disinfect with a disinfectant solution. Allow 2 min contact time then rinse and dry. Do not disinfect unnecessarily as this damages the mattress cover.
Mops (dish)	Do not use.	
Mops (dry, dust attracting)	Do not use if overloaded or for more than 1–2 days without reprocessing or washing. Alternatively a single-use disposable cover may be used and disposed of after each use.	Non-disposable dust mop covers must be vacuumed after each use. Single-use covers should be of the type which is impregnated with mineral oil to enhance dust attracting properties.
Mops (wet)	Mop heads must be changed daily. Reprocess by machine washing to thermal disinfection temperature and tumble dry.	If chemical disinfection is required, rinse in water, immerse in hypochlorite (1,000 ppm av Cl$_2$) solution for at least 30 min.
Nail brushes	Use only if essential. Heat disinfect in SSD after each use or use sterile pre-packed single-use disposable.	Do not soak in a disinfectant solution. Never use a nail brush to scrub skin.
Nebulizers	Empty in hot wash with detergent between single patient's use. Re-fill with sterile water only. Dispose of on patient discharge.	
Neurological test pins	Single-use only.	
Oxygen tents	Wash with hot water detergent solution, rinse well and dry thoroughly.	Store covered with clean plastic sheeting in a clean area.
Pillows	Use only with water impermeable cover. Treat as 'mattresses'.	Damaged pillows must be replaced immediately.

Table 6.5 *Continued*

Equipment or site	Suggested method(s)	Acceptable alternative or additional recommendations
Razors (electric)	Detach head, clean thoroughly, and immerse in 70% isopropyl alcohol for 10 min, remove and allow to dry between each patient.	Ideally each patient should have their own shaving equipment or use single-use disposable.
Razors (safety and equipment)	Use disposable or autoclave with single-use disposable head.	For clinical shaving use clipper.
Rhino/laryngoscope	Clean the blade thoroughly with detergent and hot water. Dry thoroughly and wipe with a 70% alcohol impregnated wipe.	In cases of suspected/ confirmed transmissible infection or visible blood, the blade should be sterilized before further use.
Rooms (terminal cleaning)	Wash surfaces with detergent solutions (see page 75).	*Transmissible infection:* Disinfect surface with disinfectant solution, wash with detergent, rinse and dry.
Scissors	Surface disinfection with a 70% alcohol impregnated wipe.	
Shaving brushes	Do not use for clinical shaving.	Use brushless cream or shaving foam. Patients may use their own brush for face shaves, it should be rinsed under running water and stored dry.
Sheepskins	*Synthetic:* Return to laundry department for washing in the usual way. *Natural fibre:* For individual use only.	Seek advice from the ICN.
Speculae	Single-use or clean and steam sterilize.	
Splints and walking frames	Wash and clean with detergent.	
Sputum containers	Use disposable only. Seal and discard as clinical waste daily or sooner if required.	
Stethoscope	Surface disinfect after each use.	

Table 6.5 *Continued*

Equipment or site	Suggested method(s)	Acceptable alternative or additional recommendations
Suction equipment	Following use, the reservoir should be emptied into the sluice hopper, washed with hot water and detergent, rinsed and store dried. Wear a plastic apron and non-sterile disposable for this procedure. The reservoir of the suction apparatus should be kept empty and dry when not in use.	When using a disposable system, great care is required to ensure the safe disposal of liners according to waste disposal policy. For infected patients seek advice from the ICN.
Thermometers (electronic)	Where possible use a single-use sleeve. If not possible use either single-use thermometer or clean and disinfect between use.	Do not use without sleeve or on patients with an infectious disease.
Thermometers (oral)	*Individual thermometers:* Wipe with a 70% isopropyl alcohol impregnated wipe after each use and store dry. On discharge, wash with detergent, immerse in 70% alcohol for 10 min. Wipe and store dry.	*Communal thermometers:* Wipe clean, wash in a cold neutral detergent, rinse, dry and immerse in 70% isopropyl alcohol for 10 min. Wipe and store dry.
Thermometers (rectal)	Wash in detergent solution after each use, wipe dry and immerse in 70% alcohol for 10 min. Wipe and store dry.	
Toilet seats	Wash daily with detergent and dry.	*Infected patient or if grossly contaminated:* Wash with disinfectant solution, rinse and dry. This is important in areas where soiling is more likely, i.e. gynaecology, maternity, urology department, etc.
Tooth mugs	Use disposable.	Heat disinfect in SSD, if non-disposable.
Toys	*Soft toys:* Machine wash, rinse and dry thoroughly. Do not soak toys in a disinfectant solution. *Others:* Wash with detergent, rinse and dry or wipe with an alcohol impregnated swab.	For children with infectious diseases do not use communal toys or those which cannot easily be disinfected. Heavily contaminated soft toys may have to be destroyed.

Table 6.5 *Continued*

Equipment or site	Suggested method(s)	Acceptable alternative or additional recommendations
Trolleys (dressing, patient theatre table)	Clean and surface disinfect.	Wipe trolley tops with an alcohol impregnated wipe before and after use. If contaminated, clean first, then use an alcohol impregnated wipe.
Tubing (anaesthetic or ventilator)	Reprocess by washing and sterilization in SSD.	*Infected patients:* For patients with respiratory infection, tuberculosis or patients with AIDS use disposable tubing. *Never* use glutaraldehyde to disinfect respiratory equipment.
Ultrasound	Clean and surface disinfect ultrasound head with 70% isopropyl alcohol between each patient.	
Urinals	Heat disinfect in a bedpan washer at a temperature of 80°C for 1 min or use disposables.	Disposable urinals must be disposed of in a macerator unit.
Ventilators	Cleaning and disinfecting the equipment is a procedure which is normally carried out in specified areas (i.e. ICU, special care baby unit, sterile supply department (SSD)) according to written protocol based on manufacturer's recommendations.	Contact a member of the ICT for advice if required.
Washbasin/sink	Clean with detergent, use cream cleaner for stains, scum, etc. Disinfection is not normally required.	Disinfection may be required if contaminated. Use non-abrasive hypochlorite powder or hypochlorite/detergent solution.
Wheel chairs	Clean and surface disinfect. Rinse and dry.	
X-ray equipment	Damp dust with detergent solution, do not over-wet and allow surface to dry before use.	Clean with detergent and then wipe with an alcohol impregnated wipe to disinfect. For specialized equipment, draw up local protocol for cleaning and disinfection based on the manufacturer's recommendations.

References and further reading

Alvarado CJ, Stolz SM, Maki DG. Nosocomial infections from contaminated endoscopes: A flawed automatic endoscope washer. An investigation using molecular epidemiology. *The American Journal of Medicine* 1991; **91** (Suppl. 3B): S272–S280.

Alvarado CJ, Reichelderfer M. APIC guideline for infection prevention and control in flexible endoscopy. *American Journal of Infection Control* 2000; **28:** 138–155.

American Society for Gastrointestinal Endoscopy. Ad Hoc Committee on Disinfection: Position Statement. *Gastrointestinal Endoscopy* 1996; **43:** 540–545.

Ayliffe GAJ, Babb JR, Bradley CR. Sterilization of arthroscopes and laparoscopes. *Journal of Hospital Infection* 1992; **22:** 265–269.

Ayliffe GAJ, Coates D, Hoffman PN. *Chemical Disinfection in Hospitals*, 2nd edn. London: Public Health Laboratory Service, 1993.

Ayliffe GAJ, Collins BJ, Lowbury ETL, *et al.* Ward floors and other surfaces as reservoirs of hospital infection. *Journal of Hygiene* 1967; **65:** 515.

Ayliffe GAJ. Nosocomial infections associated with endoscopy. In Mayhall CG, *Hospital Epidemiology and Infection Control*, 2nd edn. Baltimore: Lippincott Williams & Wilkins; 1999: 881–896.

Birnie GG, Quigley EM, Clements GB, Watkinson G, *et al.* Endoscopic transmission of hepatitis B virus. *Gut* 1983; **24:** 171–174.

British Society of Gastroenterology. Working party report. Cleaning and disinfection of equipment for gastrointestinal endoscopy. *Gut* 1998; **42:** 585–593.

Bronwicki JP, Venard V, Botté C, *et al.* Patient-to-patient transmission of hepatitis C virus during colonoscopy. *The New England Journal of Medicine* 1997; **4:** 237–240.

Classen DC, Jacobson JA, Burke JP, *et al.* Serious pseudomonas infections associated with endoscopic retrograde cholangiopancreatography. *American Journal of Medicine* 1988; **84:** 590–596.

Coates D, Hutchinson DN. How to produce disinfection policy. *Journal of Hospital Infection* 1994; **26:** 57–68.

Collins BJ. The hospital environment: How clean should a hospital be? *Journal of Hospital Infection* 1988; **11** (Suppl. A): 53–56.

Cooke RP, *et al.* Decontamination of urological equipment: interim report of a working group of the Standing Committee on the Urological Equipment of the British Association of Urological Surgeon. *British Journal of Urology*, 1993; **71:** 5–9.

Daschner F, *et al.* Routine surface disinfection in health care facilities: should we do it? *American Journal of Infection Control* 2002; **30**(5): 318–319.

Farina A, *et al*. Procedural residual glutaraldehyde levels in fibreoptic endoscopes: measurements and implications for patient toxicity. *Journal of Hospital of Infection* 1999; **43**: 293–297.

Favero MS, Bond WW. Chemical disinfection of medical and surgical materials. In: Block SS, ed. *Disinfection, sterilization and preservation*, 5th edn. Philadelphia: Lippincott Williams & Wilkins, 2001: 881–918.

Fraise AP. Choosing disinfectants. *Journal of Hospital Infection* 1999; **43**: 255–264.

Fraser VJ, Jones M, Murray PR, *et al*. Contamination of flexible fiberoptic bronchoscopes with *Mycobacterium chelonae* linked to an automated bronchoscope disinfection machine. *American Review of Respiratory Diseases* 1992; **145**: 853.

Hanson PJV, Clarke JR, Nicholson G, *et al*. Contamination of endoscopes used in AIDS patients. *Lancet* 1989; **2**: 86–88.

Healthcare Infection Control Practices Advisory Committee. Guidelines for Hand Hygiene in Health-Care Settings. *Morbidity and Mortality Weekly Report* 2002; **51**(RR–16): 1–45.

Hanson PJV, *et al*. Recovery of the human immunodeficiency virus from fibreoptic bronchoscopes. *Thorax* 1991; **46**: 410–412.

Infection Control Nurses Association: *Standards for Environmental Cleanliness in Hospitals*. Infection Control Nurses Association, 1999.

Larson E, Faan RN. Guideline for use of topical antimicrobial agents. *American Journal of Infection* 1988; **16**(6): 253–266.

Maki DG, Alvarado CJ, Hassemer CA, *et al*. Relation of the inanimate environment to endemic nosocomial infections. *New England Journal of Medicine* 1982; **307**: 1562.

Michele M, Cronin WA, Graham MF, *et al*. Transmission of *Mycobacterium tuberculosis* by fiberoptic bronchoscope. *Journal of American Medical Association* 1997; **278**(13): 1093–1095.

Rey JF, Halfon P, Feryn JM, *et al*. Transmission of virus Hepatitis C during endoscopic examination. *Gastroenterology Clinical Biology* 1995; **19**: 346–349.

Reeves DS, Brown NM. Mycobacterial contamination of fibreoptic bronchoscopes. *Journal of Hospital Infection* 1995; **30**: 531–536.

Rutala WA. APIC Guidelines Committee. APIC guideline for selection and use of disinfectants. *American Journal of Infection Control* 1996; **24**: 313–342.

Rutala WA, Gergen MF, Weber DJ. Comparative evaluation of the sporicidal activity of new low-temperature sterilization technologies: ethylene oxide, 2 plasma sterilization systems, and liquid peracetic acid. *American Journal of Infection Control* 1998; **26**: 393–398.

Rutala WA, Stiegel MM, Sarubbi FA, Weber DJ. Susceptibility of antibiotic-susceptible and antibiotic-resistant hospital bacteria to disinfectants. *Infection Control and Hospital Epidemiology* 1997; **18**: 417–421.

Rutala WA, Weber DJ. Clinical effectiveness of low-temperature sterilization technologies. *Infection Control and Hospital Epidemiology* 1998; **19**: 798–804.

Rutala WA, Weber DJ. Disinfection of endoscopes: review of new chemical sterilants used for high-level disinfection. *Infection Control and Hospital Epidemiology* 1999; **20**: 69–76.

Rutala WA. Weber DJ. New Disinfection and Sterilization Methods. *Emerging Infectious Diseases Journal* 2001; **7**: 348–353.

Sammartino MT, Israel RH, Magnussen CR. *Pseudomonas aeruginosa* contamination of fibreoptic bronchoscopes. *Journal of Hospital Infection* 1982; **3**: 65–71.

Satter SA, Springthorpe VS, Tetro J *et al*. Hygiene hand antiseptics: should they not have activity and label claims against viruses? *American Journal of Infection Control*. 2002; **30**: 355–372.

Spach DH, Silverstein FE, Stamm WE. Transmission of infection by gastrointestinal endoscopy and bronchoscopy. *Annals of Internal Medicine* 1993; **118**: 117–128.

Spaulding EH. Chemical disinfection of medical and surgical materials. In: Lawrence CA, Block SS (eds): *Disinfection, Sterilization and Preservation*. Philadelphia: Lea & Febiger, 1968: 517–531.

Spaulding EH. Role of chemical disinfection in prevention of nosocomial infections. In: *Proceedings of the international conference on nosocomial infections*, 1970. Brachman PS, Eickhoff TC, (eds). Chicago, IL: American Hospital Association; 1971: 247–254.

Spaulding EH. Chemical disinfection and antisepsis in hospital. *Journal of Hospital Research* 1972; **9**: 5–31.

Tanaka H, Hirakata Y, Kaku M, Yoshida R, Takemura H, Mizukane R, *et al*. Antimicrobial activity of superoxidized water. *Journal of Hospital Infection* 1996; **34**: 43–49.

UK Medical Device Agency Bulletin. *The reuse of medical devices supplied for single use only*. (MDA DB 9501). London: Medical Device Agency, 1995.

UK Medical Devices Agency. *Device bulletin: The purchase, operation and maintenance of benchtop steam sterilisers*. (MDA DB 9605). London: Medical Devices Agency, 1996.

UK Medical Devices Agency. *Device bulletin: Decontamination of endoscopes*. (MDA DB 9607). London: Medical Devices Agency, 1996.

UK Medical Devices Agency. *Device bulletin: The validation and periodic testing of benchtop vacuum steam sterilisers*. (MDA DB 9804). London: Medical Devices Agency, 1998.

UK Department of Health. Health Technical Memorandum 2010. *Sterilization* (5 parts). London: HMSO, 1994–95.

UK Department of Health. Health Technical Memorandum 2030. *Washer-Disinfectors* (3 parts). London: HMSO, 1997.

UK Department of Health. *Sterilization, Disinfection and Cleaning of Medical Equipment: Guidance on decontamination from the Microbiology Advisory Committee.* Part 1 Principles (1993), Part 2 Protocols (1996), Part 3 Procedures (1999). London: Medical Devices Agency.

UK NHS Estates. *National Standards of Cleanliness for the NHS.* Norwich: The Stationary Office, 2002.

Vandenbroucke-Grauls CM, Baars AC, Visser MR, *et al.* An outbreak of *Serratia marcescens* traced to a contaminated bronchoscope. *Journal of Hospital Infection* 1993; **23**(4): 263–270.

Walsh SE, Maillard JY, Russell AD. Ortho-phthalaldehyde: a possible alternative to glutaraldehyde for high level disinfection. *Journal of Applied Microbiology* 1999; **86**: 1039–1046.

Weber DJ, Rutala WA. Role of environmental contamination in the transmission of vancomycin-resistant enterococci. *Infection Control and Hospital Epidemiology* 1997; **18**: 306–309.

Woodcock, *et al.* Bronchoscopy and infection control. *Lancet* 1989; **2**: 270–271.

Working Party Report. Decontamination of minimally invasive surgical endoscopes and accessories. *Journal of Hospital Infection* 2000; **45**: 263–277.

Working Party Report. Rinse water for heat labile endoscopy equipment. *Journal of Hospital Infection* 2002; **51**: 7–16.

7

Isolation Precautions

In the past, in order to prevent the spread of infectious conditions, patients with communicable diseases were often segregated. However, as our understanding of the transmission of infection has improved, isolation practices have accordingly been refined and moved from an early empirical approach to become more evidence-based and targeted.

The advent of HIV/AIDS epidemic by the mid 1980s created an urgent need for new strategies to protect health care workers (HCWs) from blood-borne viral infections. In 1985, universal blood and body fluid precautions (universal precautions) were proposed by the Centers for Disease Control and Prevention (CDC). This new approach emphasized, for the first time, the universal use of blood and body fluid precautions regardless of presumed infectious status. However, the term 'universal precautions' was thought to be ambiguous, leading to universal confusion in its interpretation and a false sense of security in its application. There was also concern that the use of gloves was considered to be a substitute for hand washing, and that this perception could increase the risk of nosocomial transmission of infection.

In response to these pressures, the CDC and the Hospital Infection Control Practices Advisory Committee revised the guidelines for isolation precautions in hospitals in the US (Garner JS, 1996). However, it is important to emphasize that there are sufficient differences in the approaches and practices used in the US, Europe and other part of the world. In addition, any such 'standardised' guidelines cannot address the needs of every hospital and hence it is essential that *individual health care facilities should write policies relevant to local need.* In essence, isolation procedures can be divided into two main categories, i.e. source isolation and protective isolation.

Source isolation: The aim is to prevent the transfer of microorganisms from infected patients, who may act as a source of infection to staff or other patients.

Protective isolation: The aim is to prevent infection in severely immunocompromized patients who are highly susceptible to infection both from other persons and the environment.

Source isolation

The CDC guidelines recommend a two-tier approach. The first tier or *standard precautions* are aimed at all patients within health care facilities, regardless of their diagnosis or infectious status. The second tier or *additional precautions* are transmission-based precautions that are used for patients who are known or suspected of being colonized or infected with pathogens transmitted by contact (with skin or contaminated surface), droplet and airborne routes.

The standard precautions contain a basic level of infection control precautions that are designed for the care of all patients regardless of their diagnosis or presumed infectious status. The goal of using standard precautions is to reduce the risk of transmission of microbes from both recognized and unrecognized sources of infection. Routine practice of these precautions should become second nature for any HCW. These precautions are the primary strategy for the successful control of nosocomial infectious for the following reasons:

- Infectious patients may not show any signs or symptoms of infection that can be detected in a routine history and medical assessment.

- Infectious status is often determined by laboratory tests that cannot be completed in time to provide emergency care.

- Patients may be infectious before laboratory tests are positive or symptoms of disease are recognized.

- Patients may be asymptomatic but infectious.

The additional precautions go beyond standard precautions and are based on the transmission of infection. They are designed to supplement infection control precautions which cannot be contained by standard precautions alone. These precautions are *transmission-based* and grouped into various categories according to the mode of transmission of microorganisms.

Airborne precautions

Airborne precautions apply to patients with known or suspected infections caused by airborne pathogens such as tuberculosis, varicella (chickenpox or disseminate varicella infection), and rubella (measles). Such pathogens are transmitted when a susceptible person inhales the small droplet nuclei of particle size ≤5 μm. Such particles are dispersed by air currents and can remain airborne for long periods of time, causing infection in a susceptible person if exposed at or beyond 3 ft or 1 m of the particle source. When a susceptible person inhales dust particles that contain infectious microbes, they can reach the alveoli of the recipient to cause infection. Mechanical ventilation is helpful in diluting and removing this source of infection. *The source isolation room should be under negative pressure ventilation* (see page 21). The door should be kept closed.

A non-susceptible person, if possible, should replace a HCW who is susceptible to measles or chickenpox instead of caring for a patient with one of these diseases. If this is not possible, the susceptible worker should wear a mask. Airborne precautions require that HCWs wear respiratory protection when entering the room of a patient with known or suspected pulmonary tuberculosis (see page 137).

Droplet precautions

Droplet precautions are intended to reduce the transmission of infections spread by large particle droplets. Droplet transmission occurs when such particles come into contact with the eyes or mucous membranes of a susceptible person's nose or mouth, such as when an infected person coughs, sneezes, talks, or during procedures involving the respiratory tract such as suction, physiotherapy, intubation, or bronchoscopy. In addition, droplets are also produced when water is converted to a fine mist by a device such as an aerator or showerhead.

Large droplet transmission requires close contact with the infected person. The droplets travel only short distances (up to 3 ft or 1 m) from the source and do not remain in the air for long periods. Therefore, *special ventilation is not necessary to prevent droplet transmission.* Examples of infection caused by large droplet nuclei are meningitis caused by *Neisseria meningitidis*, pertussis, streptococcal pharyngitis, multi-drug resistant *Streptococcus pneumoniae*, influenza virus, measles, mumps, rubella virus etc.

Contact precautions

Contact is the *most important and frequent route of spread of nosocomial infections.* It occurs by either the direct or indirect route. *Direct contact* transmission involves skin-to-skin contact and physical transfer of microbes from an infected or colonized patient to a susceptible host. Direct contact may also occur between patients by means of a HCW's hand. *Indirect contact* transmission occurs when a susceptible host comes in contact with a contaminated object (such as bed scale, or commode) in the infected person's environment.

Examples of microorganisms spread by contact with secretions includes *Staphylococcus aureus* (including methicillin-resistant *Staphylococcus aureus* (MRSA)), faecal contamination from carriers of vancomycin-resistant enterococci, scabies, *Escherichia coli* 0157, *Clostridium difficile*, *Herpes simplex*, respiratory syncytial virus etc.

Protective isolation

Immunocompromised patients are generally at increased risk from both endogenous and exogenous sources of infection. They need protection from infection both from personnel and the environment. Their susceptibility to nosocomial infection may vary depending on the severity and duration of immunosuppression. *Most infections acquired by immunosuppressed patients are endogenous in origin* and isolation in a single room is not required. However, immunocompromised patients who have the greatest risk of infection include individuals who are severely neutropenic (i.e. <1,000 polymorphonuclear cells/μL for 2 weeks or <100 polymorphonuclear cells/mL for 1 week), allogeneic hematopoietic stem cell transplant patients, and those who have received intensive chemotherapy, e.g. childhood acute myeloid leukaemia. *Isolation measures are usually maximal for patients undergoing transplantation.* These patients may be particularly susceptible to environmental contaminants, such as aspergillosis or legionnaires' disease. A specialized room with positive pressure ventilation (see page 21) and high efficiency particulate air filtration is required.

In additions the following precautions should be kept in mind when dealing with immunocompromised patients:

- Where invasive medical or dental procedures are involved, it would be reasonable to place immunocompromised patients at the start of the operating schedule.

- In an outpatient waiting room, additional precautions for the control of airborne transmission of disease may be required. These patients should be seen ahead of others in the waiting room, to minimize the time for which they are exposed to other patients.

- They should be kept separate from other patients who are infected or have conditions that make the transmission of infection more likely.

Practical issues and considerations

Whenever isolation of a patient is considered, assessment of risk should be carried out and the disadvantages must be weighed against the benefits. *The placement of a patient into isolation should never be undertaken as a matter of convenience.* The patient's underlying condition is the driver for determining the provision of care and where it should be delivered. Isolation of patients may not only have a psychological impact on the patient, but isolation wards may also have an adverse influence on the quality of care by distancing the patient from specialist care. Therefore it is essential that the *need to continue isolation should be reviewed on a daily basis* and the patient should be discharged to the community or re-entered into the general hospital population at the earliest possible opportunity.

If isolation of patients is considered necessary, then it must be done at the time of admission in an appropriate single room, preferably with en suite toilet facilities.

Appropriate infection precautions must commence on clinical suspicion. If a single room is not available, then patients with the same infection or colonized with the same microorganisms may be cohorted in a designated area; this is particularly useful in an outbreak situation.

Patients with highly transmissible and dangerous infections, e.g. viral haemorrhagic fevers must be admitted or transferred to a local Infectious Diseases Unit under strict isolation.

All HCWs should be appropriately and adequately immunized against infectious diseases, both for their own protection and the protection of others. They must follow basic infection control procedures at all times. In addition, they must be given adequate education and training in all activities to prevent exposure of microorganisms to themselves and others. The education programme should be regularly updated in view of changing knowledge and work practice.

It is essential that *senior medical staff must act as role models for good infection control practice.* During the ward round they must observe all the necessary infection control precautions (esp. hand washing) and if possible, should attend the patient in source isolation last, after dealing with all non-infected patients.

Hand washing is absolutely essential to reduce the risk of infection transmission. Antiseptic hand wash preparations or alcoholic hand rub should be used. Hands must be washed or disinfected after removing gloves, between patient contacts, after touching contaminated patient care equipment, and after coming in contact with blood or body fluids.

An admissions policy to deal with potentially infectious patients, inter-hospital transfers and patients from overseas should be drawn up. The initial point of contact between a hospital and the infectious patient may be the accident and emergency (A&E) department. There is a greater risk of transfer of microorganisms in A&E as they are often crowded, may have prolonged patient stays and are usually manned by staff working under considerable pressures. In order to reduce these risks, hospitals should consider establishing a fast track or triage system through the accident and emergency department for potentially infectious patients.

Once admitted, every effort should be made to limit the movement of infectious patients for essential purpose only. Visits to other departments must be managed to limit the time out of isolation and contact with other patients. If possible, the patient should be advised of ways in which he or she can assist.

Door sign

An appropriate sign should be prominently displayed, providing sufficient information whilst ensuring that there is no breach of medical confidentiality. Care must be taken not to stigmatize the patient in isolation.

Visitors

All visitors must report to the nurse-in-charge before entering the room for instruction on protective clothing and other precautions. Effective communication by the infection control team (ICT) is necessary with visitors and staff who may need information regarding the risk of acquisition of infection.

Personal protective equipment

Gloves: Wear clean, non-sterile gloves for procedures that may involve contact with blood or body fluids, secretions, excretions, or non-intact skin or mucous membranes. Remove gloves promptly after use; *wash hands after removing gloves.* A separate pair of gloves should be used for the next patient.

Masks and eye protection: Masks and eye protection help to guard the mucous membranes of the eyes, nose, and mouth from exposure to blood or body fluids that may be splashed, sprayed, or splattered into the face. Wear such protective gear if splashing of blood or high risk body fluid is anticipated. Masks are single-use items and should be disposed of as clinical waste.

Aprons: Single-use disposable plastic aprons are recommended for general use and should be worn when there is a risk that clothing or uniform may become exposed to blood, body fluids, secretions and excretions. Plastic aprons should be worn as single-use items for one procedure or episode of patient care only. They should be removed immediately after use by tearing the neck strap and the waist tie and discarded into clinical waste bag before leaving the room. Hands must be washed immediately after removing and bagging the soiled plastic apron.

Gowns: Clean, non-sterile gowns should be worn during procedures which are likely to exposed HCWs with spraying or splashing of blood, body fluids, secretions, or excretions. Gowns should be impermeable and water repellent. If the gown is expected to become wet during the procedure and if a water repellent gown is not available, a plastic apron should be worn over the gown. Grossly soiled gowns should be promptly removed and placed in the designated leak-proof laundry bag. Hands should be washed immediately after removing and bagging of the soiled gown.

Crockery and cutlery

Crockery and cutlery used by infectious patients can be washed in the normal hospital dishwasher and represent a very low risk for the transmission of infection. The combination of hot water and detergent used by well-maintained dishwashing machines is sufficient to decontaminate crockery and cutlery. Washing by hand may not always guarantee decontamination. *Disposable utensils are not normally required.*

Linen

Wear appropriate protective equipment when handling linen contaminated with blood, body fluids, secretions, or excretions. Handle soiled linen as little as possible and place it in a appropriate laundry bag. To avoid contaminating a uniform, soiled linen should be held away from body.

Environmental cleaning

Whilst in use by a patient, the room and its equipment should be cleaned using the agreed *Standard Isolation* procedures unless the infecting microorganism or the degree of environmental contamination indicates a need for special action. Hot water and detergent are sufficient for most purposes. Thorough cleaning and adequate disinfection is particularly indicated for pathogens that can survive in the general environment for prolonged periods, e.g. the spores of *C. difficile*.

When the patient is discharged from an isolation room, before re-use, the room should be thoroughly cleaned, including all furniture and equipment (see page 75). *When dry, it may be occupied by the next patient.* The methods and frequency for these processes, and the products used, are a matter for local policy. Staff employed for these purposes should receive specific training in the relevant aspects of infection control, which includes issues for specific areas such as isolation rooms.

Spillage of blood and body fluids should be disinfected and cleaned promptly using a safe method (see page 77). Appropriate protective clothing should be worn and waste should be discarded as clinical waste.

Decontamination of items and equipment

Reusable equipment should not be used for the care of another patient until it has been cleaned and adequately decontaminated. If the equipment is soiled with blood, body fluids, secretions, or excretions, wear appropriate protective gear when cleaning or handling it. Discard single-use items after their use.

Bedpans/urinals

Excreta from infected patients should be disposed of as soon as practicable; prior soaking in disinfectant is not required. Commodes, bed pan carriers, urine measuring jugs, and toilets are a risk particularly for enteric pathogen transfer and must be regularly and adequately cleaned according to local policies.

Single-use bedpans and urinals can be employed and are disposed of in a macerator. Reusable bedpans/urinals should be cleaned and heat disinfected in a bedpan washer. *The bedpan washer must be included in a planned preventative maintenance programme.*

Clinical waste

Waste from patients with a known or suspected infection should be treated as clinical waste. It is important that the *amount of waste classified as clinical waste should be reviewed and minimized as far as possible.* All clinical waste should be put into an

Table 7.1 Summary of infection control precautions for various categories.

Activity	Standard precautions	Additional precautions		
		Airborne transmission	Droplet transmission	Contact transmission
Single room	No[a]	Yes – door closed	Yes	Yes – if possible. (cohort with patient with the same infection)
Negative pressure ventilation	No	Yes[b]	No	No
Handwashing	Yes	Yes	Yes	Yes
Gloves	For body substances	For body substances	For body substances	Yes
Gown	If soiling likely	If soiling likely	If soiling likely	If HCW's clothing will have substantial contact with the patient, environmental surfaces or items in the patient's room
Mask	Protect face if splash likely	Particulate mask for tuberculosis only. All others, regular mask.	No[c]	Protect face if splash likely
Goggles/ face-shields	Protect face if splash likely	Protect face if splash likely	Protect face if splash likely	Protect face if splash likely
Miscellaneous	Avoid contaminating environmental surfaces with gloves	Teach patient to cover nose and mouth when coughing or sneezing	Provide 1 m of separation between patients in cohort	Remove gloves and gown, wash hands before leaving patient's room

[a]Except certain circumstances determined by those responsible for infection control.
[b]Keep room vacant 1 h postdischarge of patient. 2–3 h for measles.
[c]Only for situations that may provoke contamination of mucous membrane. Procedures that are likely to create significant aerosols, e.g. suctioning, dentistry, intubation, chest physiotherapy etc.

appropriate plastic bag. All used sharps must be discarded, without re-sheathing, into an approved container. Sharps boxes should be readily accessible and must be securely fastened. Clinical waste should be segregated, stored and transported according to local policy.

Transport of pathology specimens

Collection, labelling and transportation of laboratory specimens from patients in isolation rooms should follow written policies that reflect national guidelines. *The specimens should be taken before starting antimicrobial therapy.* Laboratory specimens must be correctly labelled and packaged, i.e. the request form must be kept separate from the specimen in a self-sealing plastic bag. Specimens must be handled carefully, ensuring that the outside of the container is not contaminated. Specimens from a patient with known or suspected infectious disease should have a '*Danger of Infection – Take special care*' label both on the request form and on the specimen.

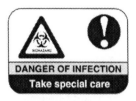

All specimens must be transported in an appropriate container to the laboratory. *The specimens from a patient with known or suspected to be infected with highly transmissible and dangerous pathogens must not be sent to the laboratory without prior arrangement with the laboratory staff.*

When a specimen pneumatic tube system exists this should only be used after appropriate consideration of the risks. Porters and others who transport specimens must be aware of the procedures for transportation and follow appropriate procedures in the event of spillage or breakage of specimen containers. Up-to-date standard operating procedures should be available for all these processes.

Commercial containers are available for safe transportation of specimens. Transportation of infectious material from one laboratory to another should follow local guidelines. International and national transport of infectious material by post, road, rail and air is subject to strict controls.

Deceased patients

As a general rule, the infection control precautions prescribed during life are continued after death. If a person known or suspected to be infected dies either in hospital or elsewhere, it is the duty of those with knowledge of the case to ensure that those who handle the body should be aware of the potential risk of infection, so that the appropriate control measures are taken. In cases where there is an infection risk from the body, a '*Danger of Infection*' label should be attached to the patient's armband.

Table 7.2 Type and duration of isolation precautions.

Disease	Category of isolation and precautions	Duration of infection control precautions	Comments
AIDS	Standard		See page 188
Actinomycosis	Standard		
Amoebiasis	Standard	As long as cysts appear in faeces	
Anthrax	Standard	Duration of hospitalization; until off antibiotics and cultures are negative	Laboratory must be informed if the specimens are sent for examination
Ascariasis	Standard		
Aspergillosis	Standard		No person-to-person transmission
Botulism	Standard		
Brucellosis	Contact	Precautions only if draining lesions(s)	Person-to-person transmission rare
Campylobacter gastroenteritis	Standard	Duration of diarrhoea	Person-to-person transmission rare
Candidiasis	Standard		Spread rare, except in high dependency units, i.e. SCBU, ICU etc
Chickenpox (Varicella)	Airborne and contact	Exclusion should continue until lesions are encrusted. Patient is infectious until 5 days after rash appears.	See page 165. Discharge patient home if clinical condition permits. HCWs should have a clear history of chicken pox or should know that they are immune. Visitors who have not had the disease to be warned of the risk.
***Chlamydia trachomatis* infection**	Standard	Duration of symptoms	
Cholera	Standard	Duration of illness	Until three cultures of stools are negative

Table 7.2 *Continued*

Disease	Category of isolation and precautions	Duration of infection control precautions	Comments
Clostridium perfringens			
Food poisoning	Standard		
Gas gangrene	Standard	Duration of illness	Usually autogenous infection. Not transmitted from person-to-person. Isolation of patient not necessary.
Clostridium difficile	Contact	Duration of diarrhoea	See page 147
Conjunctivitis			
Acute bacterial and chlamydial	Standard		
Gonococcal	Standard	Until 24 h after starting antibiotic therapy	
Acute viral haemorrhagic	Contact		
Cryptococcus	Standard	Duration of illness	
Cryptosporidiosis	Standard	Duration of diarrhoea	
Creutzfeldt-Jacob disease	Standard		No person-to-person transmission
Cytomegalovirus infection (neonates & immunocompromised)	Standard		Pregnant staff should avoid contact, particularly with patient's urine (see pages 216–217)
Diarrhoea	Standard		See page 155
Diphtheria			
Cutaneous	Contact	Until off antibiotics and three swabs are culture negative from skin lesions taken at least 24 h apart after antibiotic therapy	Throat and nasal swabs should be taken from all close contacts. Notify laboratory before swabbing contacts.
Pharyngeal	Droplet	Until off antibiotics and three consecutive swabs from nose and throat are culture negative	Culture positive carriers of toxigenic *C. diphtheria* should receive chemoprophylaxis with erythromycin

Table 7.2 *Continued*

Disease	Category of isolation and precautions	Duration of infection control precautions	Comments
			and swabs repeated after treatment. No admission of patients until contacts are bacteriologically clear.
Dysentery	Standard		
Amoebic	Standard	As long as cysts appear in faeces	
Bacillary	Contact	Duration of diarrhoea	Discharge patient home if clinical condition permits
Echinococcosis (Hydatidosis)	Standard		
Ebola virus	Contact	During hospitalization	See page 175
Encephalitis or encephalomyelitis	Contact	Until off antibiotic and cultures are negative	
Enteric fever			
Typhoid	Standard	Duration of diarrhoea	
Paratyphoid	Standard	Duration of diarrhoea	
Epiglottis (*H. Influenzae type* b)	Droplet		Close contacts should be given rifampicin as chemoprophylaxis
Gas gangrene	Contact		Usually autogenous infection. Not transmitted from person-to-person. Isolation of patient not necessary.
Gastroenteritis	Standard		See page 155
Glandular fever	Standard	Until acute phase is over	Isolation of patient not necessary
German measles (Rubella)	Droplet	From 7 days before up to 10 days from onset of rash	Discharge patients home if clinical condition permits. Exclude non-immune women (staff or visitor) of child bearing age.

Table 7.2 *Continued*

Disease	Category of isolation and precautions	Duration of infection control precautions	Comments
Gonococcal			
Ophthalmia neonatorum	Contact	For 24h after the start of effective antibiotic therapy	
Gonorrhoea	Contact	For 24h after the start of effective antibiotic therapy	
Hepatitis viral			
Type A	Standard and Contact	7 days before to 7 days after onset of jaundice	Hepatitis A is most contagious *before* jaundice and is infectious in the early febrile phase of illness. Close contacts may be given gamma globulin within 14 days to abort or attenuate clinical illness.
Type B & C	Standard		
Type E	Standard		
Herpes simplex	Contact	Until vesicles healed	Protect immunologically compromised patients. Wear gloves when hands are in contact with oral or genital secretions. Staff with cold sores should not work with compromised patients, neonates or burns patients.
Herpes zoster (Shingles)	Contact	Length of acute illness, i.e. until vesicles dry	As Herpes zoster may lead to cases of chicken pox, susceptible individuals and staff who have not had chickenpox should be excluded from contact with the patient. Visitors who have not had chickenpox should be warned of the risks.
HIV infection	Standard		Isolation required only in special

Table 7.2 *Continued*

Disease	Category of isolation and precautions	Duration of infection control precautions	Comments
			circumstances. See page 186
Hookworm disease	Standard		
Impetigo	Contact	For 24 h after start of effective antibiotic therapy	
Infectious mononucleosis (Glandular fever)	Standard	Until acute phase is over	Oral secretions precautions
Influenza	Droplet	In prodromal phase and for 5 days after onset	Immunization can be offered to a selected group
Lassa fever	Contact	Duration of hospitalization	See page 175 for details
Legionnaire's disease	Standard		Not transmitted from person-to-person; isolation of patient not necessary See page 151
Leprosy	Standard		
Leptospirosis (Weil's disease)	Standard	Duration of hospitalization	Contact precautions for urine only. Not transmitted from person-to-person; isolation of patient not necessary.
Listeriosis	Contact	Duration of hospitalization	Person-to-person spread rare
Lyme disease	Standard		
Malaria	Standard		
Marburg virus disease	Contact	Duration of hospitalization	See page 175 for details
Measles	Droplet	For 5 days start of rash, except in immunocompromized patients with whom precautions should be maintained for duration of illness	Discharge patient home if clinical condition permits. Immunoglobin for exposed immunocompromised patient. If outbreak in a paediatric ward, do not admit

Table 7.2 *Continued*

Disease	Category of isolation and precautions	Duration of infection control precautions	Comments
			children who are not immunosuppressed until 14 days after the last contact has gone home.
Meningitis			
'Coliforms'	None		
Listeria monocytogenes	None		See under Listeriosis.
Neisseria meningitidis (Meningococcal)	Droplet	For 48 h after start of effective antibiotic therapy and patient has received chemoprophylaxis	Visiting by all children should be discontinued. See page 160.
Haemophilus influenzae (type b)	Droplet	Duration of illness	Close contacts should be given rifampicin as prophylaxis.
Pneumococcal meningitis	Standard		
Tuberculosis	Standard or airborne if pulmonary TB		Isolate if patient has respiratory open pulmonary TB.
Meningitis	Droplet		
Viral	Standard	Until virus no longer present in stool	Seek advice from a member of infection control team (ICT)
Meningococcal septicaemia	Droplet	For 48 h after start of effective antibiotic therapy and patient has received chemoprophylaxis	See page 160.
MRSA	Contact	Until three swabs are negative	See page 121.
Multi-resistant Gram-negative organisms	Contact		See page 134.
Mumps	Droplet	7 days before to 9 days after onset of parotid swelling	Exclude non-immune staff. Inform visitors who are not immune. Persons with subclinical infections may be infectious.

Table 7.2 *Continued*

Disease	Category of isolation and precautions	Duration of infection control precautions	Comments
Mycoplasma	Standard		
Norcadia	Standard		
Orf	Standard		Contact precautions for exudates. Isolation of patients not necessary.
Pertussis (see Whooping cough)	Droplet		
Pinworm infection	Standard		
Plague			
Bubonic	Standard	Duration of hospitalization until culture negative	
Pneumonic	Droplet	Duration of hospitalization until culture negative	
Pneumonia	Usually none (see comments)		Isolation required with respiratory precautions for *Strep. pneumonia* resistant to penicillin MRSA, plague and psittacosis.
Poliomyelitis	Contact	Until stools negative for polio virus or 7 days from onset	Droplet spread is possible during its earliest phase first week; masks should be worn. Subsequently, faecal excretion is more important. Visitors and staff should be immunized. Gamma globulin for non-immuno contacts booster for immunized contacts. No elective surgery on non-immunized contacts. Virus shedding may follow vaccination with a live oral polio vaccine for several weeks.

Table 7.2 *Continued*

Disease	Category of isolation and precautions	Duration of infection control precautions	Comments
Psittacosis (Q fever)	Standard	For 7 days after onset	
Rabies	Standard	Duration of hospitalization	Immunize staff in close contact. See page 179 for details.
Ringworm	Standard		Isolation in a cubicle is advisable especially in paediatric ward.
Rubella	Droplet	From 7 days before up to 10 days from onset of rash	Discharge patient home if clinical condition permits. Exclude non-immune women (staff or visitor) of child bearing age.
Salmonellosis	Standard	Duration of diarrhoea	Staff (except in catering or food handler) may return to work when free of symptoms (i.e. formed stool).
Scabies	Contact	Until completion of appropriate treatment	See page 181–182 for details.
Schistosomiasis (Biliharziasis)	Standard		
Shigellosis	Standard	Until three cultures of stools are negative	
Streptococcal infection	Standard		
Group A (*Strep. pyogenes*)	Contact	Until off antibiotics and cultures are negative	
Group B	Standard		Cross-infection can occur in SCBU.
Group C	Standard		
Group G	Standard		
Staphylococcal (food poisoning)	None		
Syphilis Congenital, primary and secondary	Contact	For 48 h after start of effective therapy	Skin lesions of primary and secondary syphilis may be highly infectious.

Table 7.2 *Continued*

Disease	Category of isolation and precautions	Duration of infection control precautions	Comments
Latent (tertiary) and seopositive without lesions	Standard		
Tetanus	Standard		
Thread worm	Standard		
Toxocara	Standard		
Toxoplasmosis	Standard		
Trichomoniasis	Standard		
Trichuriasis (Whipworm)	Standard		
Tuberculosis			
Pulmonary (open)	Airborne	Two weeks after start of effective anti-TB treatment and sputum is negative for AAFB. Four weeks in neonatal and paediatric wards or if immunosuppressed patients are present.	Staff and visitors who are not immune should be warned of the risk. Face mask should be given. Refer to page 142 for details.
Closed	Standard		Isolation of patient not necessary
Typhoid/Paratyphoid fever	Standard and contact		
Vincent's angina (Trench mouth)	Standard		
Viral Haemorrhagic Fevers	Contact	Duration of hospitalization	See page 175.
VRE (Vancomycin resistant enterococci)	Contact		See page 130.
Whooping cough (Pertussis)	Droplet	Until 3 weeks after onset of paroxysmal cough or 7 days after start of effective antibiotic therapy	Discharge patient home if clinical condition permits. Visiting by children should be restricted to those who are immune. Prophylactic erythromycin to close contacts.
Yellow fever	Standard		

References and further reading

Ayliffe GAJ, Fraise AP, Geddes AM, Mitchell K (eds), Prevention of Infection in Wards II: Isolation of patients, management of contacts and infection precautions in ambulances. In: *Control of Hospital Infection – A practical handbook*. 4th edn. London: Arnold, 2000: 153–180.

Bagshawe KD, Blowers R, Lidwell OM. Isolating patients in hospital to control infection. *British Medical Journal* 1978; **2:** (Part I) 609–612, (Part II) 684–686, (Part III) 744–748, (Part IV) 808–811 and (Part V) 879–881.

Beekman SE, Henderson DK. Controversies in Isolation Policies and Practices. In: Wenzel RP (ed), *Prevention and Control of Nosocomical Infections*. 3rd edn. Baltimore: Williams & Wilkins, 1997: 71–84.

Breuer J, Jeffries DJ. Control of viral infections in hospitals. *Journal of Hospital Infection* 1990; **16:** 191–221.

Davies H, Rees J. Psychological effects of isolation nursing (1): mood disturbance. *Nursing Standard* 2000; **14:** 35–38.

Garner JS. The Hospital Infection Control Practice Advisory Committee. Guidelines for Isolation Precautions in Hospitals. *American Journal of Infection Control* 1996; **24:** 24–52.

Gopal RG, Jeanes A. A pragmatic approach to the use of isolation facilities. *Bugs and Drugs* 1999; **5:** 4.

Haley RW, Garner JS, Simmons BP. A new approach to the isolation of hospitalised patients with infectious disease: alternative systems. *Journal of Hospital Infection* 1985; **6:** 128–139.

Hospital Infection Control Working Party Report. Review of hospital isolation and infection control related precautions, July 2001. http://www.his.org.uk/

Lewis AM, Gammon J, Hosein I. The pros and cons of isolation and containment. *Journal of Hospital Infection* 1999; **43:** 19–23.

Lynch P, Jackson MM, Cummings JM, *et al.* Rethinking the role of isolation practices in the prevention of nosocomial infections. *Annals of Internal Medicine* **107:** 243–246.

Patterson JE. Isolation of Patients with Communicable Diseases. In: Mayhall CG (ed), *Hospital Epidemiology and Infection Control*. 2nd edn. Baltimore: Williams & Wilkins, 2000; 1319–1355.

Rahman M. Commissioning a new hospital isolation unit and assessment of its use over five years. *Journal of Hospital Infection* 1985; **6:** 65–70.

Rees J, Davies H, Birchall C, Price J. Psychological effects of isolation nursing (2): mood disturbance. *Nursing Standard* 2000; **14:** 32–36.

Wilson P, Dunn LJ. Risk analysis can identify those patients needing isolation. *British Medical Journal* 1997; **315:** 58.

APPENDIX I

Incubation periods

Diseases	Average period (range)
AIDS/HIV	Variable – may be years
Amoebic dysentry	2–4 weeks (few days to several months)
Anthrax	A few hours to 7 days (most cases occur within 48 h after exposure)
Ascariasis	4–8 weeks
Aspergillosis	Unknown
Botulism	12–36 h (up to several days) (Infant botulism 3 days to 2 weeks)
Brucellosis	5–60 days (highly variable may be up to several months)
Campylobacter enteritis	3–5 days (1–10 days)
Candidiasis	2–5 days
Cat-scrath disease	3–10 days to appearance of primary lesion, further 2–6 weeks to appearance of lymphadenopathy
Chancroid (*H. ducreyi*)	3–5 days (up to 14 days)
Chickenpox (Varicella)	13–17 days (10–21 days; may be prolonged after passive immunization against varicella and in the immunodeficient)
Chlamydial conjunctivitis (*Chlamydia trachomatis*)	5–12 days (3 days to 6 weeks in newborns; 6–19 days in adult)
Cytomegalovirus (CMV)	Within 3–8 weeks after transplant or transfusion with infected blood; infection acquired during first birth is demonstrable 3–12 weeks in newborn after delivery
Dengue Fever	7–10 days (3–14 days)
Dermatophytoses	See *under* Tinea
Diphtheria	2–5 days (2–7 days)
Erytherma infectiosum (Fifth disease or parvovirus)	4–10 days (variable)
Gastroenteritis (viral)	
Adenovirus	8–10 days
Astrovirus	1–2 days
Calcivirus	1–3 days
Norwalk	12–48 h
Rotavirus	1–3 days

Continued over the page

Diseases	Average period (range)
Gastroenteritis &	
food poisoning (bacterial)	
Salmonellosis	12–36 h (6–72 h)
Shigellosis (Bacillary dysentry)	1–3 days (12–96 h)
Campylobacter jejuni/coli	3–5 days (1–10 days)
Staphylococcus aureus	2–4 h (30 min to 7 h)
Clostridium difficile	5–10 days (few days to 8 weeks) after stopping antibiotics
Clostridium perfringens	10–12 h (6–24 h)
Clostridium botulinum	12–36 h (12–96 h)
Cryptosporidiosis	7 days (2–14 days)
Giardiasis (*Giardia lamblia*)	7–10 days (5–25 days)
Bacillus cereus	1–6 h where vomiting is predominant symptom 6–24 h where diarrhoea is predominant
Cholera	1–3 days (few hours to 5 days)
Escherichia coli (Entero-invasive [EIEC])	10–18 h
Escherichia coli (Enteropathogenic [EPEC])	9–12 h (probably)
Escherichia coli (Enterotoxigenic [ETEC])	1–5 days
Escherichia coli 0157:H7 (Verocyotoxin [VTEC])	1–3 days (12–60 h)
Vibrio parahaemolyticus	12–24 h (2–96 h)
Yersinia enterocolitica	24–36 h (3–7 days)
Aeromonas hydrophila	12–48 h
Listeria monocytogenes	48 h to 7 weeks
Gonorrhoea	2–7 days genito-urinary; 1–5 days ophthalmia neonatorum
***Haemophilus influenzae* type b infection**	2–4 days (probably)
Hand, foot and mouth disease	3–5 days
Hepatitis	
Hepatitis A	25–30 days (15–50 days)
Hepatitis B	75 days (45–180 days)
Hepatitis C	20 days to 13 weeks (2 weeks to 6 months)
Hepatitis D	35 days (2–8 weeks)
Hepatitis E	15–64 days (26–42 days)

Continued over the page

Diseases	Average period (range)
Herpes simplex	2–14 days (2–28 days perinatal infection)
Impetigo	
Streptococcal	7–10 days
Staphylococcal	1–10 days
Infectious mononucleosis (Glandular fever)	4–6 weeks
Influenza	1–5 days
Legionnaires' disease	5–6 days (2–10 days for pneumonia);1–2 days for pontaic fever
Leishmaniasis	
Visceral	Few weeks to 6 months
Cutaneous	Few weeks
Leptospirosis	10 days (4–19 days)
Listeriosis	3 days to 10 weeks
Lyme disease	7–10 days (3–32 days) after tick exposure
Lymphocytic choriomeningitis	8–13 days (15–21 days)
Lymphogranuloma venereum	3–30 days
Malaria	
P. falciparum	7–14 days
P. vivax	8–14 days
P. ovale	8–14 days
P. malariae	7–30 days
Measles	8–12 days (7–18 days)
Meningococcal disease	3–4 days (2–10 days)
Molluscum contagiosum	2–7 weeks (7 days to 6 months)
Mumps	16–18 days (12–25 days)
Mycoplasma pneumoniae	6–23 days
Pertussis (Whooping cough)	7–10 days (6–20 days)
Plague	
Bubonic	2–6 days
Pneumonic	2–4 days
Pneumocystis carinii	Unknown
Poliomyelitis	7–14 days (3–35 days)

Continued over the page

Diseases	Average period (range)
Psittacosis *(Chlamydia psittaci)*	1–4 weeks
Q fever *(Coxiella burnetii)*	2–3 weeks (depends on size of infecting dose)
Rabies	2–8 weeks (5 days to a year or more, depends on the site and severity of the wound; injury closer to brain has shorter incubation period)
Relapsing fever *(B. recurrentis)*	8 days (5–15 days)
Respiratory syncytial virus	4–6 days (2–8 days)
Ringworm *Tinea capitis* (scalp ringworm)	10–14 days
Tinea corporis (body ringworm)	4–10 days
Tinea pedis (athlete's foot)	Unknown
Tinea unguim	Unknown
Roseola infantum	8–10 days
Rubella (German measles)	16–18 days (14–32 days)
Salmonellosis	12–36 h (6 h to 3 days)
Scabies	2–6 weeks without previous exposure; 1–4 days re-infection
Shigellosis	1–3 days (12–96 h)
Syphilis	3 weeks (10 days to 3 months)
Tetanus	3–21 days (1 day to several months depending upon the character, extent and the location of wound)
Threadworms	Unknown
Toxic shock syndrome	2 days
Toxocariasis	Weeks to several months depending on the intensity of infection. Up to 10 years for ocular symptoms
Toxoplasmosis	7 days (4–21 days)
Tuberculosis	4–12 weeks (variable)
Typhoid and paratyphoid fevers	1–3 weeks (3–60 days)

Continued over the page

Diseases	Average period (range)
Typhus fever	12 days (1–2 weeks)
Viral haemorrhagic fevers	
Marburg	3–9 days
Ebola	2–21 days
Lassa	6–21 days
Yellow fever	3–6 days

8

Prevention of Infections Caused by Multi-resistant Organisms

Resistance to antimicrobial agents among clinically important bacteria has increased in recent decades and occurs worldwide. The impacts of resistance range from the failure of an individual patient to respond to therapy and the changes needed in empirical therapy to the economic impact of prescribing costs, hospital stay, and the social costs of morbidity and mortality from infection.

Acute health care facilities serve both as a point of origin and as a reservoir for highly resistant pathogens. This is because patients admitted to hospitals are highly susceptible and are usually subjected to intensive and prolonged antimicrobial use. In addition, failure in infection control practice can result in cross-infection and outbreak of nosocomial infections with highly resistant bacterial pathogens such as methicillin-resistant *Staphylococcus aureus* (MRSA), vancomycin-resistant enterococci (VRE) and multi-resistant Gram-negative bacilli as well as resistant fungal infections. Some of these resistant strains have now spread outside hospitals causing infections in the community. In addition, patients admitted to hospital can bring with them resistant microorganisms acquired in the community, including penicillin-resistant *Streptococcus pneumoniae*, multi-resistant salmonellae and multi-resistant *M. tuberculosis*.

The key element in minimizing the emergence of multi-resistant microorganisms and control include:

- *Active surveillance of infections and antimicrobial resistance* pattern recognition, investigation and control of outbreaks or clusters of infections.

- *Good microbiology laboratory practice* using international accepted method of antibiotic susceptibility testing is the key to the prompt identification of resistant pathogens and collection of accurate surveillance data.

- *Effective control of antimicrobial use* in health care setting by developing antibiotic policies based on local antibiotic resistance pattern and surveillance data. This should be supplemented by regular audit and feedback of date to the prescribers.

- Development and *implementation of appropriate infection control measures* including hand decontamination and isolation/cohorting of affected patients.

- *Adequate disinfection and sterilization of items and equipment,* which come into contact with patients.

- *Effective cleaning and decontamination of the hospital environment.*

- *Education and training of health care personnel* in appropriate aseptic techniques for medical and nursing procedures, infection control procedures, and antibiotic prescribing.

References and further reading

Bonten MJM, Austin DJ, Lipsitch M. Understanding the spread of antibiotic resistant pathogens in hospitals: mathematical models as tools for control. *Clinical Infectious Diseases* 2001; **33**: 1739–1746.

Goldmann DA, Weinstein RA, Wenzel RP, *et al.* Strategies to prevent and control the emergence and spread of antimicrobial-resistant microorganisms in hospitals. *Journal of American Medical Association* 1996; **275**(3): 234–240.

Nicolle L. *Infections control programmes to control antimicrobial resistance.* Geneva: World Health Organization, 2001. WHO/CDS/CSR/DRS/2001.7.

SHEA Position paper. Society for Healthcare Epidemiology of America and Infectious Disease Society of America Joint Committee on the Prevention of Antimicrobial Resistance: Guidelines for the Prevention of Antimicrobial Resistance in Hospitals. *Infection Control and Hospital Epidemiology* 1997; **18**: 275–291.

Society for Healthcare Epidemiology of America and Infectious Disease Society of America. Global Consensus Conference: Final Recommendations. *American Journal of Infection Control* 1999; **27**: 503–513.

UK Department of Health. *The Path of Least Resistance. Standing Medical Advisory Committee-Sub-Group on Antimicrobial Resistance.* London: DoH, 1998.

METHICILLIN-RESISTANT *Staph. aureus*

Staph. aureus is one of the most common pathogens well known for causing skin and soft tissue infection, e.g. impetigo, folliculitis, cellulitis etc. In addition, *Staph. aureus* may cause systemic infections such as abscesses, pneumonia, osteomyelitis, septicaemia, endocarditis and meningitis. Up to 30% of healthy people carry *Staph. aureus* in their nose and other moist and hairy areas of the body.

Methicillin (flucloxacillin or cloxacillin) resistant *Staph. aureus* (MRSA) are important in that they are resistant not only to flucloxacillin and erythromycin, the most commonly used antibiotics to treat *Staph. aureus* infection, but also to other oral antibacterial agents, leaving only intravenous (IV) antibiotics for treatment. MRSAs do not generally appear to be more virulent than sensitive strains but, because of their resistance patterns, ***they are more difficult to treat*** if infection occurs. In addition, intermediate vancomycin or glycopeptide resistant *Staph. aureus* (VISA or GISA) have been detected in some countries. In June 2002, the first clinical occurence of *Staph. aureus* fully resistant to vancomycin (VRSA) was isolated from the USA.

Despite vigorous attempts at eradication over the last 20 years, MRSA continues to be the major nosocomial pathogen worldwide. The level of hospital MRSA infection is indicative of the overall infection rate of the institution and usually reflects:

* Higher concentrations of sicker patients

* Overcrowding of wards

* Higher throughput of patients

* Heavy nursing load and under staffing, and

* Increased use of agency nursing staff unfamiliar with local infection control procedures.

There is a high patient morbidity and mortality associated with hospital-acquired MRSA especially in intensive care wards, infected vascular/orthopaedic prostheses, surgical wound infection and cases where septicaemia and pneumonia develop.

Source of infection

MRSA is common in many hospitals, and has a high propensity to become endemic. MRSA colonization precedes infection. Infected and colonized hospital patients are the major primary reservoirs in the health care setting. Colonization of hospital patients is dependent on:

* Length of hospital stay

* Severity of underlying disease

* Presence of wounds and/or invasive devices

- Recurrent or recent antibiotic treatment, and

- Nutritional status of the patient.

Community reservoirs include:

- Patients recently discharged from hospital

- Patients with chronic leg ulcer

- Nursing and residential home residents

- Patients with dermatological disease, e.g. eczema, and

- IV drug users.

Mode of transmission

The major route of transmission of MRSA within institutions is from patient-to-patient via the hands of hospital health care workers (HCWs) who acquire the organism after direct patient contact or after handling contaminated materials. *This is usually associated with inadequate handwashing.* Unfortunately it has been shown that HCWs, particularly doctors, frequently fail to wash their hands between seeing patients. Other forms of transmission, such as from colonized HCWs or from the air or environmental surfaces, are usually less important.

Control measures

It is important to ensure that a proper surveillance and monitoring system is in place. If it becomes apparent that the rate of MRSA is disproportionately high, then specific and locally appropriate preventative measures need to be developed and implemented. Although various guidelines have been published, *there are no universally agreed standards for control.* The approach of management depends on two factors:

- Endemicity of the resistant organism in the institution, and

- Vulnerability of the patients in the wards/unit where they occur.

In *non-endemic institutions,* the object should be *elimination* ('search and destroy' policy) of MRSA. Elimination involves confining the organisms to the individual(s) first identified as colonized or infected, and detecting other patients to whom the infection may have been transmitted (as for outbreak screening). Elimination is usually achieved by discharging colonized/infected patients. An alert system for readmission of these patients is required to make this fully effective, because carriage, (particularly of MRSA and VRE) can be very prolonged. The role of broader screening of risk groups on a routine basis is less clear, and costs can be considerable.

In an institution where MRSA is *endemic* the object is of *minimization* which involves ensuring that further transmission to new patients is minimized. Segregation of known colonized and infected patients still plays a useful role. In high-risk patients and clinical areas (e.g. intensive care units), some form of ongoing screening programme may be of benefit in identifying new admissions who are colonized.

In an acute health care facility, where the organisms are not endemic, rigorous application of infection control measures have been shown to be effective in containing or eliminating the problem, although this can be expensive and its cost-effectiveness is unclear.

Infection control precautions

All patients admitted from other hospitals and patients from other countries requiring medical treatment, especially with a history of previous hospital admission, should be admitted to a side ward and screened for carriage of MRSA. The patient's case notes must be identified with a warning MRSA sticker. They should also be 'flagged' on the Patient Information Services computer, if possible.

If asymptomatic patients are found to be carriers of MRSA, it is worthwhile discharging them from hospital (if clinical condition permits) on an anti-staphylococcal protocol (see page 125) for elimination of MRSA. *If the patient requires treatment in another hospital, the clinician and the member of Infection Control Team (ICT) at the receiving hospital should be informed.*

The number of staff caring for the patient should be kept to a minimum, if possible. Staff with skin lesions, eczema or superficial skin sepsis should be excluded from contact with the patient. As a general rule, patients with MRSA should be the last seen on a ward round, if at all possible.

- All patients known to be infected or colonized with MRSA should be admitted to a single room with its own bathroom facilities or cohorted with patients with the strain. The patient should be advised that there is no risk to healthy relatives or others outside the hospital. They should also be given information and a fact sheet about MRSA.

- Single-use disposable plastic aprons should be worn for activities involving contact with the patient or their environment. For extensive physical contact with the patient, non-permeable disposable gowns are required.

- The gown or plastic apron and gloves should be removed before leaving room. When disposing of protective clothing, it is essential that it should not come in contact with the environmental surfaces. Used plastic aprons/gowns should be discarded into a yellow clinical waste bag before leaving the room.

- Single-use disposable gloves should be worn for handling contaminated tissue, dressings or linen. *Hands must be decontaminated after removing gloves.*

- *High efficiency filter type masks should be used for procedures that may generate staphylococcus aerosols*, e.g. sputum suction, chest physiotherapy or procedures on patients with an exfoliative skin condition, and when performing dressings on patients with extensive burns or lesions.

- *Hands must be washed before and after contact with the patient or their immediate environment.* They should be washed thoroughly using an antiseptic chlorhexidine/detergent or alternatively, physically clean hands can be disinfected with an alcoholic hand rub.

- All single-use items must be disposed of as clinical waste. Clinical waste bags must be sealed before leaving the room. Any reusable items should be processed in accordance with the local disinfection policy.

- Use dedicated equipment, e.g. stethoscope, sphygmomanometer and thermometer. Clean and disinfect before reuse.

- Instruments used for dressing changes should not be transferred from patient-to-patient but should remain by the patient's bedside. Consider the surfaces and furniture within the rooms to be contaminated as well as the patients themselves.

- All bed linen and clothing should be changed daily. Used linen must be handled gently at all times and should be processed according to local policy. Linen bags must be sealed at the bedside and removed directly to the dirty utility area or to the collection point.

- After discharge of the patient, the room should be thoroughly cleaned using detergents. Surfaces should be disinfected using appropriate disinfectant, e.g. freshly prepared hypochlorite solution 1:100 dilution. *Once the room is dry it can be used for other patients.*

Patient's movement

Visits by patients with MRSA to other departments should be kept to a minimum. For any treatment or investigations, prior arrangements must be made with the other department. They should be seen immediately and not left in a waiting room with other patients.

Within the hospital: Transfer of infected or colonized patients to other wards or departments should be kept to a minimum. If the patient is moved to a different ward, all open lesions should be covered with an impermeable dressing during the transfer.

Inter-hospital transfer: Inter-hospital movement should be restricted where this is possible. If transfer is necessary, then the ICT of the receiving hospital should be informed. A letter should also be sent giving the relevant clinical details as to whether the patient is infected or colonized with MRSA and the details of the treatment protocol, so that a course of treatment can be completed.

Nursing or residential home: Continued *carriage of MRSA is not a contraindication for the transfer of the patient to a nursing or residential home.* If the patient is discharged to the residential or nursing home, the *owner of the nursing home should be informed.*

Decolonization therapy for MRSA

Treatment should be prescribed for 5 days at the advice of medical practitioner.

Nose: Apply 2% nasal mupirocin ointment three times a day for 5 days. A small amount of ointment (about the size of a match-head) should be placed on a cotton bud and applied to the anterior part of the inside of each nostril. The nostrils are closed by gently pressing the sides of the nose together; this will spread the ointment throughout the nares.

Body bathing: Shower: Wash vigorously with an antiseptic detergent (triclosan or chlorhexidine), beginning with and paying particular attention to the hair, around the nostrils, under the arms, between the legs (groin, perineum, and buttock area), feet and working downwards. Rinse from head to toe and dry body with a clean towel.

For the bath add antiseptic (triclosan or chlorhexidine) bath concentrate to a bath full of water immediately prior to the patient entering the water.

Body bathing or bed bathing: Patients confined to bed can be washed with an antiseptic detergent (triclosan or chlorhexidine). Wet skin, apply about 30 ml of antiseptic soap preparation directly onto the skin using a disposable cloth. Wash and rinse from head to toe. Dry body with a clean towel.

Note: Triclosan should be in contact with the skin for about 1 min and then thoroughly rinsed.

Hexachlorophane powder: Hexachlorophane 0.33% powder can be used to treat carrier sites. It should be applied to intact skin such as the perineum, buttocks, flexures and axillae three times daily for 5 days. *Do not* use hexachlorophane powder on badly excoriated or inflamed skin or during pregnancy. The product should be administered to children less than two years of age on medical advice only.

Colonized lesions: Mupirocin ointment can be applied topically three times a day to small lesions for 5 days. It should be used with caution if there is evidence of moderate or severe renal impairment. Dressing containing chlorhexidine or povidone-iodine may be applied to the infected wound.

Helpful hints

- Antiseptic detergents should be used with care in-patients with dermatitis and broken skin and must be discontinued if skin irritation develops.

- Mupirocin ointment should be reserved for the treatment of MRSA. Prolong course (more than 7 days) or repeated course (more than two courses per hospital admission) should be avoided to prevent emergence of resistant.

- Repeat swabbing is required at the advice of the ICT.

- Launder towels and cloths after use. Patient's clothes (including undergarments/nightwear) should be changed on a daily basis and washed in hot water cycle. Dry clean non-washable and woolen clothes. Bed linen should be changed at the beginning of protocol and then every day until the end of protocol.

Ambulance transportation: The ambulance service should be notified in advance. There is no evidence that ambulance staff or their families are at risk from transporting patients with MRSA. The following infection control measures should be taken:

- The patient should be given clean clothing before transport.

- A disposable plastic apron should be worn for patient contact.

- Physically clean hands can be disinfected with an alcoholic hand rub after contact with the patient or the environment.

- The patient's contact area, e.g. chair and the stretcher should be cleaned and disinfected with a large alcohol impregnated wipe or disinfectant solution after transport of an affected patient.

- Blankets and pillow cases should be placed in an appropriate bag for laundering according to local protocol.

- The vehicle should be thoroughly cleaned with detergent and disinfected with freshly prepared hypochlorite solution 1:100 dilution. The vehicle may be used when all surfaces are dry. *Fumigation and prolonged airing is not necessary. Once the ambulance is dry it can be used for other patients.*

Patient screening and microbiological surveillance

A swab moistened with sterile water should be used to sample carrier sites and lesions. The screening swabs should be taken from the nose, perineum/groin, operative and wound sites, abnormal or damaged skin, insertion sites of IV lines, catheter urine samples and sputum, if expectorating, at the advice of the ICT.

Once the patient is positive for MRSA, swabs from carrier and other sites should be taken at least 3 days after stopping the MRSA treatment protocol. Three sets of negative screening swabs are required before the patient is considered to be 'clear', as scanty colonization may not be detected with fewer screening specimens. *Advice should be taken from a member of the ICT regarding follow-up screening swabs.* It is important to note that relapses are particularly likely if the patient is receiving antibiotics and can occur after relatively long periods, such as 6–12 months. *Carriage of MRSA strains may persist for months or years* and may reappear in an apparently 'clear or cured' patient.

Clearance of MRSA carriage

If considered appropriate, clearance of MRSA carriage should be carried out as outlined on page 125. *The treatment should only be prescribed on the advice of the medical practitioner.*

Topical nasal applications of antibiotics are usually ineffective in clearing throat or sputum colonization. In addition, it is also often difficult to eradicate colonization from chronic lesions such as pressure sores or leg ulcers in elderly patients. In these situations, reliance must be placed on isolation procedures and early discharge.

Systematic therapy can be given as advised by the medical practitioner on an individual patient basis. Certain body sites are more resistant to the eradication of MRSA, e.g. tracheostomy sites, deep pressure sores and wounds, chronic leg ulcers, rectal and perineal regions and colostomy sites.

Clearance of MRSA carriage should be attempted before surgery wherever possible. These patients should be operated upon at the end of an operating list, if possible. All lesions must be covered with an impermeable dressing during the operation and the adjacent areas treated with appropriate antiseptic.

Health Care Workers

There is no evidence that MRSA poses a risk to healthy people. This includes HCWs and their families. It is essential that HCWs must adhere to the recommended infection control practice. Carriage by HCWs is usually transient, but some may harbour MRSA in the nose or on the hands (contact dermatitis or eczema), and may act as primary reservoirs. Therefore, it is important, that HCWs who have worked in a hospital or health care facility where MRSA was endemic or who have reason to believe that they may be carriers of MRSA, should inform their employer. HCWs who require treatment for MRSA carriage should be referred to the occupational health department.

References and further reading

Ayliffe GAJ, Cookson BD, Ducel G, *et al.* World health Working Group on the global control of MRSA. Geneva: World Health Organisation, 1995.

Boyce JM. MRSA patients: proven methods to treat colonization and infection. *Journal of Hospital Infection* 2001; 48 (Suppl. A): S9–S14.

Cafferkey MT (ed). *Methicillin-resistant Staphylococcus aureus: Clinical Management and Laboratory Aspects.* New York: Marcel Dekker, 1992.

Cephai C, Ashurst S, Owens C. Human carriage of methicillin-resistant *Staphylococcus aureus* linked with pet dog. *Lancet* 1994; **344:** 539–540.

Cookson BD. The emergence of mupirocin resistance: a challenge to infection control and antibiotic-prescribing practice. *Journal of Antimicrobial Chemotherapy* 1998; **41:** 11.

Cookson B. Is it time to stop searching for MRSA? *British Medical Journal* 1997; **314:** 664–666.

Duckworth GJ. Diagnosis and management of methicillin resistant *Staphylococcus aureus* infection. *British Medical Journal* 1993; **307:** 1049–1052.

Fazal BA, Telzak EE, Blum S, *et al*. Trends in the prevalence of methicillin-resistant *Staphylococcus aureus:* are we overdoing it? *Infection Control and Hospital Epidemiology* 1995; **16:** 257–259.

Fraise AP, Mitchell K, O'Brien SJO *et al*. Methicillin resistant *Staphylococcal aureus* (MRSA) in nursing homes in a major UK city: an anonymized point prevalence survey. *Epidemiology Infection* 1997; **118:** 1–5.

Gorak EJ, Yamada S, Brown JD. Community-acquired methicillin-resistant *Staphylococcus aureus* in hospitalized adults and children without known risk factors. *Clinical Infectious Diseases* 1999; **29:** 797–800.

Harstein AL. Improved understanding and control of methicillin-resistant *Staphylococcus aureus* associated with discontinuation of an isolation policy. *Infection Control and Hospital Epidemiology* 1996; **17:** 372–374.

Martin MA. Methicillin-resistant *Staphylococcus aureus:* the persistent resistant nosocomial pathogen. *Current Clinical Topics in Infectious Diseases* 1994; **14:** 170–191.

Michel M, Gutmann L. Methicillin-resistant *Staphylococcus aureus* and vancomycin-resistant enterococci: therapeutic realities and possibilities. *Lancet* 1997; **349:** 190–196.

Report of a combined working party of the British Society for Antimicrobial Chemotherapy and the Hospital Infection Society. Guidelines on the control of methicillin-resistant *Staphylococcus aureus* in the community. *Journal of Hospital Infection* 1995; **31:** 1–12.

Report of the combined working party of the British Society for Antimicrobial Chemotherapy, Hospital Infection Society and Infection Control Nurses Association: Revised guidelines for the control of epidemic Methicillin-resistant *Staphylococcus aureus* infection in hospitals. *Journal of Hospital Infection* 1998; **39:** 253–290.

Rubinovitch B, Pittet D. Screening for Methicillin-resistant *Staphylococcus aureus* in the endemic hospital: what have we learned? *Journal of Hospital Infection* 2001; **47:** 9–18.

Rampling A, Wiseman S, Davis L, *et al*. Evidence that hospital hygiene is important in the control of methicillin-resistant *Staphylococcus aureus. Journal of Hospital Infection* 2001; **49:** 109–116.

Scott GM, Thomson R, Malone-Lee J, *et al*. Cross-infection between animals and man: possible feline transmission of *Staphylococcus aureus* infection in humans? *Journal of Hospital Infection* 1998; **12:** 29–34.

Staphylococcus aureus fully resistant to vancomycin. *Morbidity and Mortality Weekly Report* 2002; **51:** 565–567.

Solberg CO. Spread of *Staphylococcus aureus* in hospitals: causes and prevention. *Scandinavian Journal of Infection* 2000; **32:** 587–595.

Tarzi S, Kennedy P, Stone S, Evans M. Methicillin-resistant *Staphylococcus aureus:* psychological impact of hospitalisation and isolation in an older adult population. *Journal of Hospital Infection* 2001; **49**: 250–254.

Vandenbroucke-Grauls CMJE. Management of methicillin-resistant *Staphylococcus aureus* in the Netherlands. *Reviews in Medical Microbiology* 1998; **9** (2): 109–116.

Wenzel RP, Reagan DR, Bertino JS, *et al.* Methicillin-resistant *Staphylococcus* outbreak: a consensus panel's definition and management guidelines. *American Journal of Hospital Control* 1998; **26**: 102–110.

VANCOMYCIN-RESISTANT ENTEROCOCCI (VRE)

The first clinical strains of vancomycin or glycopeptide resistant enterococci (VRE or GRE) were reported in 1988. Since then, the incidence of VRE (*Enterococcus faecium* or *Enterococcus faecalis*) has been rising steadily. VRE do not generally appear to be more virulent than sensitive strains but, because of their resistance patterns, are more difficult to treat if infection occurs. In addition, these microorganisms have a high propensity to become endemic.

Risk factors

The epidemiology of VRE has not been clarified. However, the following patient populations are at increased risk of colonization and infection:

- Treatment with previous vancomycin and/or multiple broad-spectrum antibiotic therapy.
- Presence of indwelling devices (peripheral IV and central lines, urinary catheters, surgical drains, endotracheal tubes).
- Critically ill patients (e.g. patients in ICU, oncology or transplant wards).
- Patients who have had intra-abdominal, cardiothoracic, orthopaedic, vascular and urology surgery.
- Severe underlying disease or immunosuppression.

Source of infection

E. faecium and *E. faecalis* are commensal bacteria in the gastrointestinal tract of healthy individuals. However, these microorganisms are selected by the use of broad-spectrum antibiotics. Most enterococcal infections have been attributed to endogenous sources. However, in an outbreak situation or when the organism is endemic in a health care institution, *patient-to-patient cross-infection can occur either through direct or indirect contact via the hands of personnel or from contaminated patient-care equipment and environmental surfaces.*

Mode of transmission

A major route of transmission of VRE within health care facilities is from patient-to-patient via the hands of HCWs that acquire the organism after direct patient contact or after handling contaminated materials. This is usually associated with inadequate hand washing.

Infection control measures

The approach to management of these organisms depends on two factors, i.e. *endemicity of the organism* in the institution, and *vulnerability of the patients*, largely determined by the presence of risk factors (see above).

Elimination is usually achieved by discharging patients (colonized/infected). Patients can remain colonized for a long time after discharge from hospital. An alert system for re-admission of these patients is required so that these patients can be promptly identified and placed on additional (contact) isolation precautions upon re-admission to the hospital. If patients require transfer to another hospital, a member of the ICT of the receiving hospital must be informed.

Where the organisms are not endemic to the institution, the object should be elimination. Rigorous application of additional precautions (contact transmission) has been shown to be effective in containing and eliminating the problem, although this can be expensive and its cost-effectiveness is unclear. Eradication of VRE from hospitals is most likely to succeed when infection or colonization is confined to a few patients on a single ward.

If the VRE has become endemic on a ward, or has spread to multiple wards, eradication becomes difficult and costly. In these cases, the object should be minimization of further transmission. Aggressive infection control measures and strict compliance by hospital personnel is required to limit nosocomial spread. Application of additional precautions (contact transmission) is useful in both settings.

In addition to infection control following infection control measures, antibiotic policy must be reviewed in an attempt to reduce use of all broad-spectrum antibiotics and glycopeptides.

- Isolate all infected or colonized patients in a single room with its own bathroom facilities or cohort them with other patients with presumed or known same strain. *Patients with VRE and diarrhoea or incontinence pose a high risk of transmission to others and must be isolated in a single room.*

- Appropriate protective clothing, i.e. gown/plastic apron should be worn when entering room.

- Wear non-sterile disposable gloves when in contact with infected or colonized patients or their environment. Hands are subsequently disinfected with an antiseptic.

- Remove gown and gloves before leaving room and wash hands with antiseptic solution or alcoholic hand rub. Ensure gown/plastic apron and gloves do not contact environmental surfaces before disposal.

- Use a mask if the patient has colonized respiratory secretions.

- Use dedicated equipment, e.g. stethoscope, sphygmomanometer, rectal thermometers.

- Use disposable equipment whenever possible. If not possible, clean and disinfect items and equipment before reuse. Standard sterilization procedures for instruments will inactivate the organisms.

- Instruments used for dressing changes should not be transferred from patient-to-patient but should remain by the patient's bedside.

- Consider the surfaces and furniture within the rooms to be contaminated as well as the patients themselves.

- Adequate cleaning and disinfection of re-usable devices should be carried out if such devices are re-used on other patients.

- Enterococci persist in the environment. Disinfection with a high-level disinfectant (e.g. freshly prepared hypochlorite solution 1:100 dilution) should be undertaken in addition to standard cleaning and this should be done on a regular basis.

- Transfer of patients to other high dependency units should be restricted, if possible.

Screening of patients

The role of broader screening of risk groups on a routine basis is less clear, and costs can be considerable. Therefore, it is not recommended as a routine procedure. However, in high-risk patients and clinical areas (e.g. in ICUs), some form of ongoing screening programme may be of benefit in identifying new admissions who are colonized. In an outbreak situation, screening swabs for culture from multiple body sites, i.e. stool or rectal swabs, perineal area, areas of broken skin (i.e. ulcer and wound), urine from catheterized patients, colostomy site should be taken to identify carriers. Since the most frequent site of colonization is the large bowel, *a faecal sample is the most useful screening specimen*. It is important to emphasize that stool carriage may persist for months or years and oral antibiotic therapy to eradicate the carriage is not successful.

References and further reading

Bowler ICJ, Storr JA, Davies GJ, *et al.* Guidelines for the management of patients colonised or infected with vancomycin-resistant enterococci. *Journal of Hospital Infection* 1998; **39**: 75–82.

Boyce JM. Vancomycin-Resistant Enterococcus: Detection, Epidemiology, and Control Measures. *Infectious Disease Clinics of North America* 1997; **11**(2): 367–384.

Hospital Infection Control Practices Advisory Committee. Recommendations for preventing the spread of vancomycin resistance entrococci. *Morbidity and Mortality Weekly Report* 1995; **44**: 1–13.

Murray BE. Vancomycin-resistant enterococcal infections. *New England Journal of Medicine* 2000; **342**: 710–721.

Nelson RRS. Intrinsically vancomycin-resistant Gram-positive organisms: clinical relevance and implications for infection control. *Journal of Hospital Infection* 1999; **42**: 275–282.

Nelson RRS. Selective isolation of Vancomycin-resistant enterococci. *Journal of Hospital Infection* 1998; **39:** 13–18.

Noshkin G, Bednarz P, Suriano T, *et al.* Persistent contamination of fabric-covered furniture by Vancomycin-resistant enterococci: implications for upholstery selection in hospitals. *American Journal of Infection Control* 2000; **28:** 311–313.

Ridwan B, Mascini E, Van Der Reijden N, *et al.* What action should be taken to prevent the spread of vancomycin-resistant enterococci in European Hospitals? *British Medical Journal* 2002; **324:** 666–668.

Spera RV, Faber BF. Multiply-resistant *Enterococcus faecium.* The nosocomial pathogen of the 1990s. *Journal of American Medical Association* 1992; **268:** 2563–2564.

Wade JJ, Uttley. Resistant enterococci – mechanisms, laboratory detection and control in the hospitals. *Journal of Clinical Pathology* 1996; **49:** 700–703.

MULTI-RESISTANT GRAM-NEGATIVE BACILLI

The first reports of extended-spectrum beta-lactamases (ESBLs) in Gram-negative bacilli came from Europe and were followed quickly by reports in the US. This type of antimicrobial resistance is now recognized worldwide. Although ESBLs are found most frequently in *Klebsiella pneumoniae*, the elements conferring this type of resistance are transferable to other genera, including *Escherichia coli* and others.

These pathogens often occur in an outbreak setting and pose a therapeutic dilemma due to resistance to multiple antimicrobials to beta-lactams and other agents, including fluoroquinolones and gentamicin. These isolates also have a propensity for spread by clonal strain-transmission from patient to patient, thereby posing an infection control dilemma. *Control interventions for these organisms involve choosing effective therapy for infected patients and instituting infection control measures and antibiotic utilization measures.*

Risk factors for colonization or infection

Reported risk factors for colonization or infection from multiple outbreaks of ESBL-producing organisms include: presence of IV catheters, emergency intra-abdominal surgery, gastrostomy or jejunostomy tube, gastrointestinal colonization, length of hospital or ICU stay, prior antibiotics (including third-generation cephalosporins), prior nursing home stay, severity of illness, presence of a urinary catheter, and ventilator assistance. In the majority of cases, these organisms affect severely ill patients in the ICU setting as well as chronically debilitated patients in the long-term care setting.

Infection control precautions

In addition to the following infection control measures, excessive use of broad-spectrum antibiotics (in particular the widespread use of ceftazidime) should be avoided. Antimicrobial prophylaxis for surgery should be restricted to a maximum of 24 h.

- Application of additional precautions (contact transmission) should be instituted. Such precautions involve use of barriers, e.g. gloves, gowns for contact with infected patients or their immediate environment. Hands must be washed after removing gloves.

- Patients should not be transferred between wards or hospital unless it is absolutely essential. If transfer is essential, the ICT of the receiving hospital should be informed in advance.

- *Bedpans and urinals should be disinfected using heat treatment.* If a bedpan disinfector breaks down, it should be repaired as an emergency. Disposable bedpans and urinals can be used, if available.

- *Communal equipment (especially if wet) may act as a source for these organisms, therefore ward equipment must be stored dry; soaking of instruments in disinfectant solution must be avoided.*

- Urinary catheters must be inserted under aseptic procedure. Urine drainage bags must be emptied by the tap, for which single-use disposable gloves should be used and hands must be washed after the procedure. Do not break the circuit and reconnect the urinary system. *A separate jug or container should be used for each patient when emptying urinary drainage bags.*

References and further reading

Garner JS. The Hospital Infection Control Practices Advisory Committee. Guideline for Isolation Precautions in Hospitals. *American Journal of Infection Control* 1996; **24:** 24–52.

Jacoby GA, Medeiros AA, O'Brien TF, Pinto ME, *et al.* Broad-Spectrum, Transmissible Beta lactamases. *New England Journal of Medicine* 1988; **319:** 723–724.

Karas JA, Pillay DG, Muckhart D, Sturm AW. Treatment Failure Due to Extended Spectrum Beta-Lactamase. *Journal of Antimicrobial Chemotherapy* 1996; **37:** 203–204.

Lucet JC, Chevret S, Decre D, *et al.* Outbreak of multiply resistant *Enterobacteriaceae* in an intensive care unit: epidemiology and risk factors for acquisition. *Clinical Infectious Diseases* 1996; **22:** 430–436.

Monnet DL, Biddle JW, Edwards JR, *et al.* Evidence of interhospital transmission of extended-spectrum beta-lactam-resistant *Klebsiella pneumoniae* in the United States, 1986 to 1993. *Infection Control Hospital Epidemiology* 1997; **18:** 492–498.

Naumovski L, Quinn JP, Miyashiro D, *et al.* Outbreak of Ceftazidime resistance due to a novel extended-spectrum beta-lactamase in isolates from cancer patients. *Antimicrobial Agents Chemotherapy* 1992; **36:** 1991–1996.

Pena C, Pujol M, Ardanuy C, *et al.* Epidemiology and successful control of a large outbreak due to *Klebsiella pneumoniae* producing extended-spectrum beta-lactamases. *Antimicrobial Agents Chemotherapy* 1998; **42:** 53–58.

Rice LB, Willey SH, Papanicolaou GB, *et al.* Outbreak of Ceftazidime resistance caused by extended-spectrum beta-lactamases at a Massachusetts chronic-care facility. *Antimicrobial Agents Chemotherapy* 1990; **34:** 2193–2199.

9

Prevention of Infection Caused by Specific Pathogens

TUBERCULOSIS (TB)

This ancient disease, characterized in 1680 by John Bunyan as the '*Caption of all these Men of Death*' – has by no means been vanquished. According to WHO estimates, 90 million new cases of TB will have occured in the 1990's causing 30 million TB-related deaths, and 90% of these will have been in developing countries. Up to 40% of patients with TB will be co-infected with HIV.

TB is an infection caused by bacterium of the *Mycobacterium tuberculosis* complex (*M. tuberculosis, M. bovis, M. africanum*). TB is usually a pulmonary disease. Extrapulmonary TB is much less common, but infection may occur in any organ or tissue including lymph nodes, meninges, pleura, pericardium, kidneys, bones, joints, larynx, skin, peritoneum, intestines and eyes, *M. tuberculosis* and *M. africanum*, primarily from humans and *M. bovis* primarily from cattle.

Clinical manifestations: Many initial infections with *M. tuberculosis* or related species are asymptomatic. Approximately 90–95% of those infected with the bacterium become latent carriers, with a lifelong risk of reactivation causing clinical (active) disease. Approximately 10% of infected adults will develop such clinical disease in their lifetime, about half of these in the first 5 years after infection (but predominantly in the first year) and the other half later in life. The risk of developing disease is much greater in infants and young children, and in those with impaired immune function.

Early clinical symptoms include fatigue, weight loss, fever and night sweats. In more advanced disease, hoarseness, cough with blood-stained sputum, and chest pain are common. Once the individual has acquired the infection it may heal spontaneously or, over weeks/months, become active disease. It may be contained and unapparent

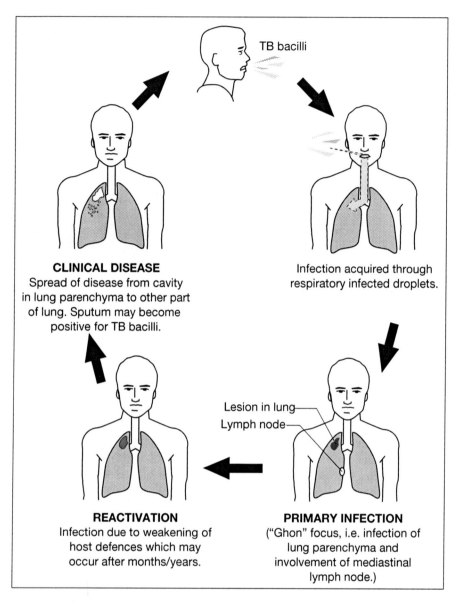

Figure 9.1 Acquisition and spread of pulmonary tuberculosis.

at the time but may cause active disease (reactivation) later in life because of old age or other events that weaken the individual's immunity.

Mode of transmission: TB is usually transmitted by exposure to airborne droplet nuclei produced by people with 'open' pulmonary TB, during expiratory efforts such as coughing and sneezing (Fig. 9.1).

The infectious person with open TB usually produces aerosolized droplets of less than 5 μm in diameter containing tuberculi bacilli. These droplets can remain afloat and viable in the environment unless removed by planned infection control procedures. When inhaled, these tuberculi bacilli can settle in the lungs, where they may result in TB infection and may remain viable for the lifetime of the new host. People with TB infection of this nature without evidence of clinical disease are not infectious and are asymptomatic.

Prolonged close exposure may lead to infection in close contacts. Direct invasion through mucous membranes or skin breaks may occur, but it is extremely rare. Extrapulmonary TB is generally not communicable apart from exceptionally rare circumstances where there is a draining abscess.

Infection by direct contact with mucous membranes or skin lesions is very rare. Bovine TB may result from drinking unpasteurized infected milk or by aerosol transmission from infected animals to farmers or animal handlers.

Either symptomatic or asymptomatic people with viable bacilli in their sputum may be infectious. Untreated, or inadequately treated, patients may be sputum-positive intermittently for many years, although children with primary TB are generally not infectious. *Patients usually become non-infectious after 2 weeks of beginning appropriate therapy.*

Risk of acquisition: The risk of acquisition is related to the degree of exposure to the aetiological agent. The greatest risk of disease occurs from 6–12 months after exposure. For people with latent infection, susceptibility to reactivation is increased in those with immunosuppression or debilitating diseases such as diabetes, cancer and renal failure and in those who engage in substance abuse or are malnourished. Reactivation of latent infection accounts for a large proportion of cases in elderly people. Risk factors for acquiring TB include extremes of age, concomitant HIV infection, ethnic group from high prevalence countries, chronic alcohol misuse, poor socio-economic background and homelessness.

Incubation period: The incubation period from exposure to demonstrable primary lesion or significant tuberculin reaction is in the range of 4–12 weeks. The subsequent risk of progressive pulmonary or extrapulmonary TB is greatest the first year or two after infection with the greatest risk in the first 6–12 months, however, latent infection may persist for a lifetime. The degree of communicability depends on the number of bacilli discharged, the virulence of the bacilli, and opportunities for exposure. Infection is transmissible from persons with TB, as long as viable tubercle bacilli are being discharged in the sputum (smear positive on Ziehl Nielsen's stain).

Treatment: The treatment of tuberculosis is complex and lengthy. *Inadequate treatment and non-compliance with medication are the main causes of relapse and of the* *emergence of drug resistant organisms.* Therefore, the treatment should be supervized by a medical practitioner with expertise in the management of TB. Compliance with treatment must be monitored. If there is any doubt, measures such as pill counts, prescription checks or urine tests may be used. Individual plans for non-compliant patients may involve arrangements for directly observed therapy. Most patients with TB can be treated at home; a few require hospital admission for severe illness, adverse effects of chemotherapy, or for social reasons. *Effective treatment with antimicrobial chemotherapy usually eliminates communicability within 2 weeks.* However, in some cases, especially in the case of multi-drug resistant tuberculosis (MDR-TB), inadequate treatment or non-compliance with treatment, the patient may remain sputum-positive or be sputum-positive intermittently for a lengthy period of time.

Infection control precautions in hospital

Although the treatment of TB should be undertaken in the patient's home whenever possible, some patients will need admission because of the severity of illness, adverse effects of chemotherapy, for social reasons, or for investigations to establish the diagnosis.

Additional precautions (airborne transmission) should be observed. Health care workers and visitors should wear a particulate filter mask when entering a TB patient's room if the patient cannot co-operate with personal risk reduction measures, or where normal risk reduction measures are not effective (e.g. disease due to drug-resistant strains of *M. tuberculosis*). Care should be taken to ensure that all people who use masks are instructed in the correct fit and wearing of the mask. When the patient is required to leave a TB isolation room (e.g. for chest X-ray), then the patient should wear a mask if their TB is considered infectious.

TB patients should be educated to cover their mouths and noses while coughing or sneezing, and to dispose of used tissue paper in a closed container to be treated as clinical waste. Medical procedures that present a particular risk of cross-contamination from an infectious patient include bronchoscopy and the use of respiratory and anaesthetic apparatus.

The following infection control measures should be observed:

- All suspected or confirmed pulmonary TB cases should initially be admitted to a single room until their sputum status is known and risk assessments are made. The door should be kept closed as much as possible.

- Adult patients with pulmonary TB with three negative smear samples and patients with non-pulmonary TB infection caused by atypical

Mycobacterium spp. (with the exception of those with infected discharging wounds) should be regarded as non-infectious and may be nursed in a general ward.

- Patients whose bronchial washings are smear-positive should be managed as if non-infectious unless the sputum is also smear-positive or becomes so after bronchoscopy or they are on a ward with immunocompromised patients, or they are known or suspected of having MDR-TB.

- No patient with suspected or confirmed respiratory TB, whatever the sputum status, should be admitted to an open ward containing immuno-compromised patients, such as HIV infected, transplant or oncology patients until their infectivity is established because of the known possibility of trans-mission of infection and the seriousness of MDR-TB.

- Patients in isolation should not visit wards, including communal washing facilities, or public areas of the hospital and should not walk or be trans-ported through open wards which may contain immunocompromised patients, unless they are wearing a mask.

- All patients should be informed that their infection is spread to others by the respiratory route. Routine surgical masks are recommended for patients with uncontrolled cough or sneezing to reduce aerosol generation. Other patients should be taught to cover the mouth and nose with dispos-able paper tissue whilst coughing and to dispose of the tissues as clinical waste.

- Visitors should, as far as possible, be limited to those who have already been in close contact before the diagnosis. Contact with staff should be kept to a reasonable minimum without compromising patient care.

- All children with TB and their visitors should be segregated from other patients until the contacts have been screened and pronounced non-infectious. It is possible that one of the visitors may have been the source of the child's infection and hence be a risk to other patients if the child is in an open ward.

- The HCW should wear a mask if a patient with active pulmonary TB is coughing and cannot be relied upon to cover his/her mouth. The patient should also be advised to wear mask if he/she leaves the room. In addition, the wearing of a mask is also recommended if direct exposure to respiratory secretions is unavoidable, e.g. during bronchoscopy or pro-longed care of a high dependency patient, after cough-inducing procedures or when performing the last offices.

The surgical masks may not be effective in preventing the inhalation of droplet nuclei. A high efficiency particulate air (HEPA) mask should be used. Masks should be close fitting and filter particles of 1–5 microns (μ). In the US, use of particulate respirators (N95) are recommended. *Use of a mask is not a substitute for good infection control practice.*

- Risk assessments for the likelihood of infectiousness and MDR-TB should be made taking into account the immune status of other patients on the ward.

- Marked crockery and separate washing up facilities are unnecessary, and no special precautions are needed for bed linen, books or other personal property.

- Sputum specimens and other respiratory specimens should be sent to a laboratory as outlined on page 103.

- *HIV infected and tuberculosis patients should not be mixed.* In settings where other patients may be infected with HIV or otherwise immunocompromised, suspected or confirmed cases of pulmonary TB should be considered as potentially infectious on every admission until proved otherwise and segregated accordingly. Patients with potentially infectious TB should be segregated from other immunocompromised patients by admission to a single room in a separate ward or to a negative pressure ventilation room (see page 21).

- For all patients in a HIV ward, aerosol generating procedures such as bronchoscopy, sputum induction, or nebulizer treatment should never be performed in an open ward or bay and appropriate environmental controls should be in place.

- When a patient is discharged home, the room should be terminally cleaned. *Fumigation of the room is not necessary.*

- *Termination of Infection Control Precautions:* Isolation of patients should commence on suspicion of infection and may only be discontinued in untreated cases where three consecutive direct smears are negative for AAFB (Acid & Alcohol Fast Bacilli). *Uncomplicated sputum positive TB will usually be non-infectious after 2 weeks compliance with standard multi-drug chemotherapy* and the patient may then be transferred to an open ward but the results of any sputum tests and/or response to treatment should be taken into account. However, in some circumstances, e.g. *where MDR-TB is suspected, three successive smear-negative sputum examinations will be required.*

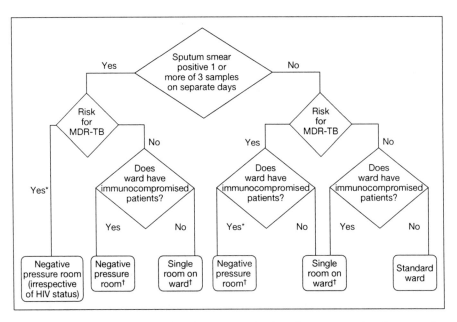

Figure 9.2 Risk assessment of infectivity and other factors. *Molecular tests for identification of *Mycobacterium tuberculosis* and rifampicin resistance strongly recommended. †If previous treatment for tuberculosis or contact with multi-drug resistant tuberculosis (MDR-TB), molecular test for rifampicin resistance mandatory; if rifampicin resistance treat/isolate as MDR-TB.

Reproduced with permission from: Control and prevention of tuberculosis in the United Kingdom: Code of Practice 2000. *Thorax* 2000; **55**: 887–901.

Multi-drug resistant tuberculosis (MDR-TB)

MDR-TB is, by definition, TB resistant to two or more of the main line anti-tuberculosis drugs (usually isoniazid and rifampicin with or without other drugs). The implications are serious both for the individual and for public health because of the limited number of the alternative anti-tuberculosis drugs available for treatment. Additional precautions may be required for patients with MDR-TB which should be considered on a case-by-case basis with the discussion of infection control team. Drug resistant disease should be considered when there is:

- A history of previous drug treatment (usually incomplete treatment or non-compliant patient).
- Contact with a patient with known MDR-TB.
- Patients infected with HIV.
- Prolonged sputum smear or culture positive while on treatment (smear positivity at 4 months or culture positivity at 5 months).

It is preferable that cases of MDR-TB be managed at facilities with expertise in such management. Because of the more serious consequences of infection, the

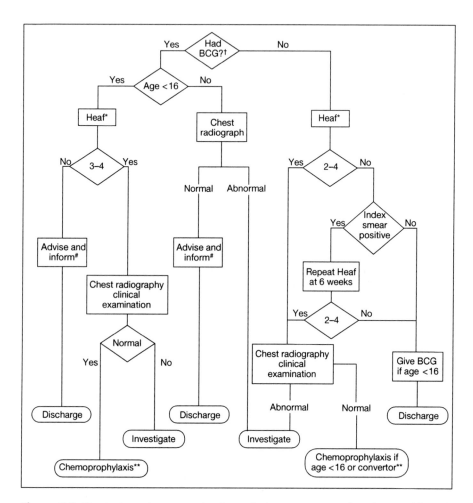

Figure 9.3 Contact tracing: examination of close contacts of patients with pulmonary tuberculosis. Contacts of patients with non-pulmonary tuberculosis need not usually be examined. Note: children under 2 years who have not had a BCG vaccination who are close contacts of a smear positive index patient should receive chemoprophylaxis irrespective of tuberculin status. †Previous BCG vaccination cannot be accepted as evidence of immunity in HIV infected subjects. *A negative test in immunocompromised subjects does not exclude tuberculosis infection. #Advise patient of tuberculosis symptoms and inform GP of contact. **Persons eligible for, but not given, chemoprophylaxis should have follow-up chest radiographs at 3 and 12 months.

Reproduced with permission from: Control and prevention of tuberculosis in the United Kindgdom: Code or Practice 2000. *Thorax* 2000; **55:** 887–901.

patient should be isolated in a negative pressure ventilation room. Their movement around the facility should be minimized. HCWs and visitors should wear a 1 μm TB particulate filter mask when entering the patient's room. Care should be taken to ensure that all people who use these masks are instructed in the correct fit and wearing of the mask. When the patient is required to leave a TB isolation room (e.g. for chest X-ray), then the patient should wear the mask if their TB is considered infectious. He/she should be educated to cover their mouth and nose while coughing or sneezing, and to dispose of used tissue paper as clinical waste. Medical procedures that present a particular risk of cross-contamination from an infectious patient include bronchoscopy and the use of respiratory and anaesthetic apparatus.

Contact tracing: Contacts should only be considered in the case of smear positive or open pulmonary TB and in the first instance should be limited to close contacts, i.e. household and close associates of patients with respiratory TB. If initial investigation reveals a number of contacts with evidence of TB, consideration should be given to widening the circle of contacts who may be offered screening. The person responsible for local contact tracing should be named in the hospital policy.

- *Staff:* Contacts should only be *considered significant if the source is smear positive on direct sputum examination or on examination of bronchial washings.* Staff undertaking mouth-to-mouth resuscitation, prolonged care of a high dependency patient or repeated chest physiotherapy should be considered as close contacts. All members of staff should be seen in the occupational health department and have their occupational health notes reviewed to ascertain whether they have had a Heaf test, BCG vaccination and BCG scar. Enquiries should be made as to any current illness or treatment that might result in their immune system being compromised. Those who have a previous history of BCG vaccination and/or were previously positive on Heaf test, do not require further investigation but should be advised of the possible symptoms of TB and the importance of reporting such symptoms promptly.

- *Patients:* If an individual on an open ward is diagnosed as having infectious TB, the risk of other patients being infected is likely to be small. Decisions about appropriate action should take into account the degree of infectivity, the length of time before the infectious individual is isolated, the proximity of contact, and whether other patients are unusually susceptible to infection.

  If the exposure of another patient is sufficiently extensive to be equivalent to a household contact, or the exposed patient is known to be particularly susceptible to infection, they should be managed in the same way as a household respiratory contact.

  In general, patients in the same bay (rather than the whole ward) should be regarded as at risk, but only if the index case was coughing and was present in the bay for more than 8 h before isolation. It is sufficient to document the possible exposure in the patient's records and the *patient's medical practitioner should also be informed.*

References and further reading

Cookson ST, Jarvis WR. Prevention of nosocomial transmission of *Mycobacterium tuberculosis. Infectious Disease Clinics of North America* 1997; 11(2): 385–409.

Crofton J, Chaulet P, Maher D. *Guidelines for the management of drug-resistant tuberculosis.* Geneva, World Health Organisation, 1997.

Harries AD, Maher D, Nunn P. Practical and affordable measures for the protection of health care workers from tuberculosis in low-income countries. *Bulletin of the World Health Organisation* 1997; 75(5): 477–489.

Horsburgh CR Jr, Feldman S, Ridzon R. Practice Guidelines for the Treatment of Tuberculosis. *Clinical Infectious Diseases* 2000; 31: 633–699.

Joint Tuberculosis Committee of the British Thoracic Society. Chemotherapy and Management of Tuberculosis in the UK: recommendations 1998. *Thorax* 1997; 53: 536–548.

Joint Tuberculosis Committee of the British Thoracic Society. Control and prevention of Tuberculosis in the UK: Code of Practice 2000. *Thorax* 2000; 55: 887–901.

McGowan JE Jr. Nosocomial Tuberculosis: New Progress in Control and Prevention. *Clinical Infectious Diseases* 1995; 21: 489–505.

Phillips MS, Fordham von Reyn. Nosocomial Infections Due to Nontuberculous Mycobacteria. *Clinical Infectious Diseases* 2001; 33: 1363–1374.

Scottish Department of Health: *The Control of Tuberculosis in Scotland.* The Scottish Office DoH, 1998.

Sepkowitz KA. How Contagious Is Tuberculosis? *Clinical Infectious Diseases* 1996; 23: 954–962.

Willeke K, Yinge Qian. Tuberculosis Control through Respirator Wear: Performance of National Institute for Occupational Safety and Health-Regulated Respirators. *American Journal of Infection Control* 1998; 26: 139–142.

UK Department of Health. *The Prevention and Control of Tuberculosis in the United Kingdom: Recommendations for the prevention and control of tuberculosis at local level.* London: DoH, 1996.

UK Department of Health. *The Prevention and Control of Tuberculosis in the United Kingdom: 1. HIV related Tuberculosis 2. Drug-resistant, including multiple-drug resistant, Tuberculosis. Recommendations for the prevention and control of tuberculosis at local level.* London: DoH, 1998.

UK Department of Health. *The Prevention and Control of Tuberculosis in the United Kingdom: Tuberculosis and homeless people.* London: DoH, 1996.

Clostridium difficile INFECTION

Clostridium difficile is an aerobic, Gram-positive bacterium that was first identified and characterized in 1935. *C. difficile* was accorded little interest until 1978 when several reports identified its association with pseudomembranous enterocolitis. Infection with *C. difficile has now become the most frequent etiologic agent for hospital-acquired diarrhoea*, and the overall frequency of this nosocomial infection appears to be increasing.

Clinical features: The symptom is mainly diarrhoea which usually starts 5–10 days (range: few days to 2 months) after commencing antibiotic therapy. It ranges from mild to severe foul smelling diarrhoea containing blood/mucus, fever, leucocytosis and abdominal pain. In the majority of patients, the illness is mild and full recovery is usual. Elderly patients may become seriously ill with dehydration. Occasionally, patients may develop a severe form of the disease called pseudomembranous colitis. Complications include pancolitis, toxic megacolon, perforation or endotoxin shock.

Risk factors: Risk factors for acquiring *C. difficile*-associated infection include:

1. Indiscriminate use and exposure to broad spectrum antibiotic therapy, particularly β-lactam agents.

2. Gastrointestinal procedures and surgery.

3. Advanced age, i.e. common in elderly and debilitated patients; outbreaks being more common in geriatric and long-stay wards.

Diagnosis: All suspected cases should be investigated by sending faecal specimens to the microbiology laboratory for detection of *C. difficile* toxin. Usually, once the diagnosis has been confirmed, repeat specimens need not be taken unless there is a relapse following treatment. This is because it is not uncommon for the faeces to remain toxin-positive for some time after the start of treatment even when the patient's symptoms have settled. *Screening and treatment of asymptomatic patients is not necessary. Routine stool culture for detection of C. difficile is not recommended* but can be considered in an outbreak situation for epidemiological investigations.

Management: Treatment of *C. difficile* enterocolitis focuses on three basic strategies.

- Firstly, the antibiotic therapy that has mediated the change in the patient's gut microflora should be discontinued or changed to an antibiotic which has less of an association with enterocolitis.

- Secondly, *antiperistaltic medication should be avoided.* Diarrhoea is the response of the infected host to expel pathogens responsible for enterocolitis. Use of opiates and antiperistaltic drugs results in the retention of pathogen, probably worsens enterocolitis-associated necrosis of the colonic mucosa, and increases the risk of toxic megacolon. Rehydration of patients usually results in rapid improvement. Loss of fluid and electrolytes must be replaced using the intravenous route until diarrhoea has ceased and effective oral intake has resumed.

- Thirdly, specific antibiotic therapy to treat the offending *C. difficile* pathogen should be initiated. ***Oral metronidazole is administered 400 mg 8 hourly for 10 days, which should be given as a first choice.*** If metronidazole is not effective then oral vancomycin 125 mg 6 hourly for 10 days should be prescribed. Vancomycin should not be prescribed as a first line therapy because of problem of emergence of vancomycin resistant enterococci (VRE). The majority of patients improve within 2–4 days. However, clinical relapse can occur in 15–25% of the cases usually within 1–3 weeks.

Control of antibiotic usage: Of all the measures that have been used to prevent the spread of *C. difficile*-associated diarrhoea, the most successful has been the restriction of the use of antimicrobial agents. Therefore it is essential that the use of inappropriate and broad spectrum antibiotics (especially oral) is avoided. The hospital should have an antibiotic policy which must be reviewed on a regular basis. Narrow spectrum antibiotics for a minimum duration are preferred if treatment is considered essential to deal with systemic infection. Antibiotics such as aminoglycosides and some fluoroquinolones appear to have little propensity to induce *C. difficile* infection, probably due to their lack of effect on the endogenous anaerobic gut bacteria.

Infection control measures: *C. difficile* is normally fastidious in its vegetative state, it is capable of sporulating when environmental conditions no longer support its continued growth. The capacity to form spores enables the organism to persist and survive in the environment (e.g. on dry surfaces) for extended periods of time. The degree to which the environment becomes contaminated with *C. difficile* spores is proportional to the number of patients with *C. difficile* associated diarrhoea. Environmental contamination can be heavy, especially if the diarrhoea is severe or accompanied by incontinence; asymptomatic patients after infection may continue to shed organisms in their stools and serve as a source of contamination.

The following infection control precautions should be taken:

- All infected patients should be segregated from non-affected patients in a single room with *en suite* toilet facilities or cohort all symptomatic patients.

- Additional (contact transmission) isolation precautions should be used.

- Hands can become contaminated by direct contact with patients who are colonized or infected with *C. difficile* or by contact with spores contaminating environmental surfaces. Therefore, strict hand hygiene before and after patient contact remains the most effective control measure to prevent cross-infection.

- Proper use of non-sterile, single-use disposable gloves is an ancillary measure that helps to further minimize transfer of these pathogens from one surface to another. *Hands must be washed after removing gloves.*

- The patient's immediate environment and other areas where spores may accumulate (e.g. sluice, commodes, toilets, bedpans, sinks, high-touch surfaces in patients' bathrooms) and other soiled areas must be cleaned and disinfected thoroughly and frequently. Separate cleaning equipment must be reserved for this purpose. Mop heads should be disposable or laundered after each use and single-use disposable cloths must be used. *C. difficile* spores are highly resistant to most disinfectants.

- The recommended approach to environmental infection control is meticulous cleaning and decontamination of surfaces. Chlorine-containing (hypochlorite) chemicals 1,600 ppm of av Cl_2 should be used for environmental surface disinfectant.

Patients discharge: Patients can remain colonized for a long time after discharge from hospital. If the patient is discharged or transfered to another hospital or long-stay health care facility, appropriate personnel at the receiving health care facility must be informed.

References and further reading

Aronsson B, Möllby, Nord C-E. Antimicrobial agents and *Clostridium difficile* in acute enteric disease: Epidemiologic data from Sweden, 1980–1982. *Journal of Infectious Disease* 1985; **151**: 476–481.

Bartlett JG. *Clostridium difficile:* History of its role as an enteric pathogen and the current state of knowledge about the organism. *Clinical Infectious Diseases* 1994; **18** (Suppl. 4): S265–S272.

Brooks SE, Veal RO, Kramer M, Dore L, Schupf N, Adachi M. Reduction in the incidence of *Clostridium difficile*-associated diarrhoea in an acute care hospital and a skilled nursing facility following replacement of electronic thermometers with single-use disposables. *Infection Control and Hospital Epidemiology* 1992; **13**: 98–103.

Cartmill TDI, Panigrahi H, Worsley MA, *et al.* Management and control of a large outbreak of diarrhoea due to *Clostridium difficile*. *Journal of Hospital Infection* 1994; **27**: 1–15.

Fekety R, Kim KH, Brown D, Batts DH, Cudmore M, Silva J Jr. Epidemiology of antibiotic-associated colitis: Isolation of *Clostridium difficile* from the hospital environment. *American Journal of Medicine* 1981; **70**: 906–908.

Gerding DN, Olson MM, Peterson LR, *et al. Clostridium difficile*-associated diarrhea and colitis in adults: A prospective case-controlled epidemiologic study. *Archive of Internal Medicine* 1986; **146**: 95–100.

Gerding DN, Johnson S, Peterson LR, Mulligan ME, Silva J Jr. *Clostridium difficile*-associated diarrhea and colitis. *Infection Control Hospital Epidemiology* 1995; 16: 459–477.

Hoffman PN. *Clostridium difficile* in hospitals. *Current Opinion in Infectious Diseases* 1994; 7: 471–474.

Johnson S, Homann SR, Bettin KM, *et al.* Treatment of asymptomatic *Clostridium difficile* carriers (fecal excretors) with vancomycin or metronidazole. A randomized, placebo controlled trial. *Annal Internal Medicine* 1992; 117: 297–302.

Johnson S, Gerding DN, Olson MM, *et al.* Prospective, controlled study of vinyl glove use to interrupt *Clostridium difficile* nosocomial transmission. *American Journal of Medicine* 1990; 88: 137–140.

Kaatz GW, Gitlin SD, Schaberg DR, *et al.* Acquisition of *Clostridium difficile* from the hospital environment. *American Journal of Epidemiology* 1988; 127: 1289–1294.

Malamou-Ladas H, Farrell SO, Nash JO, Tabaqchali S. Isolation of *Clostridium difficile* from patients and the environment of hospital wards. *Journal of Clinical Pathology* 1983; 6: 88–92.

McFarland LV, Surawicz CM, Stamm WE. Risk factors for *Clostridium difficile* carriage and *Clostridium difficile*-associated diarrhea in a cohort of hospitalized patients. *Journal of Infectious Diseases* 1990; 162: 678–684.

Pierce PF Jr, Wilson R, Silva J Jr, *et al.* Antibiotic-associated pseudomembranous colitis: An epidemiologic investigation of a cluster of cases. *Journal of Infectious Diseases* 1982; 145: 269–274.

Tabaqchali S, Jumaa P. Diagnosis and management of *Clostridium difficile* infection. *British Medical Journal* 1995; 310: 1375–1380.

Thibault A, Miller MA, Gaese C. Risk factors for the development of *Clostridium difficile*-associated diarrhoea during a hospital outbreak. *Infection Control Hospital Epidemiology* 1991; 12: 345–348.

Titov L, Lebedkova N, Shabanov A, *et al.* Isolation and molecular characterization of *Clostridium difficile* strains from patients and the hospital environment in Belarus. *Journal of Clinical Microbiology* 2000; 38: 1200–1202.

UK Department of Health and Public Health Laboratory Service. *Clostridium difficile Infection: prevention and management.* London: DoH, 1994.

Worsley MA. Infection control and prevention of *Clostridium difficile* infection. *Journal of Antimicrobial Chemotherapy* 1998; 41 (Suppl. C): 59–66.

Yannelli B, Gurevich I, Schoch PE, Cunha BA. Yield of stool cultures, ova and parasite tests, and *Clostridium difficile* determination in nosocomial diarrhoea. *American Journal of Infection Control* 1988; 16: 246–249.

Zadik PM, Moore AP. Antimicrobial associations of an outbreak of diarrhoea due to *Clostridium difficile*. *Journal of Hospital Infection* 1998; 39: 189–193.

LEGIONNAIRES' DISEASE

Legionellosis is a collective term describing infection produced by *Legionella* spp. whereas Legionnaires' disease is a multisystem illness with pneumonia. Legionnaires' disease is caused by infection with *Legionella* spp. with *Legionella pneumophila* responsible for 90% of infections. In all, about 35 species of legionella have been recognized. The incubation period of Legionnaires' disease is 2–10 days, most often 5–6 days.

Clinical features: Legionellosis is an acute bacterial pneumonia characterized initially by anorexia, malaise, myalgia and headache. Within a day, there is usually a rapidly rising fever associated with chills. A non-productive cough, abdominal pain and diarrhoea are common. Chest radiograph may show patchy or focal areas of consolidation that may progress to bilateral involvement. Severe infections may lead to respiratory failure and death. The case-fatality rate has been as high as 40% in hospitalized cases; it is generally higher in those with compromised immunity. Unrecognized infections are common.

Pontiac fever is a clinical syndrome which may represent reaction to inhaled antigen rather than bacterial invasion. It is not associated with pneumonia or death; patients recover spontaneously in 2–5 days without treatment.

Risk factors: Legionellosis may occur as sporadic cases or outbreaks, and is more frequently reported in summer and autumn. The incidence of infection increases with increasing age (i.e. persons >50 years of age) and those who smoke are at highest risk. Males are affected more commonly than females. The following groups of patients are more susceptible to infections:

- *Immunosuppressed patients*, e.g. transplant patients, cancer patients, patients receiving corticosteroid therapy, and

- *Immunocompromised patients*, e.g. surgical patients, patients with underlying chronic lung disease, dialysis patients, diabetes mellitus.

Source of infection: Reservoir and source of infection for Legionnaires' disease are hot and cold water systems (showers) particularly in hospitals and hotels, air-conditioning and wet cooling system towers, evaporative condensers, humidifiers, whirlpool and natural spas, respiratory therapy devices and decorative fountains/sprinkler systems. In several hospital outbreaks, patients were considered to be infected through exposure to contaminated aerosols generated by cooling towers, showers, faucets, respiratory therapy equipment, and room-air humidifiers. Airborne transmission in water aerosols is believed to be the major, if not sole, means of infection. *Person-to-person transmission has not been documented.*

Case definitions for Legionnaires' disease

Confirmed case: A clinical diagnosis of pneumonia with laboratory evidence of one or more of the following:

- Isolation (culture) of legionella species from clinical specimens.

- Seroconversion (a four-fold or greater increase in titre) determined using a validated indirect immunofluorescent antibody test (IFAT) incorporating a monovalent *L. pneumophila* serogroup 1 antigen.

- The presence of *L. pneumophila* urinary antigen determined using validated reagents/kits.

Presumptive case: A clinical diagnosis of pneumonia with laboratory evidence of one or more of the following:

- A single high titre of 128 using IFAT as above (or a single titre of 64 in an outbreak).

- A positive direct fluorescence (DFA) on a clinical specimen using validated monoclonal antibodies (also referred to as a positive result by Direct Immunofluorescence (DIF).

Adapted from Public Health Laboratory Services Atypical Pneumonia Working Group. Investigating a single case of Legionnaires' disease. *Communicable Disease and Public Health* 2002; 5(2): 157–162.

Diagnosis: The diagnosis of Legionellosis purely by clinical criteria can be difficult and reliance is therefore placed on laboratory tests, which include isolation of the causative organism on special media and its demonstration by direct immunofluorescence (IF) stain of involved tissue or respiratory secretions. It can also be diagnosed by detection of antigens of *L. pneumophila* in urine by RIA or by a four-fold or greater rise in IFA titre between an acute phase serum and one drawn 3–6 weeks later.

Prevention: Currently there is no vaccine against Legionellosis and since Legionella is a very widespread organism, prevention must therefore focus on reducing the risk of the organism being aerosolized. The prime aim must be to avoid creating conditions favourable for the organisms to multiply in water and be disseminated in air through droplets. Special precautions for the environment include adequate maintenance of potential reservoirs of infection, such as hot water and air conditioning systems, spa baths, humidifiers and respiratory therapy equipment.

Steps in an epidemiologic investigation for Legionellosis

- Review medical and microbiologic records.
- Initiate active surveillance to identify all recent or ongoing cases.
- Develop a line listing of cases by time, place, and person.
- Determine the type of epidemiological investigation, i.e. case-control or cohort study.
- Assess risk factors among potential environmental exposures, e.g. showers, cooling towers, respiratory therapy equipment.
- Gather and analyze epidemiological information.
- Collect water samples from environmental sources implicated by epidemiological investigation.
- Subtype strains of *Legionella* spp. cultured from both patients and environmental sources.
- Review autopsy records and include autopsy specimens in diagnostic testing.

It is important to highlight that the following factors enhance colonization and amplification of legionellae in water environments:

- Temperatures of 25–42°C [77–107.6°F]
- Stagnation of water
- Scale and sediment, and
- Presence of certain free-living aquatic amoebae that can support intracellular growth of legionellae.

Therefore it is essential that health care facilities should either maintain potable water at the outlet at >51°C (>124°F) or <20°C (<68°F) or chlorinate heated water to achieve 1–2 mg/L (1–2 ppm) of free residual chlorine at the tap.

Adequate maintenance of wet cooling towers and hot water systems is essential in control of legionella. It is important that the construction of new cooling towers in the health care facilities must be located so that the drift is directed away from the air-intake system. The cooling towers should be designed to minimize the volume of aerosol drift. Infection control procedures must be implemented for cooling towers.

Maintenance of cooling towers must be carried out according to manufacturers' recommendations. A record of detailed maintenance and infection control measures, including any environmental tests, must be kept.

If cooling towers or evaporative condensers are implicated in healthcare-associated Legionellosis, decontaminate the cooling-tower system. It is important that cooling towers should be drained when not in use. They should be mechanically cleaned to remove scale and sediment at regular intervals. Appropriate biocides should be used on a regular basis to prevent the growth of slime-forming organisms.

Tap water should not be used in respiratory therapy devices. Maintenance of hot water system temperatures at $\geq 50°C$ may reduce the risk of transmission. Decontamination of implicated sources by chlorination and/or superheating of the water supply have been shown to be effective.

Surveillance and Notification: All laboratory confirmed cases of Legionellosis should be reported to appropriate personnel. This is to ensure that appropriate control measures are taken to ensure that the source of *Legionella* is removed. In the community, cases must be reported to the appropriate local health department (CCDC in the UK). Isolated cases may be difficult to investigate. Hospital surveillance should detect healthcare-associated Legionnaires' disease.

References and further reading

Bartlett CLR, Macrae Ad, Macfarlane JT. *Legionella Infections.* London: Edward Arnold, 1986.

Brundrett GW. *Legionella and Building Services.* Oxford: Butterworth-Heinemann, 1992.

Fallon RJ. How to prevent an outbreak of Legionnaires' disease. *Journal of Hospital Infection* 1994; **27**: 247–256.

Joseph CA, Watson JM, Harrison TG, Bartlett CLR. Nosocomial Legionnaires' Disease in England and Wales, 1980–1992. *Epidemiology and Infection* 1994; **112**: 329–345.

Public Health Laboratory Services Atypical Pneumonia Working Group. Investigating a single case of Legionnaires' disease. *Communicable Disease and Public Health* 2002; 5(2): 157–162.

Sabria M, Yu VL. Hospital-Acquired Legionellosis: Solutions for a Preventable Infection. *The Lancet Infectious Diseases* 2000; **2**: 368–373.

UK Health and Safety Commission. *Legionnaires' Disease: the control of Legionella bacteria in water system: Approved Code of Practice and Guidence.* Suffolk: HSE Book, 2000.

UK Department of Health. Health Technical Memorandum 2040. *The control of legionella in healthcare premises – a code of practice.* Part 1 Management Policy, Part 2 Design Considerations, Part 3, Validation and verification, Part 4 Operational management. London: HMSO, 1994.

GASTROINTESTINAL INFECTIONS AND FOOD POISONING

Diarrhoea and vomiting may be caused by many agents, both infective and non-infective. The World Health Organization (WHO) defined food poisoning *as any disease of an infectious or toxic nature caused by or thought to be caused by the consumption of food or water.*

The definition of diarrhoea varies but generally includes the passage of liquid or watery stools, three or more times per day. In the health care setting *it is important to distinguish between infectious and non-infectious diarrhoea.* Infectious diarrhoea is caused by enteric pathogens while non-infectious diarrhoea is caused by cathartics, tube-feeding, inflammatory bowel disease, surgical resection of the gastrointestinal tract and anastomoses.

Infection control precautions: It is prudent to consider all cases of gastroenteritis as potentially infectious until appropriate investigations are completed. Patients should be isolated in a single room with toilet facilities. Contact infection control precaution should be implemented. Hand hygiene must be emphasized. Appropriate protective clothing, e.g. gloves, plastic aprons or gowns should be worn when handling contaminated material or the environment.

Clinical cases and suspected outbreaks of gastrointestinal infection among staff and patients must be reported to a member of the Infection Control Team. In the community it is normal practice to exclude a patient with gastroenteritis from work or school until the person is free of diarrhoea and vomiting and, if necessary, the appropriate clearance tests have been completed. Thereafter, it is particularly important to assess the risk of spreading infection of persons in whom special action should be considered.

In the UK, the Public Health Laboratory Services working party has defined four groups of persons in occupations or circumstances where there is a special risk of spreading gastrointestinal infection:

Group 1:	food handlers,
Group 2:	staff in health care facilities,
Group 3:	children <5 years of age, and
Group 4:	older children and adults who may find it difficult to implement good standards of personal hygiene.

The circumstances of each case, excreter, carrier or contact in these groups, should be considered individually and factors such as standards of personal hygiene be taken into account. It is important to emphasize that the agents causing gastroenteritis may infect without causing symptoms or be excreted for long periods after recovery from clinical illness. Excretion of organisms may still occur intermittently and in small numbers.

Table 9.1 Acute bacterial diarrhoeas and 'food poisoning'.

Organism	Incubation period (h)	Vomiting	Diarrhoea	Fever	Microbiology	Pathogenesis	Clinical features and treatment
Staphylococcus aureus	1–8 rarely up to 18	+++	+	–	Staphylococci grow in meats and in dairy & bakery products and produces enterotoxin.	Enterotoxin acts on receptors in gut that transmit impulses to medullary centers.	Abrupt onset, intense vomiting for up to 24 h, regular recovery in 24–48 h. Occurs in persons eating the same food. No treatment usually necessary except to restore fluids and electrolytes.
Bacillus cereus	1–8 rarely up to 18	+++	+	–	Reheated fried rice causes vomiting or diarrhoea.	Enterotoxins formed in food or in gut from growth of *B. cereus*.	After 1–6 h, mainly vomiting. After 8–16 h, mainly diarrhoea. Both self-limited to less than 1 day.
Clostridium perfringens	8–16	±	+++	–	Clostridia grow in rewarmed meat dishes and produce an enterotoxin.	Enterotoxin produced in food and in gut causes hypersecretion in small intestine.	Abrupt onset of profuse diarrhoea; vomiting occasionally. Recovery usual without treatment in 1–4 days. Many *Clostridium perfringens* in cultures of food and faeces of patients.
Clostridium botulinum	24–96	±	Rare	–	Clostridia grow in anaerobic foods and produce toxin.	Toxin absorbed from gut blocks acetylcholine at neuromuscular junction.	Diplopia, dysphagia, dysphonia, respiratory difficulty. Treatment requires clear airway, ventilation, and intravenous polyvalent antitoxin. Toxin present in food and serum. Mortality rate high.

Organism	Incubation				Epidemiology	Pathogenesis	Clinical notes
Clostridium difficile	5–10 days (up to 2 m)	−	+++	+	Associated with use of broad spectrum antibiotics.	Enterotoxin causes epithelial necrosis in colon; pseudomembranous colitis.	Abrupt onset of foul smelling diarrhoea; Toxin in stool. Oral metronidazole or vancomycin can be used for treatment.
Escherichia coli Some strain	24–72	±	+ (*E. coli* 0157; bloody diarrohea)	−	*E. coli* 0157 is associated with eating beef burger.	Enterotoxin causes hypersecretion in small intestine. Some strain invade gut mucosa.	Usually abrupt onset of diarrhoea; vomiting rare. In adults, 'traveller's diarrhoea' is usually self-limited to 1–3 days. Treatment with antibiotic is usually not recommended for infection caused by *E. coli* 0157.
Vibrio parahaemolyticus	6–96	+	+	±	Organisms grow in seafood and in gut and produce toxin or invade.	Hypersecretion in small intestine; stools may be bloody.	Abrupt onset of diarrhoea in groups consuming the same food, especially crabs and other seafood. Recovery is usually complete in 1–3 days. Food and stool cultures are positive.
Vibrio cholerae (mild cases)	24–72	+	+++	−	Organisms grow in gut and produce toxin.	Enterotoxin causes hypersecretion in small intestine. Infective dose: 10^7–10^9 organisms.	Abrupt onset of liquid diarrhoea in endemic area. Needs prompt replacement of fluids and electrolytes intravenously or orally. Tetracyclines shorten excretion of vibrios. Stool cultures positive.
Campylobacter jejuni	2–10 days	−	+++ (blood may be present)	+	Organisms grow in jejunum and ileum.	Invasion and enterotoxin production uncertain.	Fever, diarrhoea and fresh blood in stool, especially in children. Usually self-limited. Give erythromycin or fluoroquinolone in severe cases with invasion. Recovery in 5–8 days is usual.

Table 9.1 *Continued*

Organism	Incubation period (h)	Vomiting	Diarrhoea	Fever	Microbiology	Pathogenesis	Clinical features and treatment
Shigella spp.	24–72	±	+ (blood may be present)	+	Organisms grow in superficial gut epithelium and gut lumen and produce toxin.	Organisms invade epithelial cells; blood, mucus, and PMNs in stools. Infective dose: 10^2–10^3 organisms.	Abrupt onset of diarrhoea, often with blood and pus in stools, cramps, tenesmus, and lethargy. Therapy depends on sensitivity testing, but the fluoroquinolones are most effective. Do not give opiods. Often mild and self-limited.
Salmonella spp.	8–48	±	+	+	Organisms grow in gut. Do not produce toxin.	Superficial infection of gut, little invasion. Infective dose: 10^5 organisms.	Gradual or abrupt onset of diarrhoea and low-grade fever. No antimicrobials unless systemic dissemination is suspected, in which case give a fluoroquinolone. Stool cultures are positive. Prolonged carriage is common.
Yersinia enterocolitica	?	±	+	+	Fecal-oral transmission (occasionally). Food-borne.	Gastroenteritis or mesenteric adenitis. Occasional bacteremia. Enterotoxin produced.	Severe abdominal pain, diarrhoea, fever. PMNs and blood in stool; polyarthritis, erythema nodosum in children. If severe, give tetracycline or gentamicin.

Under these circumstances, transmission is unlikely providing that good personal hygiene is practised.

Members of staff suffering from gastrointestinal or food poisoning infection should inform their line manager. If the member of staff works in the kitchen or an area where food and enteral feed are prepared or handled, he or she should be taken off work and should be referred to the occupational health department.

References and further reading

Cáceres VM, Kim DK, Bresee JS, *et al.* A viral gastro-enteritis outbreak associated with person-to-person spread among hospital staff. *Infection Control and Hospital Epidemiology* 1998; **19**: 162–167.

Consultants in Public Health Medicine (Communicable Disease and Environmental Health Working Group). Scottish Centre for Infection and Environmental Health. Guidelines for bacteriological clearance following gastroenteritic infection. *Communicable Disease (Scotland) Weekly Report* 1994; **28**(26): 8–13.

Dryden MS, Keyworth N, Gabb R, Stein K. Asymptomatic food handlers as the source of nosocomial salmonellosis. *Journal of Hospital Infection* 1994; **28**: 195–208.

Guerrant RL, Van Gilder T, Steiner TS, *et al.* Practice Guidelines for the Management of Infectious Diarrhoea: Infectious Diseases Society of America. *Clinical Infectious Diseases* 2001; **32**: 331–350.

Scottish Home and Health Department. *The investigation and control of foodborne and waterborne diseases in Scotland.* Edinburgh: HMSO, 1995.

PHLS Working Group on the Control of Shigella sonnei. Revised guidelines for the control Shigella sonnei infection and other infective diarrhoeas. *Communicable Disease Report* 1993; **5**: R69–R70.

Subcommittee of the PHLS Working Group on the Vero-cytotoxin producing *Escherichia coli* (VTEC). Interim guidelines for the control if infections with Vero cytotoxin producing *Escherichia coli* (VTEC). *Communicable Disease Report* 1995; **6**: R77–R81.

The prevention of human transmission of gastrointestinal infections, infestations, and bacterial intoxication. A guide for Public Health Physicians and Environmental Health Officers in England and Wales. A Working Party of the PHLS Salmonella sub-committee. *Communicable Disease Report* 1995; **5**: R158–R172.

UK Department of Health. *Management of outbreaks of foodborne illness.* London: DoH, 1994.

MENINGOCOCCAL INFECTIONS

Meningococcal disease is caused by *N. meningitidis* or meningococci. They are Gram-negative diplococci which are divided into antigenically distinct groups. The most common are B, C, A, Y and W135. They can cause meningitis and septicaemia. Septicaemia without meningitis has the highest case fatality of 15–20% or more, whereas in meningitis alone, the fatality rate is around 3–5%. Most cases are a combination of septicaemia and meningitis. The disease can affect any age group, but the young are the most vulnerable. Cases occur in all months of the year but the incidence is highest in winter.

The nasopharyngeal carriage rate of all meningococci in the general population is about 10%, although rates vary with age; about 25% of young adults may be carriers at any one time.

Person-to-person transmission is mainly by droplets spread from the upper respiratory tract. There is no reservoir other than humans and the organism dies quickly outside the host. The incubation period is 2–10 days but most invasive disease normally develops within 7 days of acquisition. Therefore, for practical purposes 1-week period is considered sufficient to identify close contacts for prophylaxis. The incubation period is 2–3 days, and the onset of disease varies from fulminant to insidious with mild prodromal symptoms. Early symptoms and signs are usually malaise, pyrexia and vomiting. Headache, photophobia, drowsiness or confusion, joint pains and a typical haemorrhagic rash of meningococcal septicaemia may develop. In its early stages, the rash may be non-specific. *The rash, which may be petechial or purpuric, does not blanche* and this can be confirmed readily by gentle pressure with a glass slide etc, when the rash can be seen to persist. Patients may present in coma. In young infants particularly, the onset may be insidious and the classical signs are absent. The diagnosis should be suspected in the presence of vomiting, pyrexia, and irritability and, if still patent, raised anterior fontanelle tension.

Emergency action

Urgent admission to the hospital is a priority in view of the potentially rapid clinical progression of meningococcal disease. *Early treatment with benzyl penicillin is recommended* and may save life. Therefore, all general practitioners should carry benzyl penicillin in their emergency bags and give it while arranging the transfer of the case to the hospital. The only contraindication is a history of penicillin anaphylaxis. In these instances chloramphenicol (1.2 g for adult; 25 mg/kg for children under age of 12 years) may be given by injection. Immediate dose of benzyl penicillin for suspected cases are:

Adults and children (10 years or over)	1,200 mg
Children aged 1–9 years	600 mg
Children aged less than 1 year	300 mg

This dose should be given as soon as possible, ideally by intravenous injection. Intramuscular injection is likely to be less effective in shocked patients, due to reduced perfusion, but can be used if a vein cannot be found.

Management in hospital: On arrival in the hospital of a suspected case, doctors should take blood for culture and give benzyl penicillin (or suitable alternative) immediately if this has not already been done.

All patients with known or suspected meningitis must be isolated in a single room at the time of admission. The patient should be *isolated for a minimum of 24 h after the start of appropriate antibiotic and a full course of chemoprophylaxis has been given.*

Notification: In most countries, meningococcal infections are notifiable diseases. Notification to appropriate local authorities is important to ensure prompt follow up of close contacts. Close contacts should be offered chemoprophylaxis and immunization where appropriate, which can be offered up to 4 weeks after the index case became ill.

Chemoprophylaxis: Although penicillin and cefotaxime are the drugs of choice for the treatment of meningococcal infection, they have no effect on the elimination of nasopharyngeal carriage of the organism and are therefore not indicated for prophylaxis. Rifampicin, ciprofloxacin and ceftriaxone (but not cefotaxime) are effective in reducing the nasopharyngeal carriage rate and are therefore recommended for chemoprophylaxis.

Rifampicin: In the absence of contraindications, the drug of choice is rifampicin, which can be used in all age groups. It should preferably be taken at least 30 min before a meal or 2 h after a meal to ensure rapid and complete absorption. Dosages of rifampicin are as follows:

Adults:	600 mg every 12 h for 2 days.
Children:	
Over 1 year	10 mg/kg every 12 h for 2 days (up to a maximum of 600 mg per dose).
3 months to 1 year	5 mg/kg every 12 h for 2 days.

Rifampicin is contraindicated in the presence of jaundice or known hypersensitivity to rifampicin. Interactions with other drugs, such as anticoagulants, should be considered. *It also interferes with hormonal contraceptives* (family planning association advice for a 'missed' pill should be followed if rifampicin is prescribed to an oral contraceptive user) and *causes red coloration of urine, sputum and tears,* (soft contact lenses may be permanently stained). *Side effects should be explained to the patients* and the information should be supplied with the prescription.

Ciprofloxacin: Ciprofloxacin can be offered as an alternative to rifampicin and is given as a single dose of 500 mg orally in adults. It is useful when large numbers of contacts need prophylaxis, such as in the management of outbreaks in colleges or military camps or where compliance is in doubt.

Ceftriaxone: Although no drug is considered to be safe in pregnancy, all pregnant women who are contacts should be counselled carefully about risks and benefits and the option to give prophylaxis should be discussed. ***Ceftriaxone can be given as a first choice in pregnancy.*** It can also be used as an alternative to rifampicin or where compliance is in doubt. Dosages of ceftriaxone are:

Adults:	A single dose of 250 mg intramuscular injection.
Children:	A single dose of 125 mg intramuscular injection (from 6 weeks to 12 years).

Ceftriaxone is contraindicated in patients with a history of hypersensitivity to cephalosporins. It is not recommended for premature infants and full-term infants during the first 6 weeks of life.

Management of contacts

After a single case: Chemoprophylaxis should be offered to all close contacts (defined as people who had close, prolonged contact with the case) as soon as possible, i.e. within 24 h after the diagnosis of the index case. Prophylaxis is recommended to the contacts of confirmed or probable cases 7 days before the case became ill. Contacts of possible cases do not need prophylaxis unless or until further evidence emerges that changes the diagnostic category to confirmed or probable. It is recommended in the following situations:

Household: Immediate family and close contacts, i.e. people sleeping in the same house and boy/girl friends as the index case.

Kissing: Those people who have been mouth kissing contacts with the index case.

Index case: Index case should receive prophylaxis (unless they have already been treated with ceftriaxone) as soon as they are able to take oral medication.

Health care worker: HCWs are advised to reduce the possibility of exposure to large particle droplets nuclei (by wearing surgical masks and using closed suction) when carrying out airway management procedures (i.e. endotrachael intubations/ management, or close examination of orophrynx), on all patients with suspected meningococcal septicemia or meningitis.

Chemoprophylaxis is recommended only for those HCW who were in direct contact with respiratory secretions (i.e. mouth or nose is directly exposed to large particle droplets/secretions) and have not used appropriate barrier precautions. This type of exposure will only occur among staff who are working close to the face of the case without wearing a surgical mask. In practice, this implies a clear perception of facial contact with droplet secretions and is unlikely to occur unless undertaking airway management or being coughed at, directly in the face. *General medical or nursing care of cases is not an indication for prophylaxis.*

Cluster of cases: A cluster is defined as two or more cases of meningococcal disease in the same preschool group, school, or college/university within a 4-week period. If two possible cases attend the same institution, whatever the interval between cases, prophylaxis to household or institutional contacts is not indicated.

If two confirmed cases caused by different serogroups attend the same institution, they should be regarded as two sporadic cases, whatever the interval between them. Only household contacts of each case should be offered prophylaxis.

If two confirmed or probable cases who attend the same preschool group or school arise within a 4-week period and are, or could be, caused by the same serogroup, wider public health action in the institution is usually indicated.

The principle of managing such clusters is to attempt to define a group at high risk of acquiring meningococcal infection and disease, and to target that group for public health action. The target group should be a discrete group that contains the cases and makes sense to staff and parents, e.g. children and staff of the same pre-school group, children of the same school year, children who share a common social activity, or a group of friends.

It is important to emphasize that chemoprophylaxis is effective in reducing the nasopharyngeal carriage rates after treatment but does not completely eliminate transmission between household members. *Contacts should be reminded of the persisting risk of disease, whether or not prophylaxis is given,* and of the need to contact their general practitioner urgently if they develop any symptoms suggestive of meningococcal disease.

Immunization of contacts

Close contacts of cases of meningococcal meningitis have a considerably increased risk of developing the disease in the subsequent months, despite appropriate chemoprophylaxis. Therefore, *immediate family or close contacts of cases of group A or group C meningitis should be given meningococcal vaccine in addition to chemoprophylaxis.* The latter should be given first and the decision to offer vaccine should be made when the results of serotyping are available. Vaccine should not be given to contacts of group B cases. The serological response is detected in more than 90% of recipients and occurs 5–7 days after a single injection. The response is strictly group specific and confers no protection against group B organisms.

References and further reading

Cartwright K, ed. *Meningococcal Disease*. London: Wiley, 1995.

Hart CA, Rogers TRF, eds. Meningococcal disease. *Journal of Medical Microbiology* 1993; 39: 2–25.

Kaczmarski EB, Cartwright KAV. Control of meningococcal disease: guidance for microbiologist. *Communicable Disease Report* 1995; 5: R196–R198.

PHLS. Meningococcal Forum. Guidelines for public health management of meningococcal disease in the UK. *Communicable Disease and Public Health* 2002;5(3): 187–204.

PHLS Meningococcus Working Group and Public Health Medicine Environmental Group. Management of clusters of meningococcal disease. *Communicable Disease Report* 1997; 7: R3–R5.

UK Department of Health. *Immunization against infectious diseases*. London: HMSO, 1996.

VARICELLA ZOSTER VIRUS (VZV)

VZV causes chickenpox (varicella) as a primary infection. The virus persists in a latent state within the host and can subsequently reactivate years or decades later to cause shingles (zoster).

Clinical features: Chickenpox is an acute generalized illness with sudden onset of mild fever and constitutional upset and a typical skin eruption that is maculopapular for a few hours, vesicular for 3–4 days, and leaves a granular scab in 4–7 days. The vesicles are monolocular and collapse on puncture. Lesions commonly occur in successive crops, often with several stages of maturity present at the same time; they tend to be more abundant on covered than on exposed parts of the body. In some cases, the lesions may be so few as to escape observation. Mild atypical and inapparent infections may occur. The illness can result in complications such as pneumonia, encephalitis, visceral dissemination or haemorrhagic varicella.

Zoster or shingles is a local manifestation of re-activation of latent varicella infection in the dorsal root ganglia. Vesicles with an erythematous base appear, sometimes in crops, in irregular fashion on the skin to areas supplied by sensory nerves of a single or associated group of dorsal root ganglia. In the immunosuppressed or those patients with malignancies, chickenpox-like lesions may appear outside the dermatome.

Immunosuppressed patients, e.g. with cancer, especially of lymphoid tissue, with or without steroid therapy, immunodeficient patients and those on *immunosuppressive therapy may have an increased frequency and severity of zoster*, both localized and disseminated. Neonates developing varicella between ages 5–10 days, and those whose mothers develop the disease 5 days prior to or within 2 days after delivery, are at increased risk of developing severe generalized chickenpox, with a fatality rate of up to 30%. Infection in early pregnancy may be associated with congenital malformations in up to 2% of cases.

Period of infectivity: The incubation period ranges from 2–3 weeks (usually 13–17 days). In chickenpox *VZV is shed from the nasopharynx for up to 5* (usually 1–2) *days before the rash appears* and then *from the skin lesions until the vesicles have dried to a scab, usually about 4–7 days*; during this time, the patient is considered infectious. In shingles, the virus is shed from the skin lesion vesicles until they have dried to form a scab, so the patient is considered infectious for approximately 1 week after the appearance of the vesiculopustular lesions. It must be noted, however, that contagiousness may be prolonged in individuals with altered immunity.

Transmission: VZV is spread from person-to-person by direct contact or by the respiratory route (droplet or airborne) from secretions of the respiratory tract or vesicle fluid from chickenpox cases or the vesicle fluid of cases of herpes zoster. It can also be transmitted indirectly through articles freshly soiled by discharges from vesicles and mucous membranes of infected people.

About 5–8% of the adult population without a history of chickenpox do not have detectable antibody to VZV and are susceptible. Non-immune hospital staff may acquire VZV infection either in the hospital or from hospitalized patients and are at risk of developing chickenpox. Chickenpox in late pregnancy can be particularly severe, therefore *pregnant staff who have no clear history of chickenpox must avoid contact with patients and colleagues with VZV infection.* VZV vaccine should be offered to non-immune HCWs.

Infection control measures: The following measures should be considered in the control of VZV infection in health care setting:

- All suspected or clinically confirmed cases of chickenpox must be nursed in a side room with additional (airborne) isolation precautions (see page 102). The room should preferably have negative pressure ventilation. Infected patients may be cohorted together when necessary.

- Hands must be washed with antiseptic hand preparation or can be disinfected with an alcohol hand rub.

- Patients with varicella infection and susceptible (non-immune) persons exposed within the previous 21 days should not be admitted to hospital unless absolutely necessary.

- In-patients who develop varicella and susceptible patients (non-immune) exposed in hospital should be discharged as soon as possible if clinical condition permits.

- Exposed susceptible persons (non-immune), when they are hospitalized, must be isolated in a side room with appropriate infection control measures from 10 days following their earliest varicella exposure until 21 days after their most recent exposure. This period may be extended in cases where varicella zoster immunoglobin (VZIG) has been administered or in cases of immunosuppression.

- In the case of zoster infection, the patient should be nursed in a side room with infection control precautions from the first appearance of the vesiculopustular lesions until scab formation. Hands must be washed with antiseptic hand preparation or can be disinfected with an alcohol hand rub.

- In *pregnant women* the disease is more serious with a higher risk of fulminating varicella pneumonia. Therefore all pregnant patients who are admitted should be isolated in a side room with full *en-suite* facilities using the infection control precautions.

VZIG prophylaxis: VZIG prophylaxis is recommended in individuals with a significant contact with a case of varicella or zoster where the clinical condition increases the risk of severe complications of varicella. *VZIG does not prevent infection even* *when given within 72 h of exposure.* However it may attenuate disease if given up to 10 days after exposure. Severe maternal varicella may still occur despite VZIG prophylaxis. There is some evidence that the likelihood of fetal infection during the first 20 weeks of gestation is reduced in women who develop chickenpox under cover of VZIG.

A significant contact is defined as being in the same room (e.g. house or classroom or 2–4 bed hospital bay) for a significant period of time (15 min or more) or any face to face contact.

The following patients are at risk of developing severe complications of varicella and should be urgently tested for varicella immunity if significant exposure to varicella or zoster occurs:

Pregnant women: The problems of varicella infection during pregnancy relate to both the mother and fetus and also when infection takes place at term to the new born child. If varicella occurs during pregnancy, the woman should be advised of the likelihood of fetal involvement, with reference to the stages of the pregnancy that the infection took place and the providers of her antenatal care should be informed. If a pregnant woman has a significant contact with varicella or zoster and has no past history of varicella or zoster, the woman's susceptibility should be determined urgently by taking a blood sample. *If they are varicella IgG negative, they should be offered VZIG if they are within 10 days of the exposure.*

If the varicella infection occurs ≥8 days before delivery, inapparent or mild *in-utero* infection may occur. If the infection occurs 7 days before to 28 days after delivery, these women run a high risk of severe disseminated infection in the neonate and the intervention with VZIG is recommended. This should be administered to the mother before delivery and to the neonate after delivery. Varicella in the neonate should also be treated with aciclovir.

Neonates: *Babies born before 30 weeks of gestation or below 1 kg birth weight should receive VZIG if exposed to varicella, irrespective of the immune status of the mother.* It is also given to VZV antibody negative infants exposed to chickenpox or herpes zoster in the first 28 days of life. In neonates, VZIG is recommended in infants whose mother developed chickenpox (but not zoster) in the period 7 days before to 28 days after delivery. Prophylactic intravenous aciclovir should be considered for neonates whose mothers develop varicella 4 days before to 2 days after delivery as they are at the highest risk of fatal outcome despite VZIG prophylaxis. Mothers with varicella should be allowed to breast-feed. If nipple lesions are present, then milk can be expressed from the affected breast until the lesions are crusted. This expressed milk can be fed to the baby if he/she is covered by VZIG.

Patients with poor immunity: Patients with cancer, especially of lymphoid tissue, patients with leukaemia, organ transplant, AIDS and HIV infection and patients on chemotherapy for malignant disease.

Patients on systemic steroid drugs: Patients (or parents of children) at risk who use systemic corticosteroids should be advised to take reasonable steps to avoid close contact with chickenpox or herpes zoster and to seek urgent medical attention if exposed to chickenpox. Manifestations of fulminant illness include pneumonia, hepatitis and disseminated intravascular coagulation; *rash is not necessarily a prominent features.* Patients on steroids who are non-immune may require prophylactic cover with VZIG following contact with chickenpox or zoster.

VZIG is given by intramuscular injection *as soon as possible* and not later than 10 days after exposure. It must not be given intravenously. If a second exposure occurs after 3 weeks a further dose is required. VZIG does not prevent infection even when given within 72 h of exposure. However it may attenuate disease if given up to 10 days after exposure. Severe maternal varicella may still occur despite VZIG prophylaxis.

References and further reading

Enders G, Millar E, Cradock-Watson J, *et al.* Consequences of *varicella* and *herpes zoster* in pregnancy: prospective study of 1739 cases. *Lancet* 1994; **343**: 1548–1551.

Miller E. Varicella-zoster virus. In: Greenough A, *et al.* (ed). *Congenital, perinatal and neonatal infections.* London: Churchill and Livingstone, 1992: 223–232.

PHLS Joint Working Party of the Advisory Committees of Virology and Vaccines and Immunisation. Guidelines on the management of, and exposure to, rash illness in pregnancy (including consideration of relevant antibody screening programmes in pregnancy). *Communicable disease and public health* 2002; **5**: 59–71.

UK Department of Health. *Immunization against infectious diseases.* London: HMSO, 1996.

CREUTZFELDT-JAKOB DISEASE (CJD)

CJD is classified as a transmissible spongiform encephalopathy (TSE) in human; other TSEs in humans include Kuru, Gerstmann-Straussler-Scheinker syndrome, and fatal familial insomnia.

CJD is a progressive degenerative disease of the brain which causes dementia and death. At first, it was thought that the infectious agent was a virus or virus-like particle. However, in the 1980s, it became clear that a normal host protein, prion protein (PrP), was an important component of the infectious agent. The incubation period of sporadic cases of CJD is unknown, but iatrogenic cases appear to have an incubation period of 2 to 15 years or more, depending on the route of inoculation.

Mode of transmission: CJD has been transmitted accidentally in human sources including growth hormones, dura mater preparation and transplantation of a corneal graft donated by an affected patient. *CJD patients should not be accepted as blood donors, and none of their tissues used for transplant purposes.* In the case of corneal grafts, the member of the ophthalmic surgical team responsible for collecting the corneas should be instructed to make specific enquiries to exclude such cases. Corneas should not be taken from demented patients nor from those who die in psychiatric hospitals, nor from patients who die from obscure undiagnosed neurological diseases.

The PrP protein is extraordinarily resistant to standard cleaning and inactivation processes. It also has a high degree of resistance to physical and chemical procedures employed for sterilization and disinfection. Complete inactivation requires a combination of chemical and heat treatment. It also survives formalin fixation, therefore all formalin-fixed specimens should be regarded as being infective. Special care should therefore be taken to avoid accidental inoculation or other contamination while preparing the tissue for microscopy.

Clinical manifestations: New variant Creutzfeldt-Jakob Disease (vCJD) refers to a manifestation of the disease that is believed to be causally related to the Bovine Spongiform Encephalopathy (BSE) epidemic that has occurred in the UK and several other European countries. Unlike classical CJD, the initial presenting features of vCJD are usually psychiatric disturbances, such as depression and behavioural changes. Over the following months, additional symptoms such as abnormal sensation, ataxia and myoclonus develop. Although the EEG is abnormal, typical periodic complexes usually seen in classical CJD are absent in vCJD. Within about 12 months of the initial symptoms, patients enter a state of akinetic mutism, and death usually occurs within a few months. Neuropathological features differ markedly from those of classical CJD. The most consistent pathological change in vCJD, which is generally not seen in classical CJD, is the presence of PrP plaques. In most cases studied, plaques are distributed extensively throughout the cerebrum and cerebellum, with some plaques seen in the basal ganglia, thalamus and hypothalamus.

Diagnosis: There is no serological test available for the diagnosis of CJD and reliance can only be made on clinical grounds based on the history of rapidly progressive dementia, the presence of mycolonic movements and a characteristic electroencephalogram. It can be confirmed by the histological examination of brain tissue after death.

Infection control precautions: It is important to emphasize that *CJD is neither a contagious nor communicable disease, but is transmissible under certain circumstance* (see page 169). Normal social and clinical contact and non invasive procedures do not a present risk to HCWs, visitors, relatives and the wider community.

Isolation of CJD patients is not necessary. Patients can be nursed in an open ward using standard precautions. Patients may need to be placed in a single room on compassionate ground. When caring for patients with CJD, the HCW should wear single-use disposable gloves and plastic apron and gloves when carrying out procedures, e.g. lumbar punctures for radiological and other investigations, biopsies, dressing wounds and venepuncture/administration of injections etc.

Although CJD is not transmissible by the respiratory route, it is recommended to use single-use disposal instruments which are in direct contact with mouth, pharynx, tonsils and respiratory tract by a method described. Destruction by incineration of non re-usable equipment is recommended.

Surgical procedures: It is essential that the *surgical procedure should be carefully planned beforehand and appropriate personnel informed.* Where the surgical procedure involves the brain (e.g. cortical biopsy), spinal cord or eye, the following additional precautions should be taken:

- Minimum number of staff should take part in the operation.
- Disposable instruments and equipment should be used wherever possible.
- Members of the operating team should wear appropriate personal equipment, i.e. liquid repellent theatre gown over a plastic apron, gloves, mask and visor or goggles.
- Disposable drapes and dressings should be used.
- Cover all non-disposable equipment.
- One-way flow of instruments should be maintained.
- All waste should be treated as clinical waste and disposed of by incineration.
- Specimens sent to a Pathology Laboratory should be put in an appropriate container and be marked with a 'Biohazard' label.
- All surfaces should be cleaned and disinfected according to local protocol.

These precautions should also be observed when neurosurgical procedures are carried out on patients in whom the possibility of CJD enters into the differential diagnosis.

Methods of decontamination

The decision on methods of instrument decontamination should be based upon the infectivity level of the tissue and the way in which instruments will subsequently be re-used. For example, where surgical instruments contact high infectivity tissues, single-use surgical instruments are strongly recommended. If single-use instruments are not available, maximum safety is attained by destruction of re-usable instruments. Where destruction is not practical, re-usable instruments must be handled with care and must be decontaminated. *Do not mix instruments used on high and low infectivity tissues.* To avoid unnecessary destruction of instruments, *quarantine of instruments while determining the final diagnosis of persons suspected of CJD should be used.*

High-risk tissues (see Table 9.2) from high-risk patients (e.g. those with known or suspected CJD) and critical or semicritical items should be subjected to the following decontamination measures:

* These *devices must be thoroughly cleaned to ensure that all tissue is effectively removed.* To minimize drying of tissues and body fluids on the object, *instruments should be kept moist until cleaned and decontaminated.*

Table 9.2 Distribution of infectivity in the human body.

Infectivity category	Tissues, secretions and excretions	
High infectivity	Brain Spinal cord Eye	
Low infectivity	CSF Kidney Liver Lung Lymph nodes/spleen Placenta	
No detectable infectivity	Adipose tissue Adrenal gland Gingival tissue Heart muscle Intestine Peripheral nerve Prostate Skeletal muscle Testis Thyroid gland Blood	Tears Nasal mucous Saliva Sweat Serous exudate Milk Semen Urine Faeces

Adapted from Brown P, 1994 & 1996.

Notes: Assignment of different organs and tissues to categories of *high* and *low infectivity* is chiefly based upon the frequency with which infectivity has been detectable, rather than upon quantitative assays of the level of infectivity, for which data are incomplete.

- Equipment that requires special prion reprocessing should be tagged after use according to local protocol. Those instruments should be placed securely in a robust, leak-proof container labelled 'Biohazard'.

- Surgical instruments can be cleaned and then sterilized by autoclaving at 134°C for ≥18 min in a prevacuum sterilizer.

- Those devices that are impossible or difficult to clean could be discarded. Alternatively, contaminated items should be immersed in a container filled with a liquid (e.g. saline, water or phenolic solution) to minimize the adherence of material to the items. This should be followed by initial decontamination by autoclaving at 134°C for 18 min in a prevacuum sterilizer, or by soaking in 1 N NaOH for 1 h.

- Environmental surfaces (non-critical) contaminated with high-risk tissues (e.g. laboratory surface in contact with brain tissue of a person infected with CJD) should be cleaned and then spot-decontaminated with a 1:10 dilution of sodium hypochlorite (i.e. bleach). To minimize environmental contamination, disposable cover sheets could be used on work surfaces.

- *Non-critical equipment* contaminated with a high-risk tissue should be cleaned and then disinfected with sodium hypochlorite (1:10 dilution) or 1 N NaOH, depending on material compatibility. All contaminated surfaces must be exposed to the disinfectant.

Devices in contact with *low or no risk tissues* can be cleaned and either disinfected or sterilized by use of conventional protocols of heat or chemical sterilization, or high-level disinfection. Although CSF is classified as a low infectivity tissue it is recommended that *instruments contaminated by CSF should be handled in the same manner as those contacting high infectivity tissues,* that instruments used for lumbar puncture be single-use disposable and that they must be discarded and destroyed by incineration afterwards.

Post-mortem: Post-mortem examination of patients with CJD *should be done by a neuropathologist with access to a specialized mortuary.* However, a general histopathologist who has been asked to perform a necropsy on a case of possible or probable CJD must follow suitable infection control precautions based on local guidance. As few persons as possible should take part in the post-mortem. Personal protective equipment must be worn. Great care should be taken to avoid cuts and sharp injuries, particularly from contact with sharp bony edges and during sewing up. Accidental injuries or inoculation wounds should be thoroughly washed (without scrubbing) in running water immediately, and the incident should be reported according to local protocol. The bodies of patients who have died as a result of CJD must not be used for teaching anatomy or pathology.

Childbirth: CJD is not known to be transmitted from mother to child during pregnancy or childbirth. In the event that a person with CJD becomes pregnant, no particular precautions need to be taken during the pregnancy, except during invasive procedures. Childbirth should be managed using standard infection control procedures, except that precautions should be taken to reduce the risk of exposure to placenta and any associated material and fluids. These should be disposed of by incineration.

Occupational exposure

No known cases of human CJD have occurred through occupational accident or injury. In the context of occupational exposure, the highest potential risk is from exposure to high infectivity tissues through needle-stick injuries with inoculation; however, exposure to either high or low infectivity tissues through direct inoculation (e.g. needlesticks, puncture wounds, 'sharps' injuries, or contamination of broken skin) must be avoided.

Unbroken skin which has been contaminated with internal body fluids or tissues should be washed with detergent and plenty of warm water, rinsed and dried. Do not scrub. Brief exposure (1 min to 0.1 N NaOH or a 1:10 dilution of bleach) can be considered for maximum safety. If needlesticks or lacerations occur, gently encourage bleeding and wash (without scrubbing) with warm soapy water, rinse, dry and cover with a waterproof dressing. Further treatment (e.g. sutures) should be appropriate to the type of injury. Splashes into the eye or mouth should be irrigated with either saline (eye) or tap water (mouth). All occupational injuries should be reported according to local policy and protocol and the records kept for no less than 20 years.

References and further reading

Advisory Committee on Dangerous Pathogens, Spongiform Encephalopathy Advisory Committee. *Transmissible Spongiform Encephalopathy Agents: Safe Working and the Prevention of Infection*. London: The Stationery Office, 1998.

Baron H, Safar J, Groth D, DeArmond SJ, Prusiner SB. Prions. In: Block SS (ed), *Disinfection, sterilization and preservation*, 5th edn. Philadelphia: Lippincott Williams & Wilkins; 2001, 659–674.

Bell JE, Ironside JW. How to tackle a possible Creutzfeldt-Jakob Disease necropsy. *Journal of Clinical Pathology* 1993; **46**: 193–197.

Brown P, Gibbs CJ, Rodgers-Johnson P, *et al*. Human Spongiform Encephalopathy: the National Institutes of Health Series of 300 Cases of Experimentally Transmitted Disease. *Annual of Neurology* 1994; **35**: 513–529.

Brown P. Environmental Causes of Human Spongiform Encephalopathy. Baker H, Ridley RM, (eds), *Methods in Molecular Medicine: Prion Diseases*. Totowa, NJ: Humana Press, 1996: 139–154.

Brown P, Gibbs CJ Jr, Gajdusek DC, *et al.* Transmission of Creutzfeldt-Jakob Disease from formalin-fixed, paraffin-embedded human brain tissue. *New England Journal of Medicine* 1986; **315**: 1614–1615.

Consensus Group meeting between Central Sterilizing Club and Hospital Infection. Sterilization issues in vCJD – towards a consensus. *Journal of Hospital Infection* 2002; **51**: 168–174.

Dealler S. Prevention of cross infection in variant Creutzfeldt-Jakob Disease. *British Journal of Infection Control* 2001; **2**: 5–8.

Johnston L, Conly J. Creutzfeldt-Jakob disease and infection control. *Canadian Journal of Infectious Diseases* 2001; **12**(6): 332–336.

MacKnight C. Clinical Implications of Bovine Spongiform Encephalopathy. *Clinical Infectious Diseases* 2001; **32**: 1726–1731.

Painter MJ. Variant Creutzfeldt-Jakob Disease. *Journal of Infection* 2000; **41**: 117–124.

Prusiner SB. Human Prion Disease. In: Zuckerman AJ, Banatvala JE, Pattison JR (eds), *Principles and Practice of Clinical Virology*, 4th edn. London: John Wiley & Sons, 2000; 711–747.

Rutala WA, Weber DJ. Creutzfeldt-Jakob Disease: Recommendations for Disinfection and Sterilization. *Clinical Infectious Diseases* 2001; **32**: 1348–1356.

Spencer MD, Knight SG, Will RG. First hundred cases of variant Creutzfeldt-Jakob disease: retrospective case note review of early psychiatric and neurological features. *British Medical Journal* 2002; **324**: 1479–1482.

Stone DH, Jarvis S, Pless B. Iatrogenic vCJD from surgical instruments. *British Medical Journal* 2001; **322**: 1558–1559.

Will RG, Zeidler M, Stewart GE, *et al.* Diagnosis of New Variant Creutzfeldt-Jakob Disease. *Annual of Neurology* 2000; **47**: 575–582.

World Health Organization. *WHO Infection Control Guidelines for Transmissible Spongiform Encephalopathies: Report of a WHO consultation* Geneva: Switzerland, 2000. WHO/CDS/CSR/APH/2000.3.http://www.who.int/emc

VIRAL HAEMORRHAGIC FEVERS (VHFs)

VHFs are a group of viral diseases which are endemic mainly in west and central Africa. VHFs can present a significant risk to all countries due to the ease of international travel. VHFs have a significant mortality rate and there is no vaccine available. The most clinically important viruses are:

- *Lassa fever virus:* Nigeria, Sierra Leone and Liberia
- *Marburg virus:* Uganda, Kenya, Zimbabwe
- *Ebola virus:* Zaire and Sudan
- *Crimean-Congo haemorrhagic fever virus:* Former Soviet Union and east and west Africa.

Clinical manifestations: VHFs usually present as a febrile illness with headache, myalgia, sore throat, cough and vomiting. Some patients have a cough, chest pain, abdominal tenderness and skin rash. In severe cases, patients may suffer extensive haemorrhage, accompanied by a purpuric rash and bleeding from almost any part of the body, including the intestine, eyes, gums, nose, mouth, lungs and uterus. Encephalopathy and multi-organ failure are common in severe cases and the case mortality rate is high.

History of adequate malarial prophylaxis must be taken. Malaria is a common confounding diagnosis and is suspected in patients who have failed to take adequate malarial prophylaxis.

Diagnosis: A firm diagnosis is not always possible but both the clinical and the epidemiological evidence need to be considered for any patient presenting with undiagnosed fever within 3 weeks of return from an endemic area.

In the initial assessment of patients with suspected VHF, *laboratory testing should be kept to an absolute minimum to minimize the risk associated with the collection and handling of laboratory specimens.* Laboratory procedures must include a risk assessment at each stage, including risks associated with the chosen techniques, recommendations about training and surveillance measures, waste disposal and decontamination.

All patients with suspected VHF and their specimens and bodily secretions should be handled at Physical Containment Level 4. All specimens must be handled with appropriate safeguards. The specimens should not be sent through the normal courier mechanisms (human or otherwise), to ensure that accidents do not occur as a consequence of mishandling or misplacement. The laboratory staff and infection control practitioner must be alerted immediately to ensure appropriate handling of specimens.

Notification: All suspected cases of VHF must be notified to the local officer (CCDC in the UK) or other designated authority.

Incubation period: The incubation period of the infection is usually 7–10 days (ranging from 3–17 days). For infection control purposes, *if no infection has occurred in a period of up to 21 days from exposure, a contact is usually taken to be free from infection.*

Risk categories: The UK Advisory Committee on Dangerous Pathogens (1996) have categorized patients in the following risk groups:

Minimum risk: Patients for whom the possibility of a VHF has been assessed but whose history and clinical condition make the diagnosis unlikely. This category includes febrile patients who were not in known endemic or outbreak areas before they became ill, or who were in such areas but became ill more than 21 days after contact with a potential source of infection, and patients whose risk category has been revised because of their clinical condition or the results of laboratory tests. These patients can be managed using standard isolation precautions. No special ambulance transport is necessary.

Moderate risk: Febrile patients who have been in an endemic area during the 21 days before they became ill but who have no other risk factors, or who have not been in an endemic area but may have been in adjacent areas or countries during the 21 days before the onset of illness, and who have evidence of severe illness with organ failure and/or haemorrhage which could be due to a VHF and for which no alternative diagnosis is currently evident.

Few patients remain in this category for more than 48–72 h. These patients should be admitted to a designated high security infectious disease (HSID) unit or to inter-mediate isolation facilities and transported by a category ambulance. Malaria must be excluded by sending blood films to the laboratory. The appropriate local officer should be notified and contacts identified, but the contacts need not be placed under surveillance unless the patient is reclassified as high risk.

High risk: Febrile patients who have been in an endemic area during the 3 weeks before illness and have lived in or stayed in a house for more than 4 h where there were febrile people known or strongly suspected to have a VHF or have cared for a febrile patient known or strongly suspected to have a VHF, or have had contact with body fluids, tissue, or a dead person or animal known to have had a VHF, or were previously classified as moderate risk but have developed organ failure and/or haemorrhage. This category also includes febrile patients who have not been in an endemic area, but have cared for a patient or animal known or strongly suspected to have had a VHF during the 3 weeks before they themselves became ill. High-risk patients should be admitted to a HSID unit and all specimens (except the initial malaria test) must be handled in a designated laboratory. The appropriate local officer (CCDC in the UK) should be notified. All those who had close contact with the patient after the onset of illness should have their temperatures taken daily for 21 days after their last contact.

Source of infection: Patients are infectious while they are symptomatic and until the virus has been cleared from the blood and body fluids. Lassa fever virus has been found in the respiratory secretions of a symptomatic patient and in urine during the convalescent phase. Sexual transmission of Ebola virus and Lassa fever virus has been recorded, and Ebola virus has been found in seminal fluid for up to 2 months after the onset of symptoms.

Mode of transmission: Recent evidence on the mode of transmission of these viruses indicates that the *main risk of transmission in the health care settings is from mucosal or parenteral exposure to contaminated blood or other body fluids.* Lassa fever virus may also be transmitted by exposure to aerosols of contaminated body fluids, particularly nasopharyngeal secretions and urine.

Management

In general practice: If the General Practitioner has seen a patient at home and suspects a diagnosis of VHF in a patient suffering from acute atypical fevers, (especially with any accompanying superficial haemorrhages or in patients who have recently returned from endemic areas), he/she is advised not to move the patient from home and to seek specialist advice.

In hospital: It is possible that the provisional diagnosis might first be made in a patient attending hospital as an out-patient, e.g. in the Accident and Emergency department or in a patient already in a general hospital ward. It is important to emphasize that VHFs are containment 4 pathogens and appropriate procedures must be taken.

Infection control and precautions

The following action must be taken:

- The patient must be isolated in a single room with standard and contact isolation precautions. *Strict isolation precautions must be instituted.* The patient must not be moved from the suspected ward or department. It is possible that the patient may require treatment in a high security designated infectious diseases unit.

- The *absolute minimum of staff should have contact with the patient*, i.e. one doctor and one nurse. The doctor involved in making the initial diagnosis should seek advice from the consultant physician in infectious diseases. In such circumstances, no other hospital medical staff should be invited to assist in confirming suspicions to minimize the risk to HCWs.

- Instruments, dressings, documents, clothing or any other items must not be removed from the area.

- Staff already involved with the case must not resume other professional duties and should remain, as far as possible, within the department, using a designated staff room.

- Patients and their body fluids are highly infectious therefore appropriate protective clothing must be worn, e.g. scrub suit, gown, apron, two pairs of gloves, mask, headcover, eyewear, and rubber boots.

- *Disposable equipment should be used whenever possible.* Other instruments should be heat disinfected.

- The environment must be decontaminated using hypochlorite solution 1:100 dilution. Fumigation of the room is necessary after the patient has been discharged.

- *All waste must be treated as clinical waste* and must be disposed of by incineration.

- VHFs are classified as dangerous biological agents (containment 4 pathogens). Therefore, transport and handling of specimens requires special precautions.

If the diagnosis of VHF is confirmed, *staff who have been in contact with the patient may require continuing isolation and surveillance.* This should be carried out by the occupational health department. Assessment of any surveillance measures necessary for patients may be needed for other patients who may have been in contact with suspect case.

References and further reading

Cooper CB, Gransden WR, Webster M, King M, *et al.* A case of Lassa fever: experience at St Thomas' hospital. *British Medical Journal* 1982; **285**: 1003–1005.

Holmes GP, McCornick JB, Trock CC, *et al.* Lassa fever in the United States: investigations of a case and new guidelines for management. *New England Journal of Medicine* 1990; **323**: 1120.

Isaäcson M. Viral Haemorrhagic Fever hazards for travellers in Africa. *Travel Medicine, Clinical Infectious Diseases* 2001; **33**: 1707–1712.

McCormick JB, Webb PA, Krebs JW, *et al.* A prospective study of the epidemiology and ecology of Lassa fever. *Journal of Infectious Diseases* 1987; **155**(3): 437–444.

Management of patients with suspected viral haemorrhagic fever. *Morbidity and Mortality Weekly Report* 1988; 37(Suppl.): 1–16.

Notice to Readers Update: Management of Patients with Suspected Viral Haemorrhagic Fever-United States. *Morbidity and Mortality Weekly Report* 1995; **44**(25): 475–479.

UK Advisory Committee on Dangerous Pathogens. *Management and control of viral haemorrhagic fevers.* London: The Stationary Office, 1996.

UK Advisory Committee on Dangerous Pathogens. *Categorisation of biological agents according to hazard and categories of containment,* 4th edn. London: HMSO, 1995.

WHO and CDC: *Infection control for viral haemorrhagic fevers in the African health care setting.* Geneva: WHO, 1998. http://www.who.int/

RABIES

Human-to-human transmission of rabies is very rare and has been demonstrated in patients who have received infected corneal grafts. Transmission is mostly from an animal bite in countries where rabies is prevalent. The incubation period is usually 3–8 weeks, but may be as short as 9 days or as long as 7 years, depending on the severity of the wound, the site of the wound in relation to the richness of the nerve supply and its distance from the brain.

Rabies is transmitted when infected saliva contaminates mucous membrane or an open wound. The following precautions are recommended:

- The patient should be isolated in a single room with standard infection control precautions.

- The staff should wear appropriate protective clothing including gloves, gown, goggles.

- Mouth-to-mouth resuscitation should not be used.

- Staff in contact with the patient should be minimized.

- Staff with open lesions should not be allowed to have contact with the patient.

- Pregnant female staff should not attend the patient.

- Specimens from the patient should not be sent to routine diagnostic laboratories without prior consultation with the senior member of staff.

- Equipment soiled by secretions or excretions should either be single-use disposable or sterilized using heat sterilization in the Sterile Supply Department.

- Attendant staff and other close contacts should be offered immunization and sometimes rabies-specific immunoglobulin at the advice of the physician in infectious diseases.

- Post-mortem examination should not be undertaken. Where such examination may be of value, the indications and arrangements must be discussed with the histopathologist.

References and further reading

Rabies Prevention – United States 1991. Recommendations of the Immunization Practices Advisory Committee. *Morbidity and Mortality Weekly Report* 1991; **40**: 1–19.

UK Department of Health. *Memorandum on rabies*. London: HMSO, 1977.

UK Department of Health. *Immunization against infectious disease*. London: HMSO, 1996.

INFESTATIONS WITH ECTOPARASITES

Humans are the only reservoir for these parasites, which are usually localized to a specific site of the body.

Lice (Pediculosis)

There are many different species of lice but only three that are clinically important from the family pediculidae. They can be caught only by close contact, i.e. close enough for lice to walk onto another host. Lice can be found on the body, on bedding, chairs, floor etc. They are either dead, injured or dying and not able to crawl onto another host. Nits are the eggs of lice, which are firmly attached to hair and are difficult to remove.

Infestations with lice may result in severe itching and excoriation of the scalp or body. Secondary bacterial infection may occur due to severe itching resulting in regional lymphadenitis (especially cervical).

Head louse (*Pediculus humanus* var. *capitis*): This species lives on the head and eyebrow hair. The female louse lays eggs at the base of the hairs where it is warmest. Transmission to another host occurs when two heads are in direct contact, allowing lice to crawl on to a new head. Lice prefer clean hair where they can move around easily. They are invariably acquired from family members or close friends who should be checked for infection. Head lice cannot be transmitted to others on clothing or linen and therefore no precautions are necessary. Patients with head lice need not be isolated, except in paediatric wards where close contact between children may transmit the lice. Outbreaks of head lice are common among children in schools and other institutions.

Pubic or crab louse (*Phthirus pubis*): They live on coarse body hair, usually the pubic area; they may also infect facial hair (including eye lashes), axillae and body surfaces. They are transmitted by close physical contact, frequently but not always, by sexual contact. Children may acquire crab lice through close contact with their mother, e.g. axillary hair. Crab lice on clothing or bedding are not transmitted to other people and can be removed by washing clothes in a hot cycle.

Body louse (*Pediculus humanus* var. *corporis*): Body lice are still prevalent among populations with poor personal hygiene, especially in cold climates where heavy clothing is worn and bathing is infrequent. They live in clothing, rather than hair and go to the body only to feed. Transmission occurs in overcrowded conditions by contact with infested clothing. They are easy to eradicate, as they will die if the clothing is not worn for 3 days.

Infection control measures

- Carefully remove all clothing of patients with body or pubic lice and seal in a bag. As lice dislike light, clothing should be handled in bright conditions.

Single-use non-sterile disposable gloves and a plastic apron should be worn. In hospital, process linen as infected linen according to local policy.

- No special treatment of the environment is required as spread is by personal contact. Body lice are capable of surviving for a limited time in stored clothing, but head and pubic lice rapidly die when detached from their host.

- Patients with body lice do not require specific treatment but should be bathed. Infestation with head and crab lice should be referred to the medical practitioner for appropriate treatment.

- Clothing, bedding and fomites should be treated with a hot water cycle (60°C or more).

Fleas

Infestation is usually with dog, cat, or bird fleas, which will bite humans in the absence of the preferred host. The human flea is rare. Fleas are able to survive for some months in the environment without feeding. Elimination of the host or treatment of pets and the use of suitable insecticides on environment surfaces and soft furnishing is therefore essential.

Infection control measures

- Remove all clothing and bedding. All laundry should be treated as infected linen according to the local policy.

- Clothing not suitable for washing may be treated with low temperature steam. Seek advice from the SSD manager.

- The laundry bag must be removed immediately from the ward. In the laundry, the inner hot water soluble plastic bag will allow transfer to a machine without handling.

- Identify the flea, and if possible, treat or remove the host. If it is a cat flea, take steps to exclude feral cats from the site.

- Vacuum clean floors, carpets, upholstery, fabrics, etc.

- Contact your pest control officer to treat the environment, e.g. ducting, hard surfaces, and under fixtures, with a residual insecticide if necessary.

Scabies

Scabies is caused by *Sarcoptes scabiei*. The severe itching is caused by an allergic reaction to the presence of a small mite which burrows into the top layer of skin. Intense itching occurs especially at night or after a hot bath or shower. The allergic reaction does not appear immediately, but develops between 4 and 6 weeks after infection. However, symptoms may appear earlier (1–4 days) if the patient has had previous exposure.

'Norwegian' or 'crusty' scabies occurs in elderly or immunosuppressed patients, i.e. patients on immunosuppressive therapy, with AIDS and with other malignancies. Immunocompromised patients may suffer hyperinfestation. This form of scabies is highly contagious because mites multiply rapidly and large numbers of the parasites are present in the exfoliating scales.

Human beings are the only source of infection. *Spread of infection from person-to-person occurs through direct skin-to-skin contact,* which is usually prolonged and intimate.

Any person infested with either mites or eggs is infectious. In the health care setting, it is transmitted primarily through intimate direct contact with an infested person, even when high levels of personal hygiene are maintained.

Hand-holding or patient support for long periods is probably responsible for most hospital-acquired scabies. Transmission to HCWs has occurred during activities such as sponge-bathing patients or applying body lotions. Transmission between patients may also be possible when patients are ambulatory. Transmission via inanimate objects, such as clothing and bedding, is uncommon, and only occurs if contaminated immediately beforehand, as the mites do not survive very long out of contact with human skin. Spread from bedding, clothing or fomites is unlikely.

Infection control measures

- Refer members of the family and those in close physical contact to their general practitioner so that they can be treated if necessary.

- Treat bedding and clothing as infected linen according to the local policy.

- Protective long sleeved gowns and gloves should be worn. Prolonged contact should be avoided.

- No special environmental control measures are necessary.

- For hospitalized patients, institute additional isolation precautions (contact transmission) for 24 h after start of effective therapy. Consideration should be given to extending the isolation period in the case of immunocompromised or heavily infested patients. In addition, staff with scabies should be rostered to avoid patient contact for 24 h after appropriate treatment is initiated.

- Patients with 'Norwegian' scabies are highly contagious and additional isolation precautions (contact transmission) are recommended until the treatment is completed.

References and further reading

Gooch JJ, Strasius SR, Beamer B, *et al.* Nosocomial outbreak of scabies. *Archive of Dermatology* 1978; 114: 897–898.

Jimenez-Lucho VE, Fallon F, Caputo C, Ramsey K. Role of prolonged surveillance in the eradication of nosocomial scabies in an extended care Veterans Affairs medical centre. *American Journal of Infection Control* 1995; 23: 44–49.

Lettau LA. Nosocomial transmission and infection control aspects of parasitic and ectoparasitic disease. Part I. Introduction/Enteric Parasites. *Infection Control and Hospital Epidemiology* 1991; 12: 59–65.

Lettau LA. Nosocomial transmission and infection control aspects of parasitic and ectoparasitic diseases. Part II. Blood and Tissue Parasites. *Infection Control and Hospital Epidemiology* 1991; 12: 111–121.

Lettau LA. Nosocomial transmission and infection control aspects of parasitic and ectoparasitic disease. Part III. Ectoparasites/Summary and conclusions. *Infection Control and Hospital Epidemiology* 1991; 12: 179–185.

Maunder J. Treatments for eradicating lice and scabies. Prescriber 1991; April 5: 27–48.

Maunder J. The scourge of scabies. *Chemist and Druggist* 1992; 11: 54–55.

Maunder J. An update of headlice. Health Visitor 1993; 66(9): 317–318.

10

Blood-borne Hepatitis and Human Immunodeficiency Virus (HIV) Infections

Blood-borne infections are those where infectious agents in a person's blood can be transmitted to another person giving rise to infection. Since the infectious status of a patient is not always known it is essential that all *Health Care Workers adopt safe working practices at all times*. Health care facilities should implement standard infection control precautions as the primary basis of preventing transmission of infection to Health Care Workers (HCWs).

Immunization against hepatitis B infection is an effective means of protection against hepatitis B virus (HBV) but must not be used as a substitute for good clinical practice. The vaccine will protect against hepatitis B infection but will not protect against hepatitis C, HIV and other viruses transmitted through the blood-borne route.

Viral hepatitis

To date, six types of viral hepatitis have been identified, i.e. hepatitis A, B, C, D, E and most recently, hepatitis G. Hepatitis A and E are transmitted by the faecal-oral route and therefore will not be discussed; hepatitis viruses B, C, D and G are transmitted by the blood-borne route.

Hepatitis B virus (HBV)

HBV is a member of the Hepadnaviridae family of DNA viruses. The mean incubation period of acute HBV infection is 75 days but it may range from 45 to 180 days. After exposure to the virus, most infected individuals recover completely from the acute illness; however, inapparent infections are common, particularly among children. A small, and variable, proportion of individuals do not clear hepatitis B surface antigen (HBsAg), which is found circulating in blood during the latter part of the incubation period and in the acute phase of HBV. They become carriers, (i.e. individuals who shed HBsAg into the circulation for more than 6 months) following acute infection. Some of these develop chronic hepatitis, cirrhosis or hepatocellular carcinoma. The likelihood of a patient developing chronic hepatitis is inversely related to age at the time of infection.

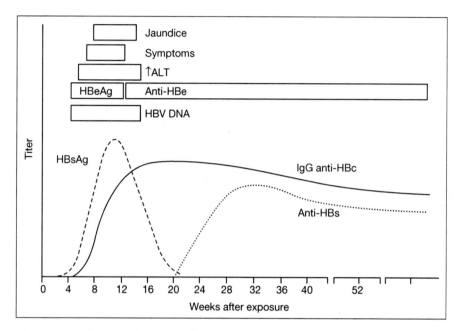

Figure 10.1 The typical course of acute type B hepatitis.
HBsAg: Hepatitis B surface antigen; anti-HBs: antibody to HBsAg; HBeAg: Hepatitis B 'e' antigen; anti-HBe: antibody to HBeAg; anti-HBc: antibody to hepatitis B core antigen; ALT: alanine aminotransferase.

Chronic infection occurs in at least 90% of cases following neonatal infection, 25% of children aged 1–10 years and 5% or less in adults. Of these, 5–10% have persistent 'e' antigenaemia *hepatitis B 'e' antigen positive (HBeAg+ve), which correlates with a high level of viral replication and heightened infectivity; these are regarded as high-grade infections.* Such high grade infections are generally associated with HBV DNA levels of greater that 10,000 genomes/ml in serum. A patient who is in the early pro-dromal or acute phase of hepatitis B should also be considered as high grade. Most carriers, however, are 'e' antigen negative and can be classified as low grade with regard to transmission of infection. However, carriers of HBV who are negative for 'e' antigen can occasionally transmit infection. Some of these low-grade carriers have been asso-ciated with the presence of a viral mutation, which stops the synthesis of 'e' antigen but still allows production of infectious virus.

Hepatitis C virus (HCV)

HCV belongs to the flaviviridae family. Incubation periods range from 20 days to 13 weeks. The acute phase of HCV infection is usually asymptomatic or mild and

Table 10.1 Interpretation of the common patterns of serological markers of HBV infection.

Interpretation	HBsAg (Hepatitis B surface antigen)	HBeAg ('e' antigen)	Anti-HBe ('e' antibody)	IgM* (to core Ag)	IgG (to core Ag)	Anti-HBs
Acute Hepatitis B	+	+ or −	+ or −	+	+	−
Recovered from HBV	−	−	Usually +	−	+	+
Chronic infection§						
High infectivity	+	+	−	−	+	−
Low infectivity	+	−	+	−	+	−
HBV immunization	−	−	−	−	−	+

HBsAg: Hepatitis B surface antigen; HBeAg: Hepatitis B 'e' antigen; Anti-HBe: Antibody to Hepatitis B 'e' antigen; Anti-HBs: Antibody to Hepatitis B surface antigen.
*Tests for IgM are usually strongly reactive during acute infection; weaker reactivity may also be present in some chronic infections.
§Someone with detectable surface antigen more than 6 months after acute hepatitis B or first detection of antigen.

patients are often unaware of the infection. Patients may complain of fatigue but a few have a history of acute hepatitis or jaundice. If it proceeds to chronic disease, progression is usually indolent and the most common complaint is fatigue. Up to 80% of people who are anti-HCV positive may continue to carry the virus, which may cause slow ongoing liver damage. It is thought that 10–20% of individuals with chronic hepatitis will go on to develop cirrhosis over 20–40 years and an significant proportion of those with cirrhosis go on to develop liver cancer.

Diagnosis of HCV is based on an enzyme immunoassay that detects antibodies to hepatitis C virus (anti-HCV). In general, the diagnosis is confirmed by use of a supplemental recombinant immunoblot assay (RIBA). However, detection of antibodies to HCV alone does not distinguish between individuals who have been previously exposed to the virus and those who continue to have viraemia. Most RIBA-positive patients are potentially infectious, as confirmed by use of a polymerase chain reaction (PCR) based-test. The PCR test detects small amounts of viral RNA and indicates if there is circulating virus (Fig. 10.2).

Hepatitis D virus (HDV)

HDV, previously known as the 'delta agent' is a defective virus that requires the presence and the helper activity of HBV to allow it to replicate. HDV virus can be co-transmitted with hepatitis B infection or can superinfect chronic HBV carriers. The mean incubation period is 35 days and transmission is mainly through parenteral routes. Hepatitis caused by HDV is usually severe and individuals with double

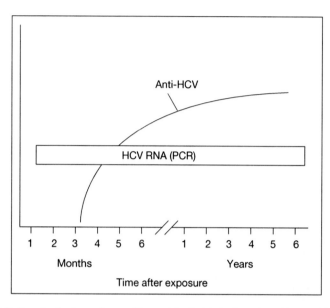

Figure 10.2 Serological markers of hepatitis C. Majority of patients with Hepatitis are asymptomatic.
Anti-HCV: antibody to hepatitis C virus by enzyme immunoassay; HCV RNA [PCR]: hepatitis C viral RNA by polymerase chain reaction.

infection, HBV and HDV, usually develop rapidly progressive disease and cirrhosis at an earlier age than those with HBV infection alone.

Hepatitis G virus (HGV)

Hepatitis G is a flavivirus that can be transmitted parenterally. At present, the epidemiology and clinical correlation of HGV infection are not well characterized.

HIV infection

HIV is a member of the retrovirus family and responsible for HIV infections and cases of acquired immunodeficiency syndrome (AIDS). It was first isolated in 1983. Two serologically distinct types, HIV 1 and HIV 2, have been recognized. HIV 2, isolated in 1986, is prevalent in certain West African countries. The two types of HIV present similar hazards and cause similar illnesses, except that there is some evidence that progression of disease is slower in a person infected with HIV 2. The term HIV used in these guidelines covers both types of virus.

Clinical features

After exposure to HIV most individuals develop antibody within 3 months. During the acute phase, (i.e. around the time when antibody first appears) there may be a self-limiting illness resembling glandular fever (infectious mononucleosis), with

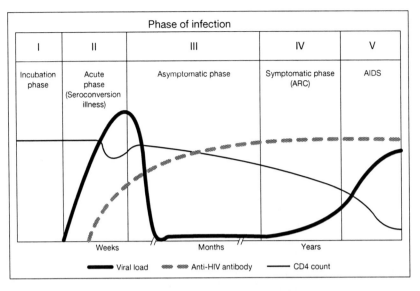

Figure 10.3 Typical course of HIV infection.

lymphadenopathy and rash. Later in the course of infection, non-specific illness (including fever, night sweats, and lymphadenopathy) is associated with progressive immune dysfunction. When AIDS develops fully it is characterized by the appearance of opportunistic infections and tumors.

Infection with yeast, *Candida* spp., may cause persistent and severe thrush in the mouth and oesophagus and there may be reactivation of common latent herpes viruses. Invasion of the lungs by *Pneumocystis carinii*, a microorganism normally of low virulence, often gives rise to a pneumonitis with shortness of breath and diffuse shadowing sometimes seen on a chest X-ray. Some individuals may be infected with *Mycobacterium* spp., i.e. *M. tuberculosis*, *M. avium-intracellulare* etc. Many other infections may supervene, caused by bacteria such as Salmonellae, viruses including cytomegalovirus and hepatitis B and protozoa such as Toxoplasma in the brain or Giardia or Cryptosporidium in the bowel. Some patients develop Kaposi's sarcoma, an unusual tumor of the skin. This appears as characteristic discrete purple patches, often affecting the extremities, although internal organs may also be involved. Still others develop lymphoma, often in the brain.

HIV testing

Routine testing of patients for unidentified HIV is not recommended. Testing should be undertaken only on the basis of clinical assessment or where it is in the interests of both patients and HCWs. The provision of patient confidentiality, privacy, and informed consent for testing are essential. The individual requiring an HIV test should be offered appropriate discussion prior to testing, which should address the specific needs of the individual. The patients should have information about HIV transmission, the significance of a positive or a negative result and be able to discuss their particular needs and concerns.

Laboratory diagnosis

HIV serology: HIV screening is undertaken by enzyme-linked immunosorbent assay (ELISA), which detects antibodies to the virus. Positive specimens are then confirmed by a series of other tests. The seroconversion or 'window period', (i.e. the time between exposure to HIV infection and the first detectable sign of antibody in blood), is usually between 10–30 days but may last several months in some cases. During this 'window period', the HIV antibody test will be negative; therefore a negative test is not an absolute exclusion of HIV infection.

CD4 lymphocyte count and HIV viral load: Several laboratory markers are available to provide prognostic information and guide decisions on starting and changing therapy. The most widely used marker is the CD4 lymphocyte count. Risk of progression to an AIDS opportunistic infection or malignancy is high with the CD4 < 200 cells/gL. While CD4 count measures immune dysfunction, it does not provide a measure of how actively HIV is replicating in the body. HIV viral load tests assess the level of viral replication and provide useful prognostic information, which is independent of the information provided by CD4 counts. Patients vary in their level of viraemia. Rapid progressors tend to have persistently high viral load whereas slow or non-progressors have low viral load. In the early stages of infection (including the 'window' period) the concentration of HIV in the bloodstream is very high. During this period the antibody test is negative, although tests for HIV RNA are positive. After the resolution of the seroconversion illness, the HIV viral load decreases due to the host immune responses and stabilizes at a lower level. As immunodeficiency progresses and AIDS develops, the HIV viral load rises again. Viral load is also influenced by antiretroviral therapy. Most patients on combination antiretroviral therapy have a low HIV viral load.

Routes of transmission

Blood-borne viruses are transmitted through transfer of blood or 'high risk' body fluids containing virus and may occur by:

- Unprotected penetrative sexual intercourse with an infected person (between men or between a man and a woman).
- Skin puncture by sharps contaminated with blood, i.e.
  - sharing used needles and syringes among intravenous drug users.
  - receipt of tattoos, ear piercing, communal hair cutting, acupuncture, dental treatment, electrolysis etc.
  - inoculation injury to HCW from an infected individual.

General principles: control of infection with blood-borne viruses

- Apply good basic hygiene practices with regular hand washing, before and after contact with each patient, and before putting on and after removing gloves. *Change gloves between patients.*

- For all clinical procedures, *cover existing wounds,* skin lesions and all breaks in exposed skin with waterproof dressings,* or with gloves if hands extensively affected.

- HCWs with chronic skin disease such as eczema should avoid those invasive procedures, which involve sharp instruments or needles when their skin lesions are active, or if there are extensive breaks in the skin surface. A non-intact skin surface provides a potential route for blood-borne virus transmission, and blood-skin contact is common through glove puncture that may go unnoticed.

- *Use protective clothing as appropriate,* including protection of the mucous membrane of the eyes, mouth, and nose from blood and body fluid splashes. Avoid wearing open footwear in situations where blood may be spilt, or where sharp instruments or needles are handled.

- Prevent puncture wounds, cuts, and abrasions and if present, ensure that they are not exposed.

- *Avoid sharps usage wherever possible* and consider the use of alternative instruments, cutting diathermy, and laser.

- *Where sharps usage is essential, exercise particular care in handling and disposal,* following approved procedures and using approved sharps disposal containers.

- Clear up spillage of blood and other body fluids promptly and disinfect surfaces.

- Follow approved procedures for sterilization and disinfection of instruments and equipment.

- Follow approved procedures for safe disposal of contaminated waste.

* Staff with larger wounds, eczema or other skin conditions that cannot be adequately protected by plastic gloves or impermeable dressings should seek advice from the Occupational Health Department.

- Childbirth from an infected mother to her baby (intrauterine and peripartum) or through breast-feeding.
- Via infected blood transfusion, blood products, donations of semen, skin grafts, and organ transplants from someone who is infected.

Transmission through contamination of open wounds and skin lesions may also occur, e.g. eczema, splashing the mucous membrane of the eye, nose or mouth and through human bites when blood is drawn.

Blood is not the only concern, as various other 'high risk' body fluids, i.e. cerebrospinal, peritoneal, pleural, pericardial, amniotic and synovial fluid, semen, vaginal secretions and any other body fluids containing visible blood, and all tissues, organs and parts of bodies which are unfixed, are also hazardous. Exposure to 'low risk' body fluids such as urine, faeces, nasal secretions, tears, saliva (except in relation to dentistry), sputum, and vomitus present a minimal risk of blood-borne virus infection unless contaminated with blood; although they may be hazardous for other reasons as they may contain other pathogenic microorganisms. When blood is mentioned, it should be taken to include blood and 'high risk' body fluids unless otherwise stated.

Occupational risks to HCWs

In the health care setting, the risk of acquiring blood-borne infection is proportional to the *prevalence of infection in the population* served and the *chance of inoculation accidents* occurring during procedures.

The risk of infection following percutaneous exposure to the blood from an infectious source from hepatitis B patients is estimated to be between 5 and 30%. The risk of hepatitis C infection after percutaneous exposure to a known infected source appears to be intermediate between the risk of HBV and HIV, i.e. between 3 and 10%. For a HCW, the average risk for HIV infection after a percutaneous needlestick injury with HIV-infected blood is estimated to be 0.3% and the risk associated with mucous membrane exposure is estimated to be about 0.09%.

Risks to patients from HCWs

Documented cases of hepatitis B and hepatitis C infections have occurred in patients operated on by hepatitis B or C infected HCWs. Internationally, there have been only two documented series of HIV transmissions from HCW to patient. One occurred in the US, where six patients became infected with HIV from a Florida dentist. This transmission was considered to be the result of a lapse in infection control procedures. A second HIV transmission occurred in one patient following prolonged orthopaedic surgery in France. No further cases of transmission of HIV from HCW to patient have been detected, despite look back studies of large numbers of patients cared for by HIV-infected HCWs.

Responsibility of HCWs

Since transmission of hepatitis B, C and HIV from infected HCWs to patients has been documented, it is essential, that *all HCWs have an overriding ethical duty to protect the health and safety of their patients.* They are strongly advised to follow basic infection control precautions scrupulously and adopt safer working practices.

All HCWs (including locum staff) who perform exposure-prone procedures should be vaccinated against HBV and their serological response checked subsequently. Any HCW who performs exposure-prone procedures and who has not yet been immunized should be tested for evidence of current infection (the presence of hepatitis B surface antigen), as soon as possible. This may mean testing before immunization has been completed. Blood specimens for testing HCWs who perform exposure-prone procedures should be collected directly by a member of the occupational health service or a person commissioned by the service.

Those who are, or have reason to believe that they may have been exposed to these infections in whatever circumstances, must seek medical advice from the occupational health department. They must not perform exposure-prone invasive procedures (see below). The occupational health department will advise the HCW on their work, which may need to be modified or restricted to protect patients. It is extremely important that the infected HCWs receive the same rights of confidentiality as any patient seeking or receiving medical care.

Provided routine infection control measures are followed scrupulously, the circumstances in which a blood-borne infection could be transmitted from the HCW to a patient are restricted to *exposure-prone procedures, which must not be performed by an infected HCW. HCWs who are infected with HIV, Hepatitis B or Hepatitis C infection* must seek advice from the occupational health department who will advise the individual about the type of work to be undertaken.

The UK Department of Health recommends that HCWs who are hepatitis B surface antigen positive (HBsAg +) and hepatitis B 'e' antigen negative (HBeAg −) and currently perform exposure-prone procedures should have their viral load (HBV DNA) measured. A HCW whose HBV DNA concentration in blood (viral load) is less than 1,000 genome equivalents per ml will not be restricted but should be advised by the occupational health department on minimizing the risk of transmission both to patients and to other close contacts and be retested every 12 months. *They should cease performing exposure-prone procedures if their viral load exceeds 1,000 copies/ml or they are shown to have transmitted HBV to a patient.*

Health Care Workers should not be allowed to perform exposure-prone procedures if they are hepatitis C RNA positive.

Exposure-prone procedures

All breaches of the skin or epithelia by sharp instruments are by definition invasive. Most clinical procedures, including many which are invasive, do not provide an opportunity for the blood of the HCW to come into contact with the patient's open tissues. Provided the general measures to prevent occupational transmission of blood-borne viruses are adhered to scrupulously at all times, most clinical procedures pose no risk of transmission of HIV from an infected HCW to a patient, and can safely be performed.

Exposure-prone procedures are those invasive procedures where there is a risk that injury to the worker may result in the exposure of the patient's open tissues to the blood of the worker (bleed-back). These include procedures where the worker's gloved hands may be in contact with sharp instruments, needle tips or sharp tissues, (e.g., spicules of bone or teeth) inside a patient's open body cavity, wound or confined anatomical space where the hands or fingertips may not be completely visible at all times. However, other situations, such as pre-hospital trauma care and care of patients where the risk of biting is predictable (e.g. with a violent patient or a patient having an epileptic fit) are also considered to be exposure-prone.

Normal vaginal delivery in itself is not an exposure-prone procedure. When undertaking a vaginal delivery, an infected HCW must not perform procedures involving the use of sharps, instruments such as infiltrating local anaesthetics or suturing of a tear or episiotomies, since fingertips may not be visible at all times and the risk of injury to the worker is greater. Neither can they perform an instrumental delivery requiring forceps or suction if infiltration of local anaesthetic or internal suturing is required. In practice, this means that an infected HCW may only undertake a vaginal delivery if it is certain that a second midwife or doctor may also be present who is able to undertake all such operative interventions as might arise during the course of delivery.

Procedures where the hands and fingertips of the worker are visible and outside the patient's body at all times, and internal examinations or procedures that do not involve possible injury to the worker's gloved hands from sharp instruments and/or tissues are considered not to be exposure-prone provided routine infection control procedures are adhered to at all times. Examples of such procedures include: taking blood (venepuncture), setting up and maintaining intravenous lines or central lines (provided any skin tunnelling procedure used for the latter is performed in a non-exposure prone manner), minor surface suturing, the incision of external abscesses, routine vaginal or rectal examinations and simple endoscopic procedures.

Surgical procedure

Each patient and each operation should be considered as a potential source of infection. Therefore, it is essential that all the operating room HCWs demonstrate their knowledge of potential risks by ensuring that a 'confine and contain' approach is implemented for every procedure. All HCWs in the surgical team should be vaccinated against HBV.

Preoperative testing of a patient for infectious agents should be on the basis of clinical indication, and medical practitioners should exercise their professional judgement in ordering any clinically relevant test, with the patient's consent. In the case of elective surgery, any testing considered relevant should be completed before admission. Discretion and patient confidentiality must be maintained in all circumstances. Surgery lists should be scheduled on the basis of clinical urgency, and in such a way as to allow ample time for adequate infection control procedures to take place. Operating room and anaesthetic HCWs who may be exposed to infectious material in the course of their duty should be informed of the patient's infectious status prior to surgery.

In addition to the basic infection control precautions (see page 191), the patient with a known blood borne viral infection may require the following additional precautions for surgical operation:

- The consultant in charge of the patient is responsible for seeing that all members of the team know of the infection hazards and appropriate measures to be taken. The *team should be limited to essential members of trained staff only*. The number of students allowed to attend the operation should be limited.

- It may help theatre decontamination if such cases are last on the list, but this is not essential.

- Depilatory creams should be used for essential hair removal.

- Unnecessary equipment should be removed from the theatre in order to reduce the amount of decontamination required after the operation. Disposable items should be used wherever possible. If any item is not disposable it must be decontaminated by the sterile supply department (SSD). Special equipment reserved for these patients is not essential.

- Disposable drapes should be used and the mattress should be protected by a plastic sheet.

- Diathermy and suction devices should be placed on the opposite side of the table to the surgeon, thereby ensuring the assistant does not reach across the table between the surgeon and nurse.

- Before any surgical procedure, the surgeon and scrub nurse should decide on the routine for passage of sharp instruments during the procedure. This may entail the designation of a 'neutral zone'. The surgeon must avoid placing his/her less dexterous hand in potential danger. *Sharp instruments should not be passed by hand.* A specified puncture-resistant sharps tray must be used for the transfer of all sharp instruments. Only one sharp must be in the tray at any one time. If two surgeons are operating simultaneously, then each surgeon needs his/her own sharps tray.

- Variations in operative technique, such as a non-touch approach, the avoidance of passing sharp instruments from nurse to surgeon and vice versa, and new techniques of cutting (e.g. with lasers) or of wound closure that obviate the use of sharp instruments and lessen the risk of inoculation are recommended. *Needles must never be picked up with the fingers*, nor the fingers used to expose and increase access for the passage of a suture in deep tissues.

- *Personal protective equipment*

  - *Gowns:* All staff in the theatre should wear a disposable plastic apron under their gowns. A water-impermeable gown should be worn if gross contamination with blood or body fluids is likely. Where waterproof aprons are worn for procedures in which there is likely to be considerable dissemination of blood, it is essential that the aprons are of sufficient length to overlap with protective footwear. This is especially important for procedures carried out in the lithotomy position, since it is common for blood accumulating in the worker's lap to be channelled down into the boots. Caps should cover the hair completely.

  - *Mask:* The **surgical team should wear a mask and two pairs of gloves and skin lesions must be covered with waterproof dressings.** Double sterile gloving, i.e. a double glove with the larger size glove on the inside is recommended for all surgeons involved in operating room procedures. If a glove is torn or a needlestick or other injury occurs, the gloves should be removed and hands washed when safety permits and new gloves put on promptly.

  - *Eye protection:* **Spectacles or goggles should be worn by those taking part in the operation** to avoid conjunctival contamination or splashing.

  - *Footwear:* Fenestrated footwear must never be worn in situations where sharps are handled. For tasks involving likely dissemination of blood it is recommended that Wellington boots or calf length plastic boots are worn rather than shoes or clogs. Contaminated footwear must be adequately decontaminated after use with appropriate precautions for those undertaking it.

- Hand-held straight needles should not be used. Where practical, blunt needles should be used to close the abdomen. When suturing, forceps or a needle holder should be used to pick up the needle and draw it through the tissue. Where practical, suture needles should be cut off before knots are tied to prevent needlestick injury. Surgeons may use a sterile thimble on the index finger of the less dexterous hand for protection when suturing. *Wire sutures should be avoided* where possible because of the high injury rate to the surgeon. After a surgical procedure, the skin should be closed with staples whenever possible.

- Hands of assisting HCWs must not be used to retract the wound on viscera during surgery. Self-retaining retractors should be used, or a swab on a stick, instead of fingers. Certain instruments should be avoided unless essential to the procedure, for example, sharp wound retractors such as rake retractors and skin hooks.

- *Closed wound drainage systems should be used*, where appropriate. Wound dressings with an impervious outer covering that will contain wound exudates should be used. If drainage is considered necessary, closed rather than open wound drainage is recommended. Blood should be cleaned off the patient's skin as far as possible at the end of the operation using suitable antiseptic/detergents solution.

- *Where practical, used instruments should be washed mechanically using an ultrasonic washer rather than by hand.* Surgical instruments and other tools used in operations should be put in a robust puncture-resistant container, labeled 'Danger of Infection' and returned to the SSD. Instruments for reuse should, as soon as possible after use, be immersed in warm water and detergent to prevent congealing or solidifying of blood and fatty materials, and must be thoroughly cleaned in the designated clean-up area before sterilization.

- Infectious waste excluding sharps must be placed in an appropriate colour coded infectious waste plastic bag, sealed and removed from the operating room. Disposal of infectious waste must comply with local regulations.

- *Needles, syringes, and disposable sharp instruments must be discarded into approved sharps boxes.* The sharps container must be closed securely when three-quarters full. Scalpel blades and needles and all other non-reusable sharps should be placed in a designated puncture-proof sharps container, which should comply with local or international standard.

- Used linen and theatre clothing should be placed in a water soluble bag which is then placed in a second plastic bag and marked as 'Infected linen'. It should be handled in accordance with local policy.

- Blood and other body fluid spills should be cleaned up immediately, using absorbent material such as paper towelling that should then be discarded into the infectious waste bag (see page 77). Gloves must be worn. The area should then be cleaned with warm water and detergent. The area may be treated with sodium hypochlorite (1% or 10,000 ppm available chlorine) or other appropriate disinfectant, in accordance with the local protocol. Disinfectant solutions should not be allowed to pool or remain on surfaces for longer than is required to effect disinfection, usually about 3–5 min.

- *Cleaning:*
  - Adequate time must be provided at the end of each case to allow for thorough cleaning of the operating theatre and the appropriate disposal of clinical waste.

- All surfaces (operating table, instrument table, equipment used and the floor) should be carefully cleaned using warm water and detergent. Walls and other surfaces do not require cleaning unless contaminated with blood.

- Large volumes of fluid should be used for cleaning and gloves and a plastic apron should be worn by the operator.

- Appropriate disinfectant, (e.g. sodium hypochlorite 1,000 ppm available chlorine) may be used after removal of gross soil. Surfaces should be cleaned and dried after applying disinfectants. Thorough rinsing is necessary to minimize damage to surfaces from the disinfectants.

Protection of the newborn

Hepatitis B infection: In high prevalence areas, hepatitis B immunization should be given to all pregnant women. In other countries, those providing antenatal care will need to take steps to identify infected mothers during pregnancy and make arrangements to ensure that babies born to these mothers receive a complete course of immunization against hepatitis B infection. This is best done by screening women early in pregnancy. Where this has not been done, it should be possible to detect carrier mothers at the time of delivery.

Specific hepatitis B immunoglobulin (HBIG) is available for passive protection while hepatitis B vaccine confers active immunity and they are normally used in combination. Babies born to mothers who are HBeAg +, who are HBsAg + without 'e' markers or where 'e' marker status has not been determined, or who have had acute hepatitis during pregnancy, *should receive specific HBIG as well as active immunization.*

The newborn should be given 200 IU HBIG at birth or as soon as possible thereafter. If immunization with the vaccine is combined with simultaneous administration of HBIG, the injection must be given at a different site.

The *first dose of vaccine should be given at birth or as soon as possible thereafter. HBIG should be given at a contralateral site* at the same time; arrangements for the supply of HBIG should be made well in advance. The complete course of Hepatitis B immunization regimen consists of a three-dose series of vaccine, with the first dose at the time of birth, the second dose one month later and the third dose at six months after the first dose. The vaccine should normally be given intramuscularly and the anterolateral thigh is the preferred site in infants.

Hepatitis C infection: Currently, there is no therapy available for the prevention of HCV infection in neonates born to mothers infected with HCV.

HIV infection: In order to prevent HIV infection in neonates, appropriate antiretroviral therapy can be given to both the mother before birth and to the neonate at birth to reduce the risk of HIV transmission. It is usually appropriate to advise against breast-feeding where the mother is known to be HIV positive.

Procedure after death

If a person known or suspected to be infected with a blood-borne virus (BBV) dies either in hospital or elsewhere, it is the duty of those with knowledge of the case to ensure that those who need to handle the body, including funeral personnel, post-mortem room and mortuary staff are aware that there is a potential risk of blood-borne viral infection. *Patients known or suspected to be infected with a BBV should not be embalmed* as embalming carries a significant risk for the operator.

The principles of safe practice for the mortuary must be adhered to irrespective of the infective state of the body. A *full post-mortem should not be done merely to confirm the cause of death.* When a post-mortem is carried out on such patients, all those concerned must be suitably informed and trained in safe procedures. They must follow local written protocol.

The body should be placed in a disposable body bag; absorbent material may be needed when there is a leakage from, e.g. surgical incisions or wounds. The bodies of children of mothers with BBV infections should be treated as infected. The discreet use of simple 'Danger of infection' labeling is appropriate and is attached in such a way that it can be read through the cadaver bag.

References and further reading

Anon. Lessons from two linked clusters of acute hepatitis B in cardiothoracic surgery patients. *Communicable Disease Review* 1996; **6**: R119.

Association of Anaesthetists of Great Britain and Ireland. *A report received by Council of the Association of Anaesthetists on Blood-borne Viruses and Anaesthesia.* London: Association of Anaesthetists of Great Britain and Ireland, 1996.

Berger A, Preiser W. Viral genome quantification as a tool for improving patient management: the example of HIV, HBV, HCV and CMV. *Journal of Antimicrobial Chemotherapy* 2002; **49**: 713–721.

BMA Board of Science and Education. *A guide to hepatitis C.* London: British Medical Association, 1996.

Breuer J, Jeffries DJ. HIV and hepatitis B virus infection in health care workers: a risk to patients? *Reviews in Medical Microbiology* 1992; **3**: 1–8.

British Orthopaedic Association. *Guidelines for the prevention of cross-infection between patients and staff in orthopaedic operating theatres with special reference to HIV and blood-borne Hepatitis viruses.* London: British Orthopaedic Association, 1992.

Centers for Disease Control and Prevention. Updated US Public Health Service guidelines for the management of occupational exposures to HBV, HCV and HIV and recommendations for post-exposure prophylaxis. *Morbidity and Mortality Weekly Report* 2001; **50**(R11): 1–42.

Centers for Disease Control and Prevention. Case-control study of HIV seroconversion in health-care workers after percutaneous exposure to HIV-infected blood – France, United Kingdom and United States, January 1988–August 1994. *Morbidity and Mortality Weekly Report* 1995; **44**: 929.

Ciesielski C, Marianos D, Ou C-Y, Dumbaugh R, *et al.* Transmission of human immunodeficiency virus in a dental practice. *Annals of Internal Medicine* 1992; **116**: 798–805.

Collins CH, Kennedy DA. Microbiological hazards of occupational needlestick and 'sharps' injuries. *Journal of Applied Bacteriology* 1987; **62**: 385–402.

Esteban JI, Gomez J, Martell M, *et al.* Transmission of hepatitis C virus by a cardiac surgeon. *New England Journal of Medicine* 1996; **334**: 555–560.

European Consensus Group on Hepatitis B Immunity. Are booster immunisations needed for life long hepatitis B immunity? *The Lancet* 2000; **355**: 561–565.

Gerberding JL. Management of occupational exposures to blood-borne viruses. *The New England Journal of Medicine* 1995; **332**: 444–451.

Healing TD, Hoffman PN, Young SEJ. The infection hazards of human cadavers. *Communicable Disease Report* 1995; **5**: R61–R68.

Health and Safety Commission. *Safe working and the prevention of infection in clinical laboratories.* London: HMSO, 1991.

Health and Safety Commission. *Safe working and the prevention of infection in the mortuary and post-mortem room.* London: HMSO, 1991.

Heptonstall J. Outbreaks of hepatitis B virus infection associated with infected surgical staff. *Communicable Disease Report* 1991; **1**: R81–R83.

Incident investigation teams and others. Transmission of hepatitis B to patients from four infected surgeons without hepatitis B e antigen. *New England Journal of Medicine* 1997; **336**: 178–84.

Lot F, Séguiner J-C, Fégueux S, *et al.* Probable transmission of HIV from an orthopaedic surgeon to a patient in France. *Annals of Internal Medicine* 1999; **130**: 1–6.

Mills PR, Thorburn D, McCruden EAB. Occupationally acquired hepatitis C infection. *Reviews in Medical Microbiology* 2000; **11**(1): 15–22.

Moloughney BW. Transmission and post exposure management of bloodborne virus infections in the health care setting: Where are we now? *Canadian Medical Association Journal* 2001; **165**(4): 445–450.

Ramsey ME. Guidance on the investigation and management of occupational exposure to hepatitis C. *Communicable Disease and Public Health* 1999; 2: 258–262.

Recommendations for follow-up of health-care workers after occupational exposure to hepatitis C cirus. *Morbidity and Mortality Weekly Report* 1997; **46**: 603–606.

Report of a WHO Consultation organized in collaboration with the Viral Hepatits Prevention Board, Antwerp, Belgium. Global surveillance and control of hepatitis C. *Journal of Viral Hepatitis* 1999; **6**: 35–47.

Report of a working group of the Royal College of Pathologists. *HIV and the practice of pathology*. London: The Royal College of Pathologists, 1995.

Report of joint working party of the Hospital Infection Society and the Surgical Infection Study Group. Risks to surgeons and patients from HIV and Hepatitis: Guidelines on precautions and management of exposure to blood or body fluids. *British Medical Journal* 1992; **305**: 1337–1343.

Rhodes RS, Bell DM, (eds). Prevention of transmission of blood-borne pathogen. *The Surgical Clinics of North America* 1995; **75**: 1047–1217.

Royal Institute of Public Health and Hygiene. *A Handbook of Mortuary Practice and Safety for Anatomical Pathology Technicians*. London: The Royal Institute of Public Health and Hygiene, 1994.

Sherman M. Management of viral hepatitis: clinical and public health perspectives – a consensus statement. *Canadian Journal of Gastroenterology* 1997; **11**: 407–416.

Society for Healthcare Epidemiology of America. (AIDS/TB Committee). Management of healthcare workers infected with hepatitis B virus, hepatitis C virus, human immunodeficiency Virus or other bloodborne pathogens. *Infection Control and Hospital Epidemiology* 1997; **18**: 349–363.

Sulkowski MS, Ray SC, Thomas DL. Needlestick Transmission of Hepatitis C. *Journal of American Medical Association* 2002; **287**: 2406–2413.

Sundkvist T, Hamilton GR, Rimmer D, Evans BG, Teo CG. Fatal outcome of transmission of hepatitis B from an e antigen negative surgeon. *Communicable Disease and Public Health* 1998; **1**: 48–50.

The European collaborative study. Caesarean section and risk of vertical transmission of HIV-1 infection. *The Lancet* 1994; **343**: 1464–1467.

UK Advisory Committee on Dangerous Pathogens. Protection against blood-borne infections in the workplace: HIV and hepatitis. London: HMSO, 1995.

UK Departments of Health. *Guidance for clinical health care workers: protection against infection with blood-borne viruses*. London: DoH, 1998.

UK Department of Health, NHS Executive. *Health Service Circular: guidance on the management of HIV/AIDS infected health care workers and patient notification*. London: DoH, 1998 (HSC 1998/226).

UK Department of Health. *Immunization against Infectious Disease*. London: HMSO, 1996.

UK Department of Health. *Guidelines for pre-test discussion on HIV testing*. London: DoH, 1996.

UK Department of Health. *AIDS/HIV-infected health care workers: guidance on the management of infected health care workers*. London: DoH, 1998.

UK Department of Health. *Protecting health care workers and patients from hepatitis B*. London: DoH, 1994 (and addendum 1996).

UK Department of Health. *Hepatitis B infected Health Care Worker*. Guidance on the implementation of Circular HSS(MD) 17/00: 2000.

UK Department of Health, NHS Executive. *Health Service Circular: hepatitis B infected health care workers*. London: DoH, 2000 (HSC 2000/020).

UK Department of Health, NHS Executive. *Guidance on the microbiological safety of human tissues and organs used in transplantation*. London: DoH, 1996.

UK Department of Health. *Hepatitis C Infected Health Care Workers*, London, 2002.

UK Public Health Laboratory Services. Occupational transmission of HIV: summary of published reports. http://www.phls.co.uk

Working Group of Royal College of Pathologists. *HIV infection: Hazards of transmission to patients and health care workers during invasive procedures*. London: The Royal College of Pathologists, 1992.

Working Party of the Royal College of Obstetricians and Gynaecologists. HIV *Infection in maternity care and gynaecology*. London: Royal College of Obstetricians and Gynaecologists Press 1997.

Zuckerman JN, Zuckerman AJ. Hepatitis – how far down the alphabet? *Journal of Clinical Pathology* 1997; **50**: 1–2.

Zuckerman JN, Zuckerman AJ. Current Topics in Hepatitis B. *Journal of Infection* 2000; **41**: 130–136.

11

Protection for Health Care Workers

Protection of health care workers (HCWs) should be an integral part of the Health and Safety programme of health care establishments. Health care facilities have a responsibility to ensure that all reasonably practicable steps are taken to ensure that the risk of infection to health workers is minimized. *Transmissible infections in HCWs must be identified quickly* so that they can be excluded from the work place or from direct patient contact until they are no longer infectious.

Occupation Health Department

The roles and responsibilities of the Occupation Health Department described below are mainly concerned with the risk of infection and are only a part of their work.

- Primary health screening of all staff by questionnaire and/or medical examination.

- Keeping accurate and up-to-date records of all members of staff.

- Immunization and vaccination of all existing staff at the required time interval.

- Training of all grades of staff in personal hygiene with special precautions for those particularly at risk of infection.

- Examination of staff returning to work after absence due to diarrhoea or other infectious conditions, to ensure that the infection has cleared and to give advice to the carrier.

- Determining staff contacts of the infectious disease, checking immunity and follow-up if necessary. Arranging tests and possibly treatment for staff with infectious diseases.

- Keeping records of all inoculation injuries, arranging post-exposure prophylaxis following inoculation injuries and counselling of staff if necessary.

- Survey potential infective and toxic hazards (e.g. chemical disinfectant) to staff in health care facilities.

Measures to protect HCWs

Measures to protect HCWs from infection fall mainly into three categories:

1. **Immunization:** All HCWs should be immunized against vaccine-preventable diseases. Chickenpox (varicella) immunization should also be offered to non-immune HCWs with no history of chickenpox or shingles. Hepatitis B immunization should also be offered to all non-immune HCWs, particularly those with potential exposure to blood or body substances, with post immunization serology testing to identify non-responders. Refusal of vaccination by any HCW should be recorded together with a reason for such refusal, if provided. Staff refusing immunizations may be prohibited from working in certain areas and their work should be reviewed.

2. **Education and training:** All HCWs must be provided with appropriate training and education in infection control as part of their orientation. This must be reinforced through a regular continuing education programme. They should be trained in the handling of blood and body fluids, chemical disinfectants and should be aware of local policies and procedures on infection control including waste disposal, dealing with contaminated sharps, etc. They should also be provided with appropriate personal protective equipment. Work practices should be developed and implemented to ensure compliance with infection control policies and procedure.

3. **Reporting:** *HCWs must report any accidents or illness to their line manager* and, if appropriate, to the occupational health department. In addition, the incident report process includes notes on remedial and follow-up action taken before the process is considered complete.

Pre-employment assessment

HCWs should be assessed before employment with the aim of preventing disease in the individual but a second and no less important function is to prevent transmission of infectious agents to patients. It is important that the employee must be given assurance of the complete confidentiality of any health questioning and their occupational health record.

It is important that all newly employed staff in the health care setting attend the occupational health department. The screening process includes assessment by a health questionnaire completed by the employee, covering questions related to general health, history of infectious diseases and immunization status. It is also important to ascertain immune status if the HCW has either had or been vaccinated against tuberculosis, rubella, measles, mumps, chickenpox and hepatitis B virus (HBV). In addition, the presence of skin disorders such as eczema, and a history of an underlying immuno-suppressive disorder might require a reassessment of the staff member's work practices.

Routine screening for staphylococcal, streptococcal and salmonella carriers is not recommended. Screening may be instituted if an outbreak or epidemic occurs and if HCWs are felt to be either at risk or potentially associated with spread of the infection. Agencies which provide temporary staff for the hospital should be informed of the staff screening policy and, wherever possible, only those agencies with an effective screening programme should be used.

Health status of HCWs

There are certain medical conditions of HCWs that increase their predisposition to infection if they come into contact with certain infectious patients, e.g. immune status, certain skin conditions and pregnancy. There are many areas within health care establishments where HCWs with these conditions can safely work and there are few tasks that such HCWs are unable to perform safely. Health care establishments have a responsibility to manage and supervise such HCWs in ways that both acknowledge their right to work, and safeguard the welfare of both patients and HCWs. This responsibility includes the need to identify such HCWs and inform them of the problems they are likely to encounter in particular circumstances. It is important that the occupational health department should liaise closely with the Infection Control Team.

Staff should not work if they have acute or chronic diarrhoeal disease or febrile respiratory illness. Catering staff need to be carefully questioned about gastrointestinal infection, history of enteric fever, skin conditions (e.g. allergic eczema, psoriasis and exfoliative dermatitis), recurrent sepsis and tuberculosis. Staff with either shedding and/or weeping skin conditions or damaged skin may readily be colonized by hospital-associated microorganisms. These HCWs may not be harmed by the acquisition of such microorganisms but may disseminate them widely. For example, placement of such HCWs in wards containing patients with multi-resistant staphylococci is not recommended. These employees should be identified by personal history screening and advised of the problems posed by their condition.

Staff who are or have reason to believe that they may have been exposed to blood-borne hepatitis (B and C) or HIV infection *must declare* this and discuss it in complete confidence with the occupational health department, either at the initial screening or when he or she first becomes aware of their infection. In general, such staff may require a work assessment and must avoid exposure-prone procedures.

Management of sharps injury

All health care establishments should develop their own infection control protocols for the management of blood-borne hepatitis (B and C) and HIV infection.

The protocols must include clear written instructions on the appropriate action to take in the event of sharps injury and blood incidents involving either patients or HCWs. The protocols must include the name of the physicians to be contacted, the laboratory that will process emergency specimens, the pharmacy that stocks pro- phylactic medication, and procedures for investigation of the circumstances of the incident and measures to prevent recurrence. The protocols should also include details for prompt reporting, evaluation, counselling, treatment and follow-up. Treatment should be available during all working hours, e.g. through the occupa- tional health department or, out of hours, the Accident and Emergency (A & E) department. *HCWs should report occupational exposures immediately after they occur.*

Occupational risks to HCWs

In the health care setting, the risk of acquiring blood-borne viral infection is pro- portional to the *prevalence of infection* in the population served and the *chance of inoculation accidents* occurring during procedures.

The risk of infection following percutaneous exposure to blood from an infectious source from HBV patients is estimated to be between 5 and 30%. The risk of hepa- titis C virus (HCV) infection appears to be intermediate between the risk of HBV and HIV, i.e. between 3–10%. For a HCW, the average risk for HIV infection after a percutaneous needlestick injury with HIV infected blood is estimated to be 0.3% and the risk associated with mucous membrane exposure is estimated to be about 0.09%.

Risk factors for acquiring blood-borne viral infections

After percutaneous exposures, the following risk factors have been associated with an increased risk for blood-borne viral infection.

1. *Type of body fluid involved:* The following body fluids pose a risk for blood- borne transmission: blood, serum, plasma and all biological fluids visibly contaminated with blood; laboratory specimens that contain concentrated virus; pleural, amniotic, pericardial, peritoneal, synovial and cerebrospinal fluids; and uterine/vaginal secretions or semen.

2. *Quantity of blood:* Larger quantities of blood, indicated by visible contam- ination of the device. Usually associated with a procedure using a hollow bore needle directly placed in a vein or artery.

3. *Type of needle:* Hollow bore needles have more risk of transmission than suture needles because of the quantity of blood they carry.

4. *Depth of injury:* A deep penetrating injury is a risk factor because it is dif- ficult to wash off blood from the wound.

5. *Infectivity of source patient:* Blood from patients with high infectivity, e.g. patients with full blown AIDS, hepatitis B 'e' antigen (HBeAg) positive and hepatitis C polymerase chain reaction (PCR) positive patients.

Management of the exposed person

Immediate care of the exposure site: In cases of exposure to blood or body fluids, the following procedures should be followed:

- Encourage the affected area of skin to bleed for few seconds.
- Do not suck the puncture site.
- Rinse immediately under running water and wash with soap and water.
- Do not scrub. Rinse and dry.

If the spillage of blood and body fluid has occurred on intact skin, contaminated clothing should be removed and the affected area should be rinsed immediately under running water and washed with soap and water. Do not scrub. Rinse and dry. Exposed mucous membrane or conjunctivae should be irrigated immediately with copious amounts of water using either running tap water or an eyewash bottle.

Immediate contact procedure: The line manager or head of the department should be informed of the incident. HCWs should be immediately referred to the Occupational Health Department or, out of hours, the A & E department, according to the local policy.

Evaluation of the exposure: The appropriate physician should assess the member of staff and initiate investigation, treatment and counselling, where required.

Evaluation and testing of the exposed person: The exposed person should have a medical evaluation, including information about medications they are taking and underlying medical conditions or circumstances. All exposed people should be assessed to determine the risk of tetanus.

The exposed person would normally be tested for HIV and hepatitis C antibody and hepatitis B surface antigen (HBsAg) at the time of the injury to establish their serological status at the time of the exposure. If the source patient is found to be HIV, HBV and HCV negative, no further follow-up of the exposed person is generally necessary, unless there is reason to suspect the source person is seroconverting to one of these viruses, or was at high risk of blood-borne viral infection at the time of the exposure. Pregnancy testing should be offered to all women of childbearing age whose pregnancy status is unknown.

In the event of seroconversion, all reasonable attempts should be made to confirm that the virus strain transmitted is identical in both patient and the source of the infected blood.

Management of occupational exposures to HIV, hepatitis B and C virus

Provide immediate care to the exposure site:

* Wash wounds and skin with soap and water.
* Flush mucous membranes with water.

Determine risk associated with exposure by:

* Type of fluid (e.g. blood, visibly bloody fluid, other potentially infectious fluid or tissue, and concentrated virus).
* Type of exposure (i.e. percutaneous injury, mucous membrane or non-intact skin exposure, and bites resulting in blood exposure).

Evaluate exposure source:

* Assess the risk of infection using available information.
* Test known sources for HBsAg, anti-HCV, and HIV antibody (consider using rapid testing).
* For unknown sources, assess risk of exposure to HBV, HCV, or HIV infection. ***Do not test discarded needles or syringes for virus contamination.***

Evaluate the exposed person:

* Assess immune status for HBV infection (i.e. by history of hepatitis B vaccination and vaccine response).

Give post-exposure prophylaxis (PEP) for exposures posing risk of infection or transmission:

HBV: PEP with hepatitis B immunoglobulin (HBIG) and/or hepatitis B vaccine series should be considered for occupational exposures after evaluation of the HBsAg status of the source and the vaccination and vaccine-response status of the exposed person.

HCV: PEP not recommended.

HIV: These steps are advised:

* ***Initiate PEP as soon as possible***, preferably within hours of exposure.
* Offer pregnancy testing to all women of childbearing age not known to be pregnant.
* Seek expert consultation if viral resistance is suspected.

- Administer PEP for 4 weeks if tolerated. Perform follow-up testing and provide counselling. Advise exposed persons to seek medical evaluation for any acute illness occurring during follow-up.

HBV exposure:

Perform follow-up anti-HBs testing in persons who receive hepatitis B vaccine. Test for anti-HBs 1–2 months after last dose of vaccine. Anti-HBs response to vaccine cannot be ascertained if HBIG was received in the previous 3–4 months.

HCV exposure:

- Perform baseline and follow-up testing for anti-HCV and alanine aminotransferase (ALT) 4–6 months after exposure.
- Perform HCV RNA at 4–6 weeks if earlier diagnosis of HCV infection desired.
- Confirm repeatedly reactive anti-HCV enzyme immunoassays (EIAs) with supplemental tests.

HIV exposure:

- Perform HIV-antibody testing for at least 6 months post-exposure (e.g. at baseline, 6 weeks, 3 months, and 6 months).
- Perform HIV antibody testing if illness compatible with an acute retroviral syndrome occurs.
- Advise exposed persons to use precautions to prevent secondary transmission during the follow-up period.

Evaluate exposed persons taking PEP within 72 h after exposure and monitor for drug toxicity for at least 2 weeks.

Adapted from Centers for Disease Control and Prevention. Updated US Public Health Service guidelines for the management of occupational exposures to HBV, HCV and HIV and recommendations for post-exposure prophylaxis. *Morbidity and Mortality Weekly Report* 2001; **50** (RR-11): 1–42.

Source patients or individual

Reasonable efforts should be made to identify the source. The source individuals should be evaluated for infection with HIV, HBV and HCV. Information available in the medical record or from the source person may suggest or rule out infection with each virus. If the source is known to have HIV infection, then information on the stage of infection and current and previous antiretroviral therapy should be gathered and used in deciding the most appropriate regimen of post-exposure prophylaxis (PEP). If the source patient refuses testing and serum storage, he/she should sign a form to that effect.

If consent cannot be obtained, for example if the patient is unconscious, then procedures should be followed which comply with guidelines in the relevant country. The source individual should be tested at the time of injury for the HIV and hepatitis C antibody and HBsAg. If the HCV antibody test is positive, then HCV PCR should be performed to test for HCV RNA. *Transmission is extremely unlikely to occur from a source that is HCV PCR negative.*

Post exposure prophylixis (PEP)

Human immunodeficiency virus (HIV)
This depends on the circumstances of exposure to HIV, and the characteristics of the source.

- *HIV PEP recommended* for percutaneous exposure to potentially infectious blood or body fluids where there is an increased risk of HIV transmission.

- *HIV PEP offered but not actively recommended* for ocular mucous membrane or non-intact skin exposure to potentially infectious blood or body fluids where there is less increased risk of HIV transmission.

- *HIV PEP not offered* for any exposure to non-bloody urine, saliva or faeces, which are not potentially infectious for HIV. As only a small proportion of occupational exposures to HIV result in transmission of the virus, the toxicity of PEP must be carefully considered against its efficacy. The exposed person should be informed of these side effects, and that there are only limited data on the efficacy of PEP. If the exposed person is pregnant, she should be informed about the available limited data on the toxicity of these drugs in pregnant women.

Antiretroviral drugs: Various antiretroviral combinations can be used. It is important that drug combinations should be guided by knowledge of the index patient's previous treatment and local knowledge and experience in treating HIV infection and disease. Prophylaxis should be given ideally within 1 h of exposure; this requires health care facilities to have a system in place to assist exposed HCWs which is available 24 h a day. The risk of toxicity in each case must be balanced against the relatively low rate of infection after the average percutaneous exposure. Therapy should be continued for 4 weeks.

Hepatitis B virus (HBV)
If the source is positive for HBsAg, then HBV PEP may be considered if the exposed person is not already immune. However, no further action is required if the person is known to be immune to HBV (antiHBsAg = 10 mIU/mL), or if testing within 48 h of the injury showed the exposed person to be immune to HBV.

If the exposed person is not immune to HBV, or is of unknown immune status, then *HBV immunoglobulin should be given within 48 h of exposure.* In addition,

Table 11.1 Recommended HIV post-exposure prophylaxis for percutaneous injuries.

Infection status of source

Exposure type	HIV-positive class 1[*]	HIV-positive class 2[*]	Source of unknown HIV status[†]	Unknown source[§]	HIV-negative
Less severe[¶]	Recommend basic 2-drug PEP	Recommend expanded 3-drug PEP	Generally, no PEP warranted; however consider basic 2-drug PEP[**] for source with HIV risk factors[††]	Generally, no PEP warranted; however, consider basic 2-drug PEP[**] in settings where exposure to HIV-infected persons is likely	No PEP warranted
More severe[§§]	Recommend expanded 3-drug PEP	Recommend expanded 3-drug PEP	Generally, no PEP warranted; however, consider basic 2-drug PEP[**] for source with HIV risk factors[††]	Generally, no PEP warranted; however, consider basic 2-drug PEP[**] in settings where exposure to HIV-infected persons is likely	No PEP warranted

[*]HIV-positive: *Class 1*: asymptomatic HIV infection or known low viral load (e.g. <1,500 RNA copies/ml). HIV-positive, *Class 2*: symptomatic HIV infection, AIDS, acute seroconversion, or known high viral load. If drug resistance is a concern, obtain expert consultation. Initiation of post-exposure prophylaxis (PEP) should not be delayed pending expert consultation, and, because expert consultation alone cannot substitute for face-to-face counselling, resources should be available to provide immediate evaluation and follow-up care for all exposures.
[†]Source of unknown HIV status, e.g. deceased source person with no samples available for HIV testing.
[§]Unknown source, e.g. a needle from a sharps disposal container.
[¶]Less severe, e.g. solid needle and superficial injury.
[**]The designation 'consider PEP' indicates that PEP is optional and should be based on an individualized decision between the exposed person and the treating clinician.
[††]If PEP is offered and taken and the source is later determined to be HIV-negative, PEP should be discontinued.
[§§]More severe, e.g. large-bore hollow needle, deep puncture, visible blood on device, or needle used in patient's artery or vein.

Reproduced from CDC Guidelines for the management of occupational exposures to HBV, HCV, and HIV and recommendations for post-exposure prophylaxis. *Morbidity and Mortality Weekly Report* 2001; **50** (RR-11): 1–42.

Table 11.2 Recommended post-exposure prophylaxis for exposure to HBV.

Vaccination and antibody response status of exposed workers*	Treatment		
	Source HBsAg⁺ positive	Source HBsAg⁺ negative	Source unknown or not available for testing
Unvaccinated	HBIG§ × 1 and initiate HB vaccine series¶	Initiate HB vaccine series	Initiate HB vaccine series
Previously vaccinated			
Known responder**	No treatment	No treatment	No treatment
Known non-responder††	HBIG × 1 and initiate revaccination or HBIG × 2§§	No treatment	If known high-risk source, treat as if source were HBsAg positive
Antibody response unknown	Test exposed person for anti-HBs¶¶ 1. If adequate,** no treatment is necessary 2. If inadequate,†† administer HBIG × 1 and vaccine booster	No treatment	Test exposed person for anti-HBs 1. If adequate,¶ no treatment is necessary 2. If inadequate,¶ administer vaccine booster and recheck titre in 1–2 months

*Persons who have previously been infected with HBV are immune to reinfection and do not require post-exposure prophylaxis.

†HBsAg: Hepatitis B surface antigen.

§HBIG: Hepatitis B immunoglobulin; dose is 0.06 mL/kg intramuscularly.

¶Hepatitis B (HB) vaccine.

**A responder is a person with adequate levels of serum antibody to HBsAg, i.e. anti-HBs ≥ 10 mIU/mL.

††A non-responder is a person with inadequate response to vaccination, i.e. serum anti-HBs < 10 mIU/mL.

§§The option of giving one dose of HBIG and reinitiating the vaccine series is preferred for non-responders who have not completed a second 3-dose vaccine series. For persons who previously completed a second vaccine series but failed to respond, two doses of HBIG are preferred.

¶¶anti-HBs: Antibody to HBsAg.

Reproduced from CDC Guidelines for the management of occupational exposures to HBV, HCV, and HIV and recommendations for post-exposure prophylaxis. *Morbidity and Mortality Weekly Report* 2001; **50** (RR-11): 1–42.

HBV vaccine should be started for HCWs who are susceptible and have not received HBV vaccine. If the exposed person is a known non-responder to HBV vaccination, then HBV immunoglobulin should be given within 48 h, with another dose in 1 month. Blood should be drawn for testing before HBV PEP is given.

Hepatitis C virus (HCV)

Current evidence suggests specific PEP for HCV is not warranted. The use of interferon is not warranted because of the high level of side effects and a lack of studies to suggest that its use in this situation is effective. However, treatment options may change in view of further studies; expert advice should be sought on this issue following a needlestick injury.

Post-exposure counselling and follow-up

It is essential that health care organizations should provide support and expert counselling on the implications of the event; post-exposure prophylaxis and appropriate long-term follow-up should be offered. Ideally, people nominated to provide support to affected individuals should have an appropriate knowledge of factors concerning transmission of HIV, HBV and HCV, and have counselling expertise. Where this is not possible, then a person with appropriate knowledge of disease transmission should be used.

Follow-up should be undertaken by a specialist with knowledge of blood-borne infections. If it is demonstrated that a person has been exposed to a blood-borne pathogen, they should not donate blood, semen, organs or tissue for 6 months, and should not share items that may be contaminated with even a small amount of blood (e.g. razors or toothbrushes). For HIV and HBV, they should be informed of the risk of transmission to sexual and injecting partners for a 6-month period, and be counselled about issues of safe sex and safe injecting. Advice should also be offered on pregnancy and breastfeeding based on an individual risk assessment.

If initial blood tests for HBV, HCV or HIV were negative, these tests should be repeated at 1, 3 and 6 months.

Protection against tuberculosis

All staff in regular contact with patients, and especially those working in chest medicine or investigation units, thoracic surgery units, infectious disease wards, laboratory staff working in microbiology, pathology and post-mortem room staff are at potential risk of contracting tuberculosis. *All staff, including agency staff and locums, should be screened and offered protection with BCG vaccine pre-employment.* Health care facilities that have contracts with agencies, should specify that the agency only supply staff that meets this requirement.

It is important that all prospective staff should undergo pre-employment health screening. Enquiries about symptoms suggestive of tuberculosis should form part of the pre-employment health questionnaire, which should be checked by the

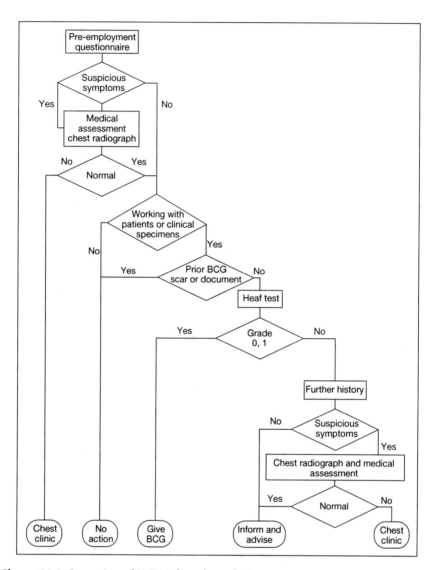

Figure 11.1 Screening of HCWs for tuberculosis.
Reproduced with permission from: Control and prevention of tuberculosis in the United Kingdom: Code of Practice 2000. *Thorax* 2000; **55**: 887–901.

occupational health department. The results of Heaf testing and BCG vaccination should be obtained when feasible.

The recommendations for new staff are summarized in figure 11.1. A Heaf test should be carried out on those prospective employees who do not have a definite BCG scar. A negative or grade 1 Heaf test in the absence of a definite BCG scar is an indication for BCG vaccination. Those without a definite BCG scar should have Heaf testing and those with a positive response (grades 2–4) should undergo clinical examination and chest X-ray. Those with strongly positive Heaf tests (grade 3 or 4) and/or relevant clinical findings should be referred to a respiratory physician for further management. Asymptomatic individuals who have no BCG scar and on Heaf testing have grade 2, 3 or 4 results should be advised that they have encountered *M. tuberculosis* in the past and do not require BCG vaccination. Careful enquiries must be made to ensure that they are truly asymptomatic and they must be advised of the relevant symptoms and the need to report these immediately.

Staff with symptoms compatible with tuberculosis: It is the ethical duty of all HCWs to protect the health of their patients. Staff with symptoms compatible with tuberculosis should seek advice either from the occupational health department or from their own medical practitioner so that they do not expose patients to infection.

Post-exposure follow-up: Following exposure of staff to a patient with open pulmonary (positive sputum smear for AAFB) tuberculosis, a list of staff at risk should be drawn by the line manager (see page 145). This list should only include staff that have had direct contact. The list should be sent to the occupational health department who will assess the circumstances of the exposure incident and review the HCWs.

Pregnant HCWs

Certain infections can be a problem during pregnancy, some of which may, potentially, be acquired at the workplace: for example cytomegalovirus (CMV), hepatitis viruses, human immunodeficiency virus, parvovirus (erythrovirus) B19, rubella and varicella. In general, adherence to standard precautions and maintaining high standards of general hygiene in the workplace will provide the HCWs with the necessary protection against infection.

It is the responsibility of the pregnant HCW to advise their medical practitioner and employer of their pregnancy. The employer should advise pregnant HCWs of the special risks associated with pregnancy and give them an opportunity to avoid patients with specific infections. All women of childbearing age should be counselled regarding their immune status and, if necessary, should be offered immunization before they become pregnant. All information about immune status and pregnancy of HCWs must remain confidential.

The following information relates to infections that are both significant in pregnancy and have some possibility of being acquired through patient care. It is not meant to be a comprehensive account of all infections having relevance to pregnant women.

Rubella

Confirming rubella immunity is part of routine antenatal screening. However, serious congenital abnormalities most commonly follow rubella infection occurring in the first trimester. For this reason, *rubella antibody status should be checked at employment in all HCWs, particularly women of childbearing age.* If rubella antibody is absent or below protective levels, then the HCW should be offered vaccination on beginning employment. Rubella vaccination should be avoided in early pregnancy, and conception should be avoided for 2 months following vaccination, although no case of congenital rubella syndrome has been reported following inadvertent vaccination shortly before or during pregnancy. Where necessary, those vaccinated can be tested for seroconversion 2 months after vaccination, and be revaccinated if necessary.

PEP with normal immunoglobulin will not prevent infection in non-immune contacts and is therefore of little value in the protection of pregnant women exposed to rubella. It may, however, prolong the incubation period, which in turn may marginally reduce the risk to the fetus. It may also reduce the likelihood of clinical symptoms in the mother. Normal immunoglobulin should only be used if termination of pregnancy due to confirmed rubella infection is unacceptable. In such cases, it should be given soon after exposure. Serological follow-up of recipients is essential, and should continue for up to 8 weeks.

Hepatitis B

Routine antenatal screening to determine HBV immune status is commonly performed in some countries. All HCWs should be screened by medical history and if in any doubt about previous infection/immunization, they should be tested for antibodies to HBsAg. All non-immune HCWs should be offered HBV vaccination as soon as possible at the start of employment and should be tested for antibodies to HBsAg 3 months after the third dose of vaccine. Those who do not respond should be offered a fourth dose or a further three doses depending upon the antibody level. Persistent non-responders should be informed about the need for HBIG with 48 h of parenteral exposure to HBV. If a HCW has not been vaccinated or is not known to be immune to HBV, then HBIG should be offered within 48 h of significant exposure to blood or potentially blood-contaminated secretions from a known HBV carrier or an unknown source. HBV vaccination should be offered at the same time. While the safety of the HBV vaccine for the developing fetus has not yet been confirmed by a large-scale trial, HBV infection in a pregnant woman may result in severe disease for the newborn. Pregnancy should therefore not be considered a contraindication to the administration of HBIG or HBV vaccination.

Cytomegalovirus (CMV)

While CMV may commonly be encountered in urine and saliva, surprisingly there is little evidence that this virus has been acquired by women HCWs and, in particular, has then resulted in fetal infection. However, *infection of HCWs is largely preventable by applying standard precautions, including the use of gloves and regular hand washing.* Generally, CMV infection in HCWs, even those working in high-risk areas such as neonatal units, transplant units and caring for HIV positive patients, is not significantly more common than that in the general community.

After primary infection, young children excrete CMV in urine and saliva in larger amounts and for longer periods than adults. There is a high incidence of asymptomatic excretion of CMV among infants and toddlers. For this reason, isolation of children known to be excreting CMV is not recommended. *To avoid CMV infection, washing hands after all patient contact and after contact with urine and saliva is essential.* Avoidance of direct contact with saliva (e.g. kissing toddlers on the mouth) is also important. Pregnant HCWs should be informed of the risks of CMV infection and provided with an opportunity to determine their susceptibility by performing antibody testing. They should be counselled about hygiene to minimize contact with known CMV-infected patients. Pregnant HCWs, or those contemplating pregnancy, should be counselled regarding mode of transmission of CMV and safe work practices. Routine antenatal screening is not recommended even in HCWs in high-risk areas, but can be offered on an individual basis. The implications of screening test results should be clearly explained.

Evidence of past CMV infection is a good indicator that symptomatic infection or congenital defects in the infant are unlikely to occur. However, it does not totally exclude the possibility of congenital infection, because reactivation of a past infection can occur during pregnancy. Conversely, if a HCW is antibody negative, avoidance of high-risk work areas will not eliminate the risk of primary CMV infection during pregnancy, especially if the HCW has close contact with children or other sources outside work. CMV seronegative women who care for children over the age of 2 years have a lower risk of infection. Redeploying seronegative pregnant employees to care for older children may further minimize the risk of working in high-risk areas. CMV immunoglobulin is available for the prevention and treatment of CMV infection in certain individuals at high risk of infection. However, its value is unclear.

Varicella-zoster virus (chickenpox and shingles)

Primary infection with varicella-zoster virus (VZV) causes chickenpox. The *infection is highly contagious and is spread via the respiratory route or by direct contact with skin vesicles.* The contagious period extends from 2 days before to approximately 5 days after the onset of rash. Crusted vesicles are no longer infectious. Infection of adults is generally more severe than infection of children.

There is some evidence that the infection may be more severe in pregnant than in non-pregnant women. Less than 5% of women of childbearing age do not have immunity to VZV. Even individuals who cannot recall having had chickenpox have an 80% chance of having had VZV infection. If chickenpox occurs during the first 20 weeks of gestation, intra-uterine fetal infection and occasionally fetal damage can occur. The fetal varicella syndrome is rare (<2% of affected pregnancies) and clues to its presence may be found at a 20-week ultrasound scan. The most dangerous time in pregnancy to acquire chickenpox is at term or immediately after term. This is because there is a high chance that the newborn infant may be exposed and may have little or no immunity. The newborn may then become seriously ill with VZV infection. For these reasons, non-immune pregnant women should not care for patients who are infectious, such as patients with chickenpox or shingles.

An enzyme-linked immunosorbent assay (ELISA) test reliably detects the presence of serum antibodies to VZV after natural infection. If a HCW has a history of clinical chickenpox, testing is not necessary since they will be immune. If the HCW is unsure whether or not they have had chickenpox and they are pregnant or contemplating pregnancy, then they may have their VZV antibody status checked. VZV vaccine is recommended for non-immune HCWs, but is not recommended during pregnancy. Vaccinees should not become pregnant for 1 month after vaccination. Pregnant HCWs who are not immune should not care for patients with chickenpox or shingles. If inadvertent exposure occurs, VZV immunoglobulin (ZIG) may be given to the pregnant HCW as soon as possible but up to 7 days after exposure to the virus. Aciclovir can be used for the treatment of acute VZV infection.

Parvovirus (erythrovirus) B19

Human parvovirus B19 is *usually transmitted via the respiratory route*, but the virus is very resistant in the environment and in biological materials such as blood or plasma. Diagnosis is by serology and/or viral DNA detection. At present there is no vaccine. Nosocomial outbreaks of B19, involving infection of patients and HCWs, including pregnant HCWs, have been reported. Infection early in pregnancy may affect the fetus, causing aplastic anaemia that later becomes manifest as hydrops fetalis. Pregnant HCWs should therefore avoid contact with patients who are infected with human Parvovirus (erythrovirus) B19.

Table 11.3 Summary of suggested work restrictions for HCWs exposed to or infected with infectious diseases.

Disease	Work restrictions	Duration
Conjunctivitis	Restrict from patient contact and contact with patients' environment.	Until discharge ceases.
Cytomegalovirus infection	No restriction.	
Diarrhoeal diseases Acute stage	Restrict from patient contact, contact with patient's environment, and food handling.	Until symptoms resolve.
Convalescent stage (*Salmonella* spp.)	Restrict from care of high-risk patients.	Until symptoms resolve; refer to local guidelines regarding need for negative stool culture.

Table 11.3 *continued*

Disease	Work restrictions	Duration
Diphtheria	Exclude from duty.	Until antimicrobial therapy completed and two cultures obtained ≥24 h apart are negative.
Enteroviral infections	Restrict from care of infants, neonates or immunocompromised patients and their environments.	Until symptoms resolve.
Hepatitis A	Restrict from patient contact, contact with patients' environment, and food handling.	Until 7 days after onset of jaundice.
Hepatitis B HCW with acute or chronic hepatitis B (HBsAg positive) who does *not* perform exposure-prone procedures.	No restriction; standard precaution should always be observed.	
HCW with acute or chronic hepatitis B (HBsAg positive) who *performs* exposure-prone procedures.	Do not perform exposure-prone invasive procedures. Seek advice from Occupational Health Department who will review and recommend procedures (see page 193).	
Hepatitis C	Do not perform exposure-prone invasive procedures. Seek advice from Occupational Health Department who will review and recommend procedures (see page 193).	
Herpes simplex Genital	No restriction.	
Hands (herpetic whitlow)	Restrict from patient contact and contact with patient's environment.	Until lesions heal.
Orofacial	Evaluate for need to restrict from care of high-risk patients.	
HIV infection	Do not perform exposure-prone invasive procedures. Seek advice from Occupational Health Department who will review and recommend procedures (see page 193).	
Measles Active	Exclude from duty.	Until 7 days after the rash appears.
Post-exposure (susceptible HCW)	Exclude from duty.	From 5th day after first exposure through 21st day after last exposure and/or 4 days after rash appears.

Table 11.3 *continued*

Disease	Work restrictions	Duration
Mumps		
Active	Exclude from duty.	Until 9 days after onset of parotitis.
Post-exposure (susceptible HCW)	Exclude from duty.	From 12th day after first exposure through 26th day after last exposure or until 9 days after onset of parotitis.
Pediculosis	Restrict from patient contact.	Until treated and observed to be free of adult and immature lice.
Pertussis		
Active	Exclude from duty.	From beginning of catarrhal stage through 3rd week after onset of paroxysms *or* until 5 days after start of effective antibiotic therapy.
Post-exposure (asymptomatic HCW)	No restriction, prophylaxis recommended (see page 105).	
Post-exposure (symptomatic HCW)	Exclude from duty.	Until 5 days after start of effective antibiotic therapy.
Rubella		
Active	Exclude from duty.	Until 5 days after rash appears.
Post-exposure (susceptible HCW)	Exclude from duty.	From 7th day after first exposure through 21st day after last exposure.
Scabies	Restrict from patient contact.	Until cleared by medical evaluation.
***Staphylococcus aureus* infection**		
Active, draining skin lesions	Restrict from patient contact, contact with patient's environment, and food handling.	
Carrier state	No restriction, unless HCW is epidemiologically linked to transmission of the organism.	
Streptococcal infection, group A (*Strep. pyogenes*)	Restrict from patient contact, contact with patients' environment, and food handling.	Until 24 h after antibiotic therapy.
Tuberculosis		
Active	Exclude from duty.	Until proven non-infectious (see page 143).
PPD converter	No restriction.	

Table 11.3 *continued*

Disease	Work restrictions	Duration
Varicella		
Active	Exclude from duty.	Until all lesions dry and crust.
Post-exposure (susceptible HCW)	Exclude from duty.	From 10th day after first exposure through 21st day (28th day if VZIG given) after last exposure.
Zoster		
Localized in healthy person	Cover lesions, restrict from care of high-risk patients[1].	Until all lesions dry and crust.
Generalized or localized in immunosuppressed person	Restrict from patient contact.	Until all lesions dry and crust.
Post-exposure (susceptible HCW)	Restrict from patient contact.	From 8th day after first exposure through 21st day (28th day if VZIG given) after last exposure or, if varicella occurs, until all lesions dry and crust.
Viral respiratory infections, acute febrile	Consider excluding from the care of high-risk patients or contact with their environment during community outbreak of RSV and influenza.	Until acute symptoms resolve.

HBsAg: Hepatitis B surface antigen; HIV: human immunodeficiency virus; VZIG: varicella zoster immunoglobin; RSV: respiratory syncytial virus.
[1]Those susceptible to varicella or at increased risk of complication of varicella, e.g. neonates and immunocompromised persons (see pages 167–168).

Modified from Bolyard EA, Tablon OC, Williams WN, *et al.* CDC Guideline for infection control in healthcare personnel, 1998. *American Journal of Infection Control* 1998; **26** (3): 289–354.

Table 11.4 Post-exposure prophylaxis against infectious disease.

Disease	Prophylaxis	Indications	Comments
Hepatitis A	One IM dose normal immunoglobulin given within 2 weeks of exposure.	HCW exposed to faeces of infected persons during outbreaks.	Persons with IgA deficiency, if administered within 2 weeks after MMR (Measles-Mumps-Rubella) or within 3 weeks after varicella vaccine then the immune response to these vaccines is likely to be inadequate.
Hepatitis B	See Table 11.2	HCW exposed to blood or body fluids containing HBsAg and who are not immune to HBV infection.	
HIV infection	See Table 11.1		
Varicella zoster	Varicella zoster immunoglobulin	HCW known or likely to be susceptible (especially those at high risk for complications, e.g. pregnant women) who have close and prolonged exposure to a contact case or an infectious HCW/patient.	See pages 217–218

Disease	Prophylaxis	Indication	Reference
Diphtheria	Benzathine penicillin 1.2 megaunit IM single dose or erythromycin 1 g per day orally for 7 days.	HCW exposed to diphtheria or identified as carrier.	
Meningococcal disease	Rifampicin 600 mg orally every 12 h for 2 days, or Ceftriaxone 250 mg IM single dose or Ciprofloxacin 500 mg orally single dose.	HCW with direct contact with respiratory secretions from infected persons without the use of proper precautions, e.g. mouth-to-mouth resuscitation, endotracheal intubation, endotracheal management, or close examination of oropharynx.	See page 162
Pertussis	Erythromycin 500 mg 6 hourly orally for 14 days after exposure.	HCW with direct contact with respiratory secretions or large aerosol droplets from respiratory tract of infected persons.	

References and further reading

AIDS/TB Committee of the Society for Healthcare Epidemiology of America. Management of healthcare workers infected with hepatitis B virus, hepatitis C virus, human immunodeficiency virus or other blood-borne pathogens. *Infection Control and Hospital Epidemiology* 1997; **18**: 349–363.

Alter HJ, Seeff LB, Kaplan PM, *et al.* Type B hepatitis: the infectivity of blood positive for e antigen and DNA polymerase after accidental needlestick exposure. *New England Journal of Medicine* 1976; **295**: 909–913.

Bell DM. Occupational risk of human immunodeficiency virus infection in healthcare workers: an overview. *American Journal of Medicine* 1997; **102**: 9–15.

Bell DM, Shapiro CN, Ciesielski CA, *et al.* Preventing blood-borne pathogen transmission from healthcare workers to patients. The CDC perspective. *Surgical Clinic of North America* 1995; **75**: 1189–1203.

Bronowicki JP, Venard V, Botte C, *et al.* Patient-to-patient transmission of hepatitis C virus during colonoscopy. *New England Journal of Medicine* 1997; **337**: 237–240.

Bolyard EA, Tablon OC, Williams WN, *et al.* CDC guideline for infection control in healthcare personnel, 1998. *American Journal of Infection Control* 1998; **26**(3); 289–354.

Cardo DM, Bell DM. Bloodborne pathogen transmission in health care workers: risks and prevention strategies. *Infectious Disease Clinics of North America* 1997; **11**: 331–346.

Centers for Disease Control and Prevention. Recommendations for follow-up of health-care workers after occupational exposure to hepatitis C virus. *Morbidity and Mortality Weekly Report* 1997; **46**: 603–606.

Centers for Disease Control and Prevention. Public Health Service guidelines for the management of healthcare worker exposures to HIV and recommendations for post-exposure prophylaxis. *Morbidity and Mortality Weekly Report* 1998a; **47**: 1–33.

Centers for Disease Control and Prevention. Recommendations for prevention and control of hepatitis C virus (HCV) infection and HCV-related chronic disease. *Morbidity and Mortality Weekly Report* 1998b; **47**: 1–39.

Centers for Disease Control. Case-control study of HIV seroconversion in health care workers after percutaneous exposure to HIV infected blood – France, United Kingdom and United States, January 1988–August 1994. *Morbidity and Mortality Weekly Report* 1995; **44**: 929–933.

Centers for Disease Control and Prevention. Updated US Public Health Service guidelines for the management of occupational exposures to HBV, HCV and HIV and recommendations for post-exposure prophylaxis. *Morbidity and Mortality Weekly Report* 2001; 50(RR-11): 1–42.

Ciesielski CA, Metler RP. Duration of time between exposure and seroconversion in healthcare workers with occupationally acquired infection with human immunodeficiency virus. *American Journal of Medicine* 1997; **102**: 115–116.

Ciesielski CA, Bell DM, Marianos DW. Transmission of HIV from infected healthcare workers to patients. *AIDS* 1991; **5**: S93–S97.

Collins CH, Kennedy DA. Microbiological hazards of occupational needlestick and 'sharps' injuries. *Journal of Applied Bacteriology* 1987; **62**: 385–402.

Doebbeling BN. Protecting the Healthcare Worker from Infection and Injury. In: Wenzel RP, ed. *Prevention and Control of Nosocomial Infections*, 3rd edn. Baltimore: Williams & Wilkins 1997: 397–435.

European Consensus Group on Hepatitis B Immunity. Are booster immunisations needed for life long hepatitis B immunity? *The Lancet* 2000; **355**: 561–565.

Gerberding JL. Management of occupational exposures to blood-borne viruses. *New England Journal of Medicine* 1995; **332**: 444–451.

Healing TD, Hoffman PN, Young SEJ. The infection hazards of human cadavers. *Communicable Disease Report* 1995; **5**: R61–R68.

Herwaldt LA, Pottinger JM, Carter CD, *et al*. Exposure workshops. *Infection Control and Hospital Epidemiology* 1997; **18**: 850–871.

Joint Tuberculosis Committee of the British Thoracic Society. Control and prevention of tuberculosis in the United Kingdom: Code of Practice 2000. *Thorax* 2000; **55**: 887–901.

Mills PR, Thorburn D, McCruden EAB. Occupationally acquired hepatitis C infection. *Reviews in Medical Microbiology* 2000; **11**(1): 15–22.

Moloughney BW. Transmission and post exposure management of bloodborne virus infections in the health care setting: Where are we now? *Canadian Medical Association Journal* 2001; **165**(4): 445–450.

Pomeroy C, Englund JA. Cytomegalovirus: epidemiology and infection control. *American Journal of Infection Control* 1987; **15**: 107–119.

Public Health Laboratory Services. Hepatitis subcommittee. Exposure to hepatitis B virus: guidance on post-exposure prophylaxis. *Communicable Disease Report* 1992; **2**: R97–R101.

Public Health Laboratory Services. Working party of the PHLS salmonella. The prevention of human transmission of gastrointestinal infections, infestations and bacterial intoxications. *Communicable Disease Report* 1995; **5**: R158–R172.

Ramsey ME. Guidance on the investigation and management of occupational exposure to hepatitis C. *Communicable Disease and Public Health* 1999; **2**: 258–262.

Rhodes RS, Bell DM. Prevention of transmission of blood-borne pathogens. *The Surgical Clinics of North America* 1995; **75**(6): 1047–1241.

Sherman M. Management of viral hepatitis: clinical and public health perspectives – a consensus statement. *Canadian Journal of Gastroenterology* 1997; **11**: 407–416.

UK Advisory Committee on Dangerous Pathogens. *Infection risks to new and expectant mothers in the workplace: A guide to employers*. Suffolk: HSE Books, 1997.

UK Department of Health. *Guidance for clinical health care workers. Protection against infection with bloodborne viruses.* London: DoH, 1998.

UK Department of Health. *Protecting health care workers and patients from hepatitis B.* London: DoH, 1994.

UK Department of Health. *HIV post-exposure prophylaxis: Guidance from the UK chief medicals officers' expert advisory group on AIDS.* London: DoH, 2000.

UK Department of Health. *Immunization against Infectious Disease.* London: HMSO, 1996.

UK Department of Health. *The prevention and control of tuberculosis in the United Kingdom: Recommendations for the prevention and control of tuberculosis at local level.* London: DoH, 1996.

UK Department of Health. *Hepatitis C Infected Health Care Workers.* London, 2002.

Yeager AS. Longitudinal, serological study of cytomegalovirus infections in nurses and in HCWs without patient contact. *Journal of Clinical Microbiology* 1975; **2**: 448–452.

Zuckerman AJ. Occupational exposure to hepatitis B virus and human immunodeficiency virus: a comparative risk analysis. *American Journal of Infection Control* 1995; **23**: 286–289.

12

Hand Hygiene and Personal Protective Equipment

More than 150 years ago Ignaz Semmelweis (1818–1865) demonstrated that puerperal fever was a contagious disease caused by infectious organisms, which were spread from patient to patient by the hands of health care workers (HCWs). This led to the introduction of hand dips with chlorinated lime at Vienna General Hospital. Since then, many studies have demonstrated that contaminated hands are responsible for transmitting infections.

It has been estimated that up to 30% of nosocomial infections could be prevented if HCWs thoroughly wash their hands before and after contact with body substances. Therefore, *importance of regular hand hygiene must be emphasized as one of the most crucial interventions in the prevention of cross-infection* in health care facilities.

It is the responsibility of health care establishments to ensure that adequate numbers of hand washing facilities are readily available in all clinical areas (see page 20). They should be of suitable types and be located in areas where there is significant patient contact. The supply of soap and disposable towels should be readily available.

Microorganisms present on the hands may be divided into two categories:

Resident organisms: These microorganisms are normal flora of the skin and include coagulase-negative staphylococci (mainly *Staphylococcus epidermidis*), members of the genus *Corynebacterium* (commonly called diphtheroids) and *Propionibacterium* spp. They are usually deep seated in the epidermis and are not easily removed by a single hand washing procedure. They rarely cause infection apart from during implant surgery and at intravenous sites.

Transient organisms: These microorganisms are those that are not part of the normal flora and represent recent contamination, usually surviving only for a limited period of time. They are acquired during contact with the infected/colonized patient or the environment and are easily removed by hand washing. The transient flora includes most of the organisms responsible for cross-infection, e.g. Gram-negative bacilli (*Escherichia coli*, *Klebsiella* spp. and *Pseudomonas* spp.), *Salmonella* spp., *Staph. aureus* and viruses, e.g. rotaviruses.

Methods of hand decontamination

Choice of method of hand decontamination will depend upon assessment of what is appropriate for the episode of care, what is practically possible and, to some degree, personal preference based on the acceptability of preparations or materials.

Hands must be decontaminated before every episode of care that involves direct contact with patients' skin, their food, invasive devices or dressings. The choice of method is based on an assessment of the degree of risk which depends on the following factors:

- Level of anticipated contact with patient or object.
- Extent of contamination that may occur with that contact.
- Patient care activities being performed.
- Susceptibility of the patient.

Routine hand washing: Routine hand washing will render the hands socially clean and remove transient microorganisms provided that an effective technique is used.

Procedure

1. Wet hands and forearms.
2. Apply sufficient plain, non-microbial (bar or liquid) soap to the hands to obtain good lather.
3. Rub vigorously to form lather on the surface of the hands for at least 10 seconds.
4. The hands should then be thoroughly rinsed under running water for a further 10 seconds.
5. Dry thoroughly using good quality paper towels.

Hands should be washed:

- Before and after a work shift.
- Before and after each nursing contact.
- After contact with blood, body fluids, secretions and excretions.
- After handling soiled or contaminated equipment or linen.

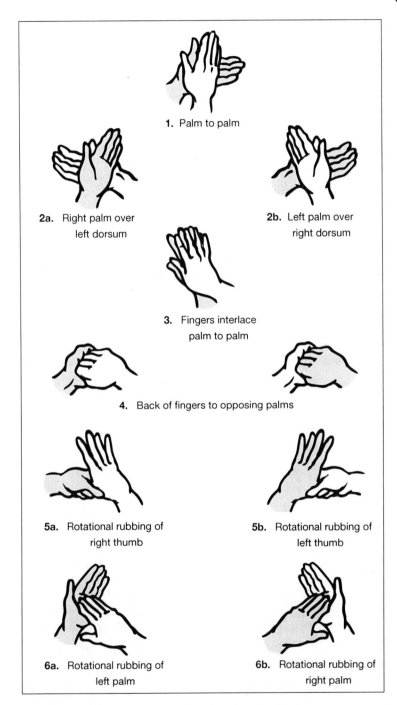

1. Palm to palm

2a. Right palm over left dorsum

2b. Left palm over right dorsum

3. Fingers interlace palm to palm

4. Back of fingers to opposing palms

5a. Rotational rubbing of right thumb

5b. Rotational rubbing of left thumb

6a. Rotational rubbing of left palm

6b. Rotational rubbing of right palm

Figure 12.1 Figures showing steps in hand washing technique.

eating, drinking or handling food (including serving meals) or
or administering drugs.

ing the toilet.

Hygienic hand disinfection: Hygienic hand disinfection will remove and kill most transient microorganisms. An antiseptic hand wash preparation is used.

Procedure

1. Wet hands and forearms.

2. Apply 3–5 ml of antiseptic solution into cupped hands.

3. Rub vigorously to form lather on all surfaces of the hands and forearms for at least 1 minute.

4. The hands should then be thoroughly rinsed under running water for 10–15 seconds, applying friction over all hand surfaces.

5. Rinse and then dry thoroughly.

Hands should be disinfected:

- During outbreaks of infection where contact with blood and body fluids or in situations where microbial contamination is likely to occur.

- In high-risk areas, e.g. patients in isolation, Intensive Care and Special Care Baby Units.

- Before performing an invasive procedure.

- Before and after touching wounds, urethral or IV catheters.

- Before wearing and after removing gloves.

Hygienic hand rub: An alternative method of hand disinfection is the application of 3–5 ml of a fast-acting antiseptic alcoholic hand rub into cupped hands. Hands are rubbed until they are dried using the defined technique. Alcoholic hand rub containing an emollient (e.g. glycerol) should be used to prevent excessive drying of hands. Alcoholic hand rubs do not cleanse and therefore it is important that hands should be cleaned first in the presence of visible contamination. The hygienic hand rub method is convenient, rapid and effective alternative to hand washing method and is useful in areas where a hand washbasin is not readily available, e.g.

- Emergency situations where there may be insufficient time and/or facilities.

- When hand washing facilities are inadequate.

- In the community or when return to a hand washbasin is impractical.

- During a ward round where there is a need for rapid hand disinfection.

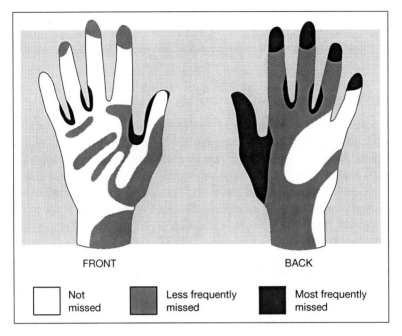

Figure 12.2 Parts of the hands most frequently missed during hand washing.

Reproduced with permission from Taylor LJ. An evaluation of handwashing techniques. *Nursing Times* 1978; **74:** 54–55.

Surgical hand disinfection: The first surgical scrub for the day should be for 3–5 minutes. Subsequent washes for 3 min between consecutive operations or application of alcoholic-based products to clean the hands for 3 min (see page 252) should suffice.

Hand washbasin

The health care facilities should have adequate numbers of hand washbasins (see page 20). They should be located conveniently (i.e. preferably near an entrance) for easy access to the HCW.

Hand washbasin should be supplied with both hot and cold water, preferably with a mixer tap to achieve correct temperature. The tap should be fitted with hands-off control (e.g. elbow operated) to avoid contamination. Hand washbasin should ideally be fitted with a soap dispenser. The water should be turned off using a paper towel rather than bare fingers or hands to avoid recontamination of hands. Plugs are not necessary, since hands should be washed only under running water.

Hand drying

Only good quality paper should be used. It should be within easy reach of a sink. *Cloth/fabric towels are not recommended* for use in health care facilities as they are recognized as a source of cross-infection. However if they are used, then they *must be single-use* and sent to the laundry. Use of hot air dryers in health care facilities is not recommended as they are noisy and slow and can be used by only one individual at a time.

Hand cleaning preparations

Hand cleaning preparations are mainly available in three forms, i.e. plain soap (bar or liquid), antimicrobial hand washes, and alcohol hand rubs. Various studies have been published concerning the effectiveness of various hand cleaning preparations in removing microorganisms from hands. Overall there was no evidence to favor the use of one antimicrobial agent over another. The choice of which hand decontamination preparation to use must take into consideration the need to remove transient and/or resident hand flora. Preparations with a residual effect are not normally necessary for everyday clinical practice.

The acceptability of agents and techniques is an essential criterion for the selection of preparations for hand hygiene. Acceptability of preparations is dependent upon ease of use combined with their dermatological effects.

Soap: It is important to emphasize that soap and water is as effective as preparations containing antimicrobial agents for decontaminating hands and removing *transient* microorganisms. Therefore, for general patient care, a plain neutral pH soap (without added substances that may cause irritation or dryness) should be used for routine hand washing.

If *bar soap* is used then the bar should be small in size to allow frequent changing. The *soap should be kept dry* (in a soap rack or on a magnet or ring) to promote drainage of water and avoid contamination with microorganisms which grow in moist conditions.

Liquid soap products should be stored in closed containers and dispensed from disposable containers. The *dispensers should be regularly cleaned and maintained*. If liquid soap is dispensed from reusable containers, these must be cleaned when empty and dried before refilling with fresh soap to avoid contamination. Special attention should be taken to clean pump mechanisms as these have been implicated as sources of infection.

Antiseptics: Preparations containing antimicrobial agents are more effective in removing resident microorganisms than those without an antimicrobial agent. Preparations containing antimicrobial agents have different effects on specific microorganisms (see Table 6.2, page 62).

A range of products is available, but chlorhexidine, povidone iodine, alcohol and triclosan are commonly used. Examples include 4% chlorhexidine gluconate-detergent, povidone iodine solution containing 0.75% available iodine, 0.5%

chlorhexidine gluconate with 70% isopropyl alcohol or 2% triclosan in a tenside base. A similar concentration of the antiseptic agent in different products does not necessarily imply similar effectiveness, therefore *new products should be tested before introduction.* Any *preparation used for hand washing or hand disinfection must be acceptable to the user* and must not damage the skin on repeated use. If staff do not accept the preparation, it will not be used. Therefore, it is recommended that a trial be undertaken before introduction of a new product in some areas to assess the acceptability by staff.

Alcohol based hand rubs: Alcohol based hand rubs are more effective in decontaminating hands than soap and water and antimicrobial handwashing agents. Their use gives a greater initial reduction in hand flora. However *they are not effective in removing physical dirt or soiling and should be used to disinfect physically clean hands.*

Nailbrushes

Routine use of nailbrushes is not recommended because frequent and vigorous use of a nail brush may damage the skin, encouraging the proliferation and persistence of microorganisms on the skin. Soft nailbrushes may be used for cleaning the nails and subungual spaces prior to the first operation of the day. In such circumstances, they must either be sterile single-use disposable, or be supplied sterilized by the hospital sterile service department. *Nailbrushes must never be soaked in a disinfectant solution.*

Hand care

Skin damage is generally associated with the detergent base of the preparation and/or poor hand washing technique. Hand care is important, because *intact skin is a natural defense against infection.* Damaged skin may result in increased carriage of pathogens responsible for hospital-acquired infection. In addition, the irritant and drying effects of hand preparations have been identified as one of the reasons that health care practitioners fail to adhere to hand hygiene guidelines. Therefore hand preparations that contain emollients and moisturizers should be used. The following points should be kept in mind:

- To minimize chapping of hands, use warm water and pat hands dry rather than rubbing them.

- Apply an emollient hand cream regularly to protect skin from the drying effect of preparations.

- *Nails should be kept short* to allow thorough cleaning of the hands and to prevent tears in gloves. *Artificial nails should be discouraged* as they contribute to increased bacterial counts.

- *Cuts and abrasions should be covered by water-resistant occlusive dressings* that should be changed as necessary.

- HCWs who have skin problems such as exudative lesions or weeping dermatitis must seek medical advice and should be removed from direct patient care until the condition resolves.

- Repeated hand washing and wearing of gloves can cause irritation or sensitivity, leading to dermatitis or allergic reactions. This can be minimized by early intervention, including assessment of hand washing technique and the use of suitable individual use hand care product.

Hand care products are used to help prevent excessive dryness. Some are also responsible for skin sensitization. Therefore, only suitable hand creams or lotions should be used and the following points should be considered in their choice:

- They should be supplied in small, individual use containers that are not refilled.

- Some types of hand creams and lotions may interact with antiseptics (e.g. chlorhexidine) and affect the integrity of gloves.

- Aqueous-based hand creams should be used before wearing gloves as oil-based preparations may cause latex gloves to deteriorate.

Compliance

Although hand washing is considered to be the most important single intervention for preventing nosocomial infections, studies have repeatedly shown poor compliance with hand washing by hospital personnel. The problem has been highlighted especially among doctors who frequently fail to wash their hands between patients. Failure to comply is a complex problem that includes elements of lack of motivation and lack of knowledge about the importance of hand washing. It may also be due to real or perceived obstacles, such as understaffing, inconveniently located hand washing facilities, an unacceptable hand washing product or dermatitis caused by previous hand washing. A number of strategies have been suggested to improve compliance. Long-term success will require development of programmes and sustained efforts at promoting compliance with hand washing. Effective interventions will probably be multidimensional, and will require the application of behavioural science theory combined with engineering and/or product innovation.

PERSONAL PROTECTIVE EQUIPMENT

The primary use of protective clothing in health-care settings is:

- To protect the skin and mucous membranes of HCWs from exposure to blood/body fluid.

- To prevent contamination of clothing and reduce the opportunity of spread of organisms from patients or fomites to other patients or environments.

The decision to use and select appropriate personal protective equipment must be based upon an assessment of the level of risk associated with contamination of clothing and skin by blood and body fluids from a specific patient care activity or intervention. The HCW must complete a similar exercise for all personnel visiting a patient in isolation. When protective wear is considered necessary, he or she is responsible for educating visitors and supervizing its use. Protective clothing which conforms to appropriate standards should be used.

Gloves

Provided gloves are correctly used, they can perform the following functions:

- Provide a protective barrier and prevent gross contamination of the hands when touching blood and body fluids, secretions, excreta, mucous membranes and non-intact skin.

- Reduce the likelihood that organisms from the hands of personnel will be transmitted to patients during invasive or other patient care procedures that involve touching mucous membranes and non-intact skin.

- Reduce the likelihood that the hands of personnel contaminated with organisms from a patient or a fomite can transmit these microorganisms to another patient.

- Protect the skin against hazardous substances, e.g. chemicals.

HCWs need to be aware that the inappropriate use of gloves can be a hazard and has been associated with cross-infection. Defects in gloves may be present and hands may be contaminated during their removal. Therefore, it is important that hands must always be decontaminated after using gloves. The *use of gloves should never be viewed as a substitute for appropriate hand washing.*

Types of gloves

As with all items of personal protective equipment, the need for gloves and the selection of appropriate materials must be subject to careful assessment of the task to be carried out and its related risks. Having decided that gloves should be used, HCWs must make a choice between the use of sterile or non-sterile gloves depending on the tasks being undertaken.

Donning technique

- Remove jewellery (wrist watches and rings) which may puncture the gloves.
- Open the protective paper package containing the sterile gloves onto a sterile surface.
- Unfold packaging by touching the corners only.
- Pick up the inside cuff using the non-dominant hand. *Do not touch the outside of the glove.*
- Slide the dominant hand inside the glove with correct alignment of thumb and fingers.
- Slip the fingers of the gloved hand under the cuff of the remaining glove.
- Slide the hand inside the glove with fingers and thumb correctly aligned.
- Avoid touching any part of the exposed hand with the gloved hand.
- Interlock fingers after the gloves are in place to ensure a comfortable fit and free movement.

Note: No special technique is necessary for use of non-sterile gloves. Pull gloves on in a convenient manner. Gloves should cover wrists.

Glove removal technique

- Grasp the palm of the first glove just below the wrist.
- Roll the glove towards the fingertips so that it turns inside out.
- Hold the removed glove by the fingertips of the remaining gloved hand.
- Place two fingers of the bare hand inside the cuff of the remaining glove.
- Roll the second glove towards the fingertips with the bare hand until the first glove is inside the second glove.
- Continue to remove until both gloves are inside out.
- Dispose of used gloves into a yellow clinical waste bag.
- Wash and dry hands thoroughly.

Note: It is the outside of the glove which is in contact with potentially infected material and the possibility of exposure to unprotected skin is at its greatest when the gloves are removed.

1. Single-use gloves

Sterile gloves: Single-use disposable *sterile gloves should be used during aseptic procedures* to prevent patients acquiring infection. They should not be washed or disinfected and re-used.

Non-sterile gloves: Non-sterile gloves should be used for procedures involving contact with blood, body fluids, excretions and secretions or non-intact skin or mucous membranes where there is a risk of infection to the HCW.

Gloves must be changed both between patient contacts and between separate procedures on the same patient. They should be changed if torn or punctured. *Hands should be decontaminated following the removal of gloves.* Gloved hands should neither be wiped with any form of alcoholic substance nor washed. Single-use gloves should be removed carefully to avoid contamination of hands or other surfaces. Keep in mind that gloves may develop defects or tears after extended use; that is why it is so important to wash your hands after removing your gloves. Gloves contaminated with blood and/or body fluids must be treated as clinical waste and disposed of accordingly.

2. General-purpose utility gloves

The use of heavy duty or household type gloves is required for environmental cleaning and decontamination procedures because they are robust and offer greater protection to the HCW. They should be washed in detergent and stored dried after each use. They should be replaced if punctured, torn, cracked, or showing signs of deterioration.

Glove materials

A number of materials are used in the manufacture of gloves. It is important that the most appropriate material for the purpose should be selected (see Table 12.1). Latex gloves are the most widely used, especially when dexterity is required, as they are the most sensitive. Recently the quality of vinyl gloves has improved and providing the type chosen reaches the specified standards, they can be considered suitable for barrier protection. Polythene gloves are not suitable for clinical use due to their permeability and tendency to damage easily. Synthetic materials are generally more expensive than latex and due to certain properties may not be suitable for all purposes. The problem of patient or HCW sensitivity to latex proteins must be considered when deciding on glove materials.

Latex allergy

Latex protein is a natural component of rubber which tends to produce an immediate hypersensitivity reaction (Type I) whilst other chemicals used in processing latex products can cause delayed hypersensitivity responses (Type IV). The usual route of exposure is the skin. *To minimize the risk of allergy, latex gloves should have low levels of extractable proteins and residual accelerators.* Evidence

Table 12.1 Types of gloves and suggested uses.

⌐ type	Features	Suggested use
⌐ner	• Cheap • Tear easily and often fit poorly	• Not recommended as there are no agreed specific indication for infection control use
.e)	• Strong • Good fit • Risk of sensitization	• Use when delicate manipulation is required • Use for protection against blood and body fluids
⌐ x (sterile)	• Strong • Good fit • Prone to sensitization	• Use for invasive procedures requiring high levels of patient and user protection or prolonged contact with body fluids
Vinyl	• Less sensitive as fit is not as good as latex gloves	• Use for handling cytotoxic agents
Rubber	• Expensive • Strong	• Use for environmental cleaning
Nitrile	• More expensive than latex • Not available as a surgical glove	• For individuals working with glutaraldehyde or sensitive to latex
Neoprene	• More expensive than latex • Available as a surgical glove	• For individuals sensitive to latex

Adapted from Hospital Infection Control Working Party Report. Review of hospital isolation and infection control related precautions, July 2001.

indicates that cornstarch glove powder aerosolizes latex proteins causing the allergens to be inhaled by both the glove wearer and others in the immediate environment. It is recommended that *all latex gloves should be non-powdered* and that all patient-admission processes should establish whether there is a history of allergy to latex. In addition to latex allergy, it is also associated with adhesions and increasing risks of infection associated with invasive devices. Therefore it is strongly recommended that powdered gloves should not be used in the health-care setting.

Nitrile gloves have the same chemical range as latex and therefore may lead to sensitivity problems. In order to minimize latex allergy it is important that *gloves should be worn only when necessary and be removed as soon as the activity is completed.* HCWs who develop sensitivity or allergy to latex should use another type of glove, e.g. neoprene.

Protective eyewear

The aim of protective eyewear (glasses, goggles or face-shields) is to help guard the mucous membranes of the eyes, nose, and mouth of the HCW from exposure to blood or body fluids that may be splashed, sprayed, or splattered into the face during the clinical procedures. *Protective eye wear must be worn during procedures that are likely to generate droplets of blood or high-risk body fluids.* They should comply with approved standards. They must be close fitting, optically clear, antifog and distortion free, and shielded at the side.

Face mask

Masks in conjunction with eyewear should be worn during procedures that are likely to generate aerosols or splashes of blood and body fluids to prevent contamination of mucous membranes of the mouth, nose and eyes. The type of mask best suited to a particular situation depends on the body substances likely to be encountered and the nature of the activity. *Wearing of masks during routine ward procedures such as wound dressing or invasive medical procedures is not necessary.*

Surgical masks may not be effective in preventing the inhalation of droplet nuclei. When caring for patients with known or suspected infectious pulmonary or laryngeal tuberculosis, it is recommended that a high efficiency particulate air (HEPA) mask should be used. Masks should be close fitting and filter particles of 1–5 μm. In the US, use of particulate respirators (N95) are recommended. *Use of a mask is not a substitute for good infection control practice.*

Dental procedures can generate large quantities of aerosols of 3 μm or less, and therefore *dental HCWs should wear masks or facial barriers* that block particles of this size. Masks should be changed after 20 minutes of continuous exposure to aerosols in the environment or as soon as practicable after they become moist or visibly soiled. If the masks are used then they should:

- Be fitted according to the manufacturer's instructions.
- Be used only *once* and *changed when moist or grossly contaminated.*
- Not be touched by hand while being worn.
- Be removed by untying and handled only by the ties and never by the face covering part which may be heavily contaminated with the microorganisms.
- *Not be worn loosely around the neck,* but be removed and discarded as soon as practicable after use.

Aprons and gowns

Apron: Single-use disposable plastic aprons are recommended for general use and should be worn when there is a risk that clothing or uniforms may become exposed to blood, body fluids, secretions and excretions. Plastic aprons should be worn as single-use items for one procedure or episode of patient care only. They should be removed immediately after use by tearing the neck strap and the waist tie and discarded into clinical waste bag before they leave the room. Hands must be washed immediately after removing and bagging the soiled plastic apron.

Gowns: Clean, non-sterile gowns should be worn during procedures which are likely to expose HCWs with spraying or splashing of blood, body fluids, secretions, or excretions. Gowns should be impermeable and water repellent. If the gown is expected to become wet during the procedure and if a water repellent gown is not available, a plastic apron should be worn over the gown. Grossly soiled gowns should be promptly removed and placed in a designated leak proof laundry bag. Hands should be washed immediately after removing and bagging of the soiled gown.

Plastic overshoes

The *use of overshoes is not recommended,* as it is an ideal way of transferring microorganisms from floor and shoes to hands.

References and further reading

Albert RK, Condie F. Hand-washing patterns in medical intensive care units. *New England Journal of Medicine* 1998; **24**: 1465–1466.

Archibald LK, Corl A, Shah B, *et al. Serratia marcescens* outbreak associated with extrinsic contamination of 1% chlorxylenol soap. *Infection Control Hospital Epidemiology* 1997; **18**: 704–709.

Ayliffe GA. Masks in surgery? *Journal of Hospital Infection* 1991; **18**: 165–166.

Ayliffe GA, Babb JR, Davies JG, Lilly HA. Hand disinfection: a comparison of various agents in laboratory and ward studies. *Journal of Hospital Infection* 1988; 11(3): 226–243.

Ayliffe GA, Babb JR, Quoraishi AH. A test for 'hygienic' hand disinfection. *Journal of Clinical Pathology* 1978; 31(10): 923–928.

Belkin NL. Use of scrubs and related apparel in health care facilities. *American Journal of Infection* 1997; **25**: 401–404.

Berger SA, Kramer M, Nagar H, *et al.* Effect of surgical mask position on bacterial contamination of the operative field. *Journal of Hospital Infection* 1993; **23**: 51–54.

Bischoff WE, Reynolds TM, Sessler CN, *et al.* Handwashing compliance by health care workers. The impact of introducing an accessible, alcohol based hand antiseptic. *Archive of Internal Medicine* 2000; **160**: 1017–1021.

Boyce JM. Using alcohol for hand antisepsis: dispelling old myths. *Infection Control and Hospital Epidemiology* 2000; **21**: 438–441.

Casewell M, Phillips I. Hands as route of transmission for *Klebsiella* species. *British Medical Journal* 1977; **2**: 1315–1317.

Dave J, Wilcox MH, Kellett M. Glove powder: implications for infection control. *Journal of Hospital Infection* 1999; **42**: 283–285.

Doebbeling BN, Pfaller MA, Houston AC, *et al.* Removal of nosocomial pathogens from the contaminated glove: implications for glove re-use and handwashing. *Annals of International Medicine* 1988; **109**: 394.

Doebbeling BN, Stanley GL, Sheetz CT, *et al.* Comparative efficacy of alternative hand-washing agents in reducing nosocomial infections in intensive care units. *New England Journal of Medicine* 1992; **327**(2): 88–93.

Donowitz LG. Failure of the overgown to prevent nosocomial infection in a paediatric intensive care unit. *Pediatrics* 1986; **77**: 35–38.

Garner JS. The Hospital Infection Control Practices Advisory Committee: Guidelines for Isolation Precautions in Hospitals. *Infection Control and Hospital Epidemiology* 1996; **17**: 53–80.

Gerberding JL, Quebbeman EJ, Rhodes RS. Hand protection. *Surgical Clinics of North America* 1995; **75**: 1133–1139.

Graham M. Frequency and duration of handwashing in an intensive care unit. *American Journal of Infection Control* 1990; **18**: 77–80.

Infection Control Nurses Association. *Glove Usage Guidelines.* ICNA, 1999.

Infection Control Nurses Association. *Protective clothing.* ICNA, 2001.

Infection Control Nurses Association. *Hand decontamination guidelines.* ICNA, 2002.

Haque KN, Chagla AH. Do gowns prevent infection in neonatal intensive care units? *Journal of Hospital Infection* 1989; **14**: 159–162.

Harbarth S, Sudre P, Dharan S, *et al.* Outbreak of Enterobacter cloacae related to under-staffing, overcrowding and poor hygiene practices. *Infection control and Hospital Epidemiology* 1999; **20**: 598–603.

Healthcare Infection Control Practices Advisory Committee. Guideline for Hand Hygiene in Health-Care Settings. *Morbidity and Mortality Weekly Report* 2002; **51**(RR-16):1–45.

Humphreys H, Marshall RJ, Ricketts VE, *et al.* Theatre over-shoes do not reduce operating theatre floor bacterial counts. *Journal of Hospital Infection* 1991; **17**: 117–123.

Jarvis W, Bolyard E, Bozzi C. Respiratory recommendations and regulations. The controversy surrounding protection of health-care workers from tuberculosis. *Annals of Internal Medicine* 1995; **122**: 142–146.

Kramer A, Rudolph P, Kampf G, Pittet D. Limited efficacy of alcohol-based hand gels. *The Lancet* 2002; **359**: 1489–1490.

Kretzer EK, Larson EL. Behavioral interventions to improve infection control practices. *American Journal of Infection Control* 1998; **26**: 245–253.

Labadie JC, Kampf G, Lejeune B, *et al.* European Guidelines. Recommendations for surgical hand disinfection – requirements, implementation and need for research. A proposal by representatives of the SFHH, DGHM and DGKH for a European discussion. *Journal of Hospital Infection* 2002; **51**: 312–315.

Lagier F, Vervolet D, Lhermet I. Prevalence of latex allergy in operating room nurses. *Journal of Allergy and Clinical Immunology* 1992; **21**(90): 319.

Larson E. A causal link between hand washing and risk of infection? Examination of the evidence. *Infection Control and Hospital Epidemiology* 1988; **9**: 28–36.

Larson E. Skin hygiene and infection prevention: More of the same or different approaches? *Clinical Infectious Diseases* 1999; **29**: 1287–1294.

Larson E, Killien M. Factors influencing handwashing behavior of patient care personnel. *American Journal of Infection Control* 1982; **10**: 93–99.

Larson E, Kretzer EK. Compliance with handwashing and barrier precautions. *Journal of Hospital Infection* 1995; **30**(Suppl.): 88–106.

Larson E, McGinley KJ, Grove GL, *et al.* Physiologic, microbiologic, and seasonal effects of handwashing on the skin of health care personnel. *American Journal of Infection Control* 1986; **14**: 51–59.

Larson EL. APIC guideline for hand washing and hand antisepsis in health care settings. *American Journal of Infection Control* 1995; **23**: 251–269.

Larson EL, Bryan JL, Adler LM, Blane C. A multifaceted approach to changing hand washing behavior. *American Journal of Infection Control* 1997; **25**: 3–10.

Lilly HA, Lowbury EJL. Transient skin flora. *Journal of Clinical Pathology.* 1978; **31**: 919–922.

Lovitt SA, Nichols RL, Smith JW, *et al.* Isolation gowns: A false sense of security. *American Journal of Infection Control* 1992; **20**: 185–191.

Lowbury EJL, Lilly HA, Bull JP. Disinfection of hands: removal of transient organisms. *British Medical Journal* 1964; **2**: 230–233.

Mitchell NJ, Hunt S. Surgical face masks in modern operating rooms – a costly and unnecessary ritual? *Journal of Hospital Infection* 1991; **18**: 239–242.

Olsen RJ. Lynch P. Coyle MB. Examination gloves as barriers to hand contamination in clinical practice. *Journal of the American Medical Association* 1993; **270**: 350–353.

Pittet D. Improve compliance with hand hygiene in hospitals. *Infection Control and Hospital Epidemiology* 2000; **21**: 381–386.

Pittet D, Hugonnet S, Harbarth S, *et al.* Effectiveness of a hospital-wide programme to improve compliance with hand hygiene. *The Lancet* 2000; **356**: 1307–1312.

Poole CJM. Hazards of powdered surgical gloves. *The Lancet* 1997; **350**: 973.

Reybrouck G. Hand washing and hand disinfection. *Journal of Hospital Infection* 1986; **8:** 5–23.

Reybrouk G. Role of the hands in the spread of nosocomial infections. *Journal of Hospital Infection* 1983; **4:** 103–110.

Richmond PW, McCabe M, Davies JP, Thomas DM. Perforation of gloves in an accident and emergency department. *British Medical Journal* 1992; **304:** 879–880.

Rotter ML. Hand Washing and Hand Disinfection. In: Mayhall CG, ed. *Hospital Epidemiology and Infection Control*, 2nd edn. Baltimore: Lippincott Williams & Wilkins, 1999: 1339–1355.

Rotter ML. Hand Washing, Hand Disinfection, and Skin Disinfection. In: Wenzel RP (ed.), *Prevention and Control of Nosocomial Infections*, 3rd edn. Baltimore: Williams & Wilkins 1997: 691–709.

Rutala WA, Weber DJ. A review of single-use and reusable gowns and drapes in health care. *Infection Control and Hospital Epidemiology* 2001; **22:** 2248–2257.

Satter SA, Springthorpe VS, Tetro J *et al.* Hygiene hand antiseptics: should they not have activity and label claims against viruses? *American Journal of Infection Control* 2002; **30:** 355–372.

Semmelweis I. Die Aetiologie, der Begiriff und die Prophylaxis des Kindbettfiebers. Pest, Wien und Leipzig: CA Hartleben's Verlag Expedition; 1861.

Simmons B, Bryant J, Neiman K, *et al.* The role of hand washing in prevention of endemic intensive care unit infections. *Infection Control Hospital Epidemiology* 1990; **11:** 589–594.

Taylor LJ. An evaluation of hand washing techniques. *Nursing Times* 1978; **74:** 54–55 (Part I), 108–110 (part II).

Teare EL, Cookson B, French G, *et al.* UK Hand washing Initiative. *Journal of Hospital Infection* 1999; **43:** 1–3.

Tunevall TG. Post-operative wound infections and surgical face masks: A controlled study. *World Journal of Surgery* 1991; **15:** 383–388.

Turjanmaa K. Incidence of immediate allergy to latex gloves in hospital personnel. *Contact Dermatitis* 1987; **17:** 270–275.

UK Department of Health. Standard principles for preventing hospital-acquired infections. *Journal of Hospital Infection* 2001; **47**(Suppl.): S21–S37.

UK Department of Health. Expert Advisory Group on AIDS and the Advisory Group on Hepatitis. *Guidance for clinical health care workers: Protection against infection with blood-borne viruses.* London: DoH; 1998.

UK Medical Devices Agency. *Latex Sensitisation in the Health-care Setting: Use of Latex Gloves* 1996. Device Bulletin No MDA DB 9601.

Voss A, Widmer AF. No time for handwashing: Handwashing versus alcoholic rub: can we afford 100% compliance? *Infection Control and Hospital Epidemiology* 1997; **18**: 205–208.

Wake D, Bowry AC, Crook B, Brown RC. Performance of respirator filters and surgical masks against bacterial aerosols. *Journal of Aerosol Science* 1997; **28**: 1311–1329.

Ward V, Wilson J, Taylor L, Cookson B, Glynn A. *Preventing Hospital-Acquired Infection: Clinical Guidelines*. London: Public Health Laboratory Service; 1997.

Widmer AF. Replace hand washing with use of a waterless alcohol hand rub? *Clinical Infectious Disease* 2000; **31**: 136–143.

Yassin MS, Lierl MB, Fischer TJ. Latex allergy in hospital employees. *Annals of Allergy* 1994; **72**: 245–249.

13

Prevention of Surgical Site Infections

Despite advances in operative techniques and a better understanding of the pathogenesis of wound infection, post-operative wound infection continues to be a major source of morbidity and mortality for patients undergoing operative procedures. It can account for up to 15% of all nosocomial infections.

The most critical factors in the prevention of post-operative infections, although difficult to quantify, are the sound judgement and proper technique of the surgeon and surgical team, as well as the general health and disease state of the patient. In order to minimize post-operative surgical wound infection, it is important to create a safe environment by controlling four main sources of infection, i.e. personnel, equipment, the environment and patient's risk factors.

Surveillance

Surveillance of surgical site infection (SSI) is a useful tool to demonstrate the magnitude of the problem. Regular feedback of SSI to the surgeon has been shown to provide strong motivation and a reduction in infection rates in clinical practice.

For surveillance of SSI, it is important that internationally *agreed definitions should be followed, which must be agreed with the surgical team prior to embarking on the surveillance programme.* The most widely used definition of SSI (see pages 246–247) is that employed by the Center for Disease Control's National Nosocomial Infections Surveillance (NNIS) system. They *must be risk adjusted* so that they can be compared amongst surgeons or among facilities.

In recent years, the surveillance of SSIs has been complicated by changes in surgical practice, the short duration of post-operative stay, outpatient procedures, and laparoscopic procedures. *SSIs are considered to be nosocomial if the infection occurs within 30 days the operative procedure or within 1 year if a device or foreign material is implanted.*

CDC criteria for defining a surgical site infection (SSI)*

Superficial incisional SSI

Infection occurs within 30 days after the operation, *and* infection involves only skin or subcutaneous tissue of the incision, *and* at least one of the following:

1. Purulent drainage, with or without laboratory confirmation, from the superficial incision.

2. Organisms isolated from an aseptically obtained culture of fluid or tissue from the superficial incision.

3. At least one of the following signs or symptoms of infection: pain or tenderness, localized swelling, redness or heat and the superficial incision is deliberately opened by surgeon, *unless* incision is culture-negative.

4. Diagnosis of superficial incisional SSI by the surgeon or attending physician.

Do *not* report the following conditions as SSI:

1. Stitch abscess (minimal inflammation and discharge confined to the points of suture penetration).

2. Infection of an episiotomy or newborn circumcision site.

3. Infected burn wound.

4. Incisional SSI that extends into the fascial and muscle layers (see deep incisional SSI).

Note: Specific criteria are used for identifying infected episiotomy and circumcision sites and burn wounds.**

Deep incisional SSI

Infection occurs within 30 days after the operation if no implant¶ is left in place or within 1 year if implant is in place and the infection appears to be related to the operation. Infection involves deep soft tissues (e.g. fascial and muscle layers) of the incision and at least one of the following:

1. Purulent drainage from the deep incision but not from the organ/space component of the surgical site.

2. A deep incision spontaneously dehisces or is deliberately opened by a surgeon when the patient has at least one of the following signs or

symptoms: fever (>38°C), localized pain or tenderness, unless site is culture-negative.

3. An abscess or other evidence of infection involving the deep incision is found on direct examination, during reoperation, or by histopathologic or radiologic examination.

4. Diagnosis of a deep incisional SSI by a surgeon or attending physician.

Notes:

1. Report infection that involves both superficial and deep incision sites as deep incisional SSI.

2. Report an organ/space SSI that drains through the incision as a deep incisional SSI.

Organ/space SSI

Infection occurs within 30 days after the operation if no implant[1] is left in place or within 1 year if implant is in place and the infection appear to be related to the operation *and* infection involves any part of the anatomy (e.g. organs or spaces) other than the incision which was opened or manipulated during an operation *and* at least *one* of the following:

1. Purulent drainage from a drain that is placed through a stab wound[§] into the organ/space.

2. Organisms isolated from an aseptically obtained culture of fluid or tissue in the organ/space.

3. An abscess or other evidence of infection involving the organ/space that is found on direct examination, during reoperation, or by histopathologic or radiologic examination.

4. Diagnosis of an organ/space SSI by a surgeon or attending physician.

*Horan TC, Gaynes RP, Martone WJ, Jarvis WR, Emori TG. CDC definition of nosocomial surgical site infections. 1992: a modification of CDC surgical wound infections. *Infection Control Hospital Epidemiology* 1992; **13**(10): 606–608.
**Gaynes RP, Horan TC. Surveillance of nosocomial infections. In: Mayhall CG, ed. *Hospital Epidemiology and Infection Control*, Baltimore: Williams & Wilkins; 1996, 1017–1031.
¹National Nosocomial Infection Surveillance definition: a non-human-derived implantable foreign body (e.g. prosthetic heart valve, non-human vascular graft, a mechanical heart, or hip prosthesis) that is permanently placed in a patient during surgery.
§If the area around a stab wound becomes infected, it is not an SSI. It is considered a skin or soft tissue infection, depending on its depth.

The traditional classification of surgical wound infection was based on the exposure of the incision to bacterial contamination (see Table 13.1). In 1992, the NNIS system (Horan TC, *et al.* 1992) attempted to redefine surgical wound infection. This system has provided a greater discrimination for the patients at risk of developing wound infection. The NNIS system includes:

- Contaminated or dirty wound class.

- High pre-operative risk as defined by the American Society of Anesthesiologists (ASA) pre-operative assessment score.

- Duration of operation exceeding the 75th percentile for a given procedure.

Additional risk factors of developing SSI are summarized in Table 13.2.

Microbiology

The pathogens isolated from infections differ, primarily depending on the type of surgical procedure. For example, in clean surgical procedures, *Staphylococcus aureus* from the exogenous environment or the patient's skin flora is the usual cause of infection. In other categories of surgical procedures, including clean-contaminated, contaminated, and dirty, the polymicrobial aerobic and anaerobic flora closely resembling the normal endogenous microflora of the surgically resected organ are the most frequently isolated pathogens.

According to data from the NNIS, there has been little change in the incidence and distribution of the pathogens isolated from infections during the last decade. However, more of these pathogens show antimicrobial-drug resistance, especially methicillin-resistant *S. aureus* (MRSA).

Pre-operative patient care

Patient's risk factors

These include extreme age, obesity, malnutrition, certain concurrent disease or conditions, i.e. diabetes, malignancy, chronic chest or heart disease, and immunosuppression. Patients with pre-existing skin lesions or infection in another site, and treatment with steroids and immunosuppressive drugs, are more prone to get surgical wound infection due to impaired host defense mechanisms. These should be corrected or treated before an elective operation is planned. Cessation of tobacco use 30 days before surgery is also recommended.

Pre-operative showers

Pre-operative showers or baths on the night before an operative procedure using antimicrobial agents have been suggested as a means of reducing SSI in certain categories of patients. Several studies observed lower infection rates when the patient showered preoperatively with antiseptic agents while other studies have failed to

Table 13.1 Wound classification based on estimation of bacterial density, contamination and risk of subsequent infections.

Surgical procedure	Definition	Expected infection rate (%)
Clean	Non-traumatic, uninfected operative wounds in which no inflammation is encountered; there is no break in technique; and the respiratory, alimentary, or genitourinary tracts or the oropharyngeal cavities are not entered.	1–3
Clean contaminated	Operation in which the respiratory, alimentary or genitourinary tracts are entered under controlled conditions and without unusual contamination.	8–10
Contaminated	Operation associated with: • Open, fresh trauma wounds • Major breaks in a sterile technique or gross spillage from the gastrointestinal tract • Acute, non-purulent inflammation	15–20
Dirty and infected	Operation involving old trauma wounds with retained devitalized tissue, foreign bodies, or faecal contamination, and those with existing infection.	25–40

Table 13.2 Risk factors associated with surgical site infections.

	Risk factors	
	Host-related	Procedure-related
Definite	• Age • Obesity • Disease severity • ASA (American Society of Anesthesiologists) Score • Nasal carriage of *Staph. aureus* • Remote infection • Duration of pre-operative hospitalization	• Pre-operative hair removal • Type of procedure • Antibiotic prophylaxis • Duration of surgery
Likely	• Malnutrition and low serum albumin • Diabetes mellitus	• Multiple procedures • Tissue trauma • Foreign material • Blood transfusion
Possible	• Malignancy • Immunosuppressive therapy • Breast size in women	• Pre-operative showers • Emergency surgery • Drains

Reproduced from Smyth ETM, Emmerson AM. *Journal of Hospital Infection* 2000; **45**: 173–184.

Table 13.3 Antibiotics prophylaxis for surgical procedures.

Surgical procedures	Antibiotics
Cardiac surgery	Cefuroxime or cefazolin (three doses)
Neurosurgery	Cefuroxime or cefazolin (single dose)
Head and neck (operation involving the mucous membranes and deep tissue)	Cefuroxime or cefazolin ± metronidazole (up to three doses)
Biliary tract surgery	Cefuroxime or cefazolin or gentamicin (single dose)
ERCP	Cefuroxime or cefazolin (single dose)
Gastroduodenal	Cefuroxime or cefazolin (single dose)
Appendectomy (simple)	Cefuroxime or cefazolin or gentamicin + metronidazole (single dose)
Colorectal surgery	Cefuroxime or cefazolin or gentamicin + metronidazole (single dose)
Orthopaedic surgery • Insertion of prosthetic joints, open operation	Cefuroxime or cefazolin. Substitute vancomycin if history of penicillin or cephalosporin allergy (single dose)
• Lower limb amputation	Benzylpenicillin 2 mega units IV 6 hourly. Metronidazole or clindamycin for patient allergic to penicillin. All antibiotics should be given for 24 h duration
Peripheral vascular surgery	Cefuroxime or cefazolin (three doses)
Urological surgery	IV antibiotic cover depends on sensitivity testing of screening urine. In an emergency situation, give gentamicin 2–3 mg/kg body weight (single dose)
Hysterectomy	Cefuroxime or cefazolin + metronidazole or co-amoxiclav alone (single dose)
Caesarean section	Cefuroxime or cefazolin or co-amoxiclav after umbilical cord is clamped (single dose)

Helpful hints

- All antibiotics should be administered at the induction of anaesthesia. Repeat dose of antibiotic should be given for the operations when the duration of operation exceeds 3 h or in the case of massive haemorrhage ($\geq$2 litres of blood is lost in an adult). **Do not give prophylactic antibiotic for more than 24 h.**

- Prophylactic antibiotic dosage for adults: cefuroxime, 1.5 g IV (750 mg if body weight <50 kg); cefazolin 1–2 g; clindamycin 600 mg IV; metronidazole 500 mg IV and co-amoxiclav 1.2 g IV.

show a reduction in the wound infection rate. Even though pre-operative showers may reduce the skin's microbial colony count, they have *not definitively been shown to reduce the infection rates.*

Pre-operative hospitalization

Pre-operative stay in hospital *should be kept to a minimum* before operations because the longer the patient stays in the hospital before an operation, the greater becomes the likelihood of succeeding wound infection.

Pre-operative shaving

Pre-operative shaving should be avoided because shaving can cause small nicks and breaks leaving the skin bruised and traumatized which increases the risk of colonization and infection. If hair is to be removed from the operative site, only the area needing to be incised should be shaved. This should preferably be done using depilatory cream the day before operation. Depilatory cream should be used with caution as it can cause serious skin irritation and rashes, which may lead to wound infection. Alternately hair can be removed with clippers in the anaesthetic room immediately before the operative procedure. If clippers are used, then the head must be sterile. *Razors and shaving brushes should not be used.*

Antibiotic prophylaxis

The use of antibiotic prophylaxis before surgery has evolved greatly in the last 20 years. Improvements in the timing of initial administration, the appropriate choice of antibiotic agents, and shorter duration of administration have defined more clearly the value of this technique in reducing post-operative wound infections. It is generally recommended that a single dose of cephalosporin, e.g. cefuroxime or cefazolin (see Table 13.3) *should be administered intravenously with the induction of anaesthesia.* For caesarean sections, IV antibiotic should be given immediately after cord is clamped. *Prophylaxis should not exceed 24 h following surgery.* Use of third generation cephalosporins for surgical prophylaxis is not recommended because they are costly and promote emergence of bacteria resistance. *Routine use of vancomycin as surgical prophylaxis should be avoided.* Repeat doses of IV cefuroxime or cefazolin should be given in the case of massive haemorrhage ($\geqslant 2$ litres of blood is lost in an adult) or when the duration of operation exceeds 3 h.

Before elective colorectal operations, in addition to parenteral agent, mechanically prepare the colon by use of enemas and cathartics. Administer non-absorbable oral antimicrobial agents in divided doses on the day before the operation. Three regimens of oral agents combine neomycin with erythromycin base, metronidazole, or tetracycline. Mechanical cleansing for pre-operative preparation before elective colon resection should be used.

Operative factors

The principles of surgical asepsis, which is the prevention of access of infectious agents to a surgical field, must be used for all operating room procedures. This is achieved by methods that destroy microorganisms (by use of disinfectants and sterilization procedures) or that prevent them from contaminating objects that come into contact with the surgical field (by use of barrier protection).

Modern surgery is aseptic in the use of sterile instruments, sutures and dressings and in the wearing of sterile gowns and gloves by the operating team. *All articles used in an operation must be 'sterile'*. All members of the operating team who are 'sterile' must touch only sterile articles: persons who are 'unsterile' must touch only unsterile articles. All sterile packs should be opened using a technique that will prevent contamination of sterile instruments.

The surgeon in charge of the patient, the anaesthetist and the scrub nurse should be responsible for ensuring that all members of the operating team know the operating room procedures and infection control precautions that are to be taken, including any additional precautions that may be required. Staff involved in cleaning and sterilizing instruments and equipment used in the operating theatre should also be informed of the need for any additional precautions.

Surgical hand scrub

Before surgical procedures, hands, nails and forearms should be washed thoroughly with an appropriate skin disinfectant to reduce the number of microorganisms that could be transferred from personnel to the patient. Rings, watches and bracelets should be removed and fingernails should be kept short and clean. The hands and forearms should be free of open lesions and breaks in the skin.

The application time and volume of antiseptic used for surgical scrub must be in accordance with the efficacy of antiseptic solution used. Any agent or method of skin decontamination that causes skin abrasions (e.g. use of a brush on skin) must be avoided. The first wash of the day should include a thorough clean under the fingernails; a brush or a stick can be used if necessary.

There is no universal agreement either on the type of antiseptic or the optimum duration of surgical scrub. From evidence, it appears that the first surgical scrub of the day should be for 3–5 min with subsequent washes for 3 min between consecutive operations; alternatively, apply alcohol-based products to clean hands for 3 min. A European guideline recommends that the total application for surgical scrub time must not be shorter than 2 min and a minimum of *two applications* are necessary (Labadie JC, *et al.* 2002). Hands should be air dried before gloves are put on. Care should be taken to ensure there is no hand contact with any non-sterile object.

Theatre wear

Outside clothing must be changed for clean, laundered operating room attire of loosely woven material. An impermeable, cuffed-wrist, sterile gown should be worn by scrubbed health care workers (HCWs). Operating room gowns should be made of waterproof fabric with an ability to breathe, and should be comfortable to wear. Alternatively, plastic aprons should be worn under gowns and should be of sufficient length to overlap with footwear.

Procedure for surgical scrub

Rings, watches and bracelets should be removed before surgical scrub. The first surgical scrub for the day should be for 3–5 min with subsequent washes for 3 min between consecutive operations.

1. Turn the taps on using the elbows and adjust the flow of water and temperature of the water.

2. Wet hands and forearms.

3. Apply an antiseptic (e.g. chlorhexidine or povidone iodine)/detergent preparation from an elbow operated pump dispenser.

4. Lather hands, wrists and forearms, keeping them above elbow level and rinse thoroughly under running water. Clean finger nails and remove ingrained dirt with a manicure stick held under running water. Sterile nail brush can be used to clean nails and subungual spaces but *not* the skin to prevent skin damage. This should only be done at the beginning of the operation list.

5. Repeat the handwashing procedure. Rinse the hands, wrists and fore-arms thoroughly under running water, making sure that fingertips always point upwards, with elbows down, to avoid recontamination of clean fingers and hands by water running down from contaminated proximal areas.

6. The technique of drying is very important. Use a separate, sterile towel for each arm, moving from fingertips to elbow using a dabbing action.

7. Discard the towel and repeat the procedure for the other arm.

8. When hands, wrists and forearms are thoroughly dry, the individual is ready to gown and glove.

Theatre gowns: The operating team should wear sterile gowns at surgery. Operating suite/operating room clothing should not be worn outside the operating room environment. Clothing contaminated with blood or body substances should be removed as soon as possible and bagged for laundering.

Surgical face mask: *All members of staff scrubbed and assisting at the operating table must wear fluid repellent high efficiency filter masks.* Wearing of masks by other members of staff not assisting the operation is not necessary. A fresh mask must be worn for each operation and care must be taken when the mask is discarded. It should be tied securely to cover the nose and mouth, and should be changed frequently.

Eye protection: Masks and protective eye wear or face shields should be worn during procedures which are likely to generate droplets of blood or body fluids to prevent exposure of the mucous membranes of the mouth, nose and eyes. Eye protection and face shields are essential to avoid blood splashes to the conjunctiva.

Gloves: Using gloves during surgery serves two purposes: it protects the surgical team from contamination by blood and exudates from the patient and prevents transfer of microorganisms from the surgeon's hands to patient. Single-use sterile disposable gloves should be used. They should not be washed or disinfected and re-used.

Hair/beard cover: All members of staff entering the theatre must wear their hair in a neat style. Long hair should be tied in such a way that when the head is bent forward, hair does not fall forward. Hair must be completely covered by a close fitting cap made of synthetic material. Beards should be fully covered by a mask and a hood of the balaclava type, which is tied securely at the neck.

Footwear: This should be enclosed and capable of protecting HCWs from accidentally dropped sharps and other contaminated items. If there is constant risk of spillage then ankle length, antistatic waterproof overboots should be worn. Open footwear must never be worn in the operating room.

Plastic overshoes: Plastic shoe covers can be replaced by ordinary shoes dedicated exclusively to the operating theatre as no difference exists in floor contamination whether personnel wear shoe covers or not.

Skin disinfection

It is essential that the operating site is well disinfected before incision. This is achieved by application of skin disinfectants, e.g. 70% ethanol or 60% isopropanol, preferably with 0.5% chlorhexidine or 10% povidone iodine. The use of antiseptic with alcohol increases the risk of burns to the patient during diathermy, especially if the alcohol is not allowed to dry and drapes are soaked with alcoholic disinfectant. Therefore, if *an alcohol preparation is used the area must be allowed to dry before operating.* Alternatively, 7.5% povidone iodine or 0.5% aqueous chlorhexidine may be used.

The *antiseptic skin preparation should be applied with friction in concentric circles moving away from the proposed incision site to the periphery* and well beyond the operation site to accommodate an extension to the incision or new incisions or drain site to be made.

Draping

To restrict the transfer of microorganisms to the wound and to protect the sterility of the instruments, equipment, supplies, and gloved hands of personnel, a sterile field must be established by placing sterile drapes around the wound. The use of plastic incisional adhesive drapes is controversial and is not associated with a reduction in infection rate. Sterile drapes used in operating rooms should be impervious. Drapes should incorporate systems for the containment of blood and irrigation fluids.

Wound drains

It is generally accepted that wound drains provide access for bacterial entry via colonization and hands. *Drains should not be used as an alternative to good haemostasis.* The closed system of wound drainage is indicated where drainage is essential; open wound drains are not considered appropriate.

Staff movement

Excessive presence and movement of staff contributes to an increase in airborne bacterial particles. Staff with bacterial skin infections may cause dispersal of *Staph. aureus* or *Streptococcus pyogenes*. Therefore it is advisable to **keep operating theatre staff to the essential minimum.** Additional personnel who wish to view the operation can be accommodated in surgical viewing suites, where available. *Staff with a boil or septic lesion of the skin or eczema colonized with Staph. aureus should not be allowed in the theatre.* The door to the operating room should be closed at all the times to avoid mixing corridor air with the operating room air, which would increase the number of microorganisms present.

Surgical technique

The skill of the surgeon has a central role in minimizing surgical wound infection. Bad surgical practice must not be 'covered up' with antibiotics. Expeditious surgery, gentle handling of tissue, reduction of blood loss or haematoma formation, elimination of dead tissue, debridement of devitalized tissue, removal of all purulent material by irrigation or suction, and removal of all foreign materials from the wound are essential to minimize surgical wound infections in all patients.

Duration of operation

There is a direct link between the length of the operation and the infection rate with a clean wound, which doubles every hour. This is because bacterial contamination increases over time and the operative tissues are damaged by drying and other surgical manipulations, i.e. use of retractor, diathermy, etc.

Post-operative factors

Wound dressing

Staff should be trained in the appropriate method of dressing the wound. Frequency of dressing should be kept to a minimum and dressings should not be opened for 48 h after the operation unless infection is suspected. The longer a wound is open, and the longer it is drained, the greater the risk of contamination.

Clean, undrained wounds seal within 48 h and are unlikely to be infected in the ward. Ward-acquired infection is less common than intra-operative infection and is often superficial. On the other hand, *theatre-acquired post-operative infections are usually deep-seated and often occur within 3 days of the operation or before the first dressing.* Many infections, particularly after prosthetic surgery, may not be recognized for weeks or months.

Post-operative stay

Avoid post-operative stay and overcrowding in the ward and discharge the patient as soon as possible. If this is necessary for medical reasons, keep the patient in a clean environment to protect them from colonization with bacteria from infected patients.

Other factors

In addition, the following practices do not reduce surgical wound infection:

- Provision of a transfer area in the operating theatre where patients are transferred from ward trolleys to clean operating room trolleys.

- *Routine microbiological sampling of the operating room or environment is not recommended* as inanimate objects and surfaces are seldom the cause of surgical wound infection. Settle plates used to evaluate air-borne contaminants are not useful for the same reason.

- *Routine screening of theatre personnel is not necessary,* unless an outbreak clearly links personnel to infected cases. Staff who are carriers/dispersers of *Staph. aureus* (including MRSA) or with septic lesions should not work in the theatre until the condition resolves.

- Scheduling 'dirty' cases at the end of the day is preferable but not necessary.

- *Using tacky mats and plastic overshoe* covers in operating rooms and other patient-care areas does little to minimize the overall degree of contamination of floors, and *has little impact on the incidence rate of nosocomial infections.*

Environmental cleaning of operating theatre

The floor of the operating theatre should be cleaned at the end of each session and scrubbed daily. *Routine use of disinfectant is not required* apart from their use in removal and disinfection of blood and other high-risk body fluids. Spillages on the floor should be disinfected and removed as soon as possible (see page 77). Walls and ceilings are rarely heavily contaminated and for general housekeeping purposes they should be cleaned twice a year. *Lint free cloth is recommended for all operating theatre cleaning.*

References and further reading

Agarwal M, Hamilton-Stewart P, Dixon RA. Contaminated operating room boots: the potential for infection. *American Journal of Infection Control* 2002; **30**: 179–183.

Alexander JW, Fischer JE, Boyajian M, *et al.* The influence of hair-removal methods on wound infections. *Archives of Surgery* 1983; **118**: 347–352.

Ayliffe GAJ. Role of environment of the operating suite in surgical wound infection. *Reviews of Infectious Diseases* 1991; **13** (Suppl. 10): S800–S804.

Belkin NL. The evolution of the surgical mask: filtering efficiency versus effectiveness. *Infection Control and Hospital Epidemiology* 1997; **18**: 49–57.

Bruce J, Russell EM, Mollison J, Krukowski ZH. The quality of measurement of surgical wound infection as the basis for monitoring: a systematic review. *Journal of Hospital Infection* 2001; **49**: 98–108.

Cruse PJE, Foord R. A five-year prospective study of 23,649 surgical wounds. *Archives of Surgery* 1973; **107**: 206–210.

Classen DC, Evans RS, Pestotnik SL, *et al.* The timing of prophylactic administration of antibiotics and the risk of surgical-wound infection. *New England Journal of Medicine* 1992; **326**: 281–286.

Cruse PJE, Ford R. The epidemiology of wound infections: a 10 year prospective study of 62,939 wounds. *Surgical Clinics of North America* 1980; **60**: 27–40.

Dharan S, Pittet D. Environmental controls in operating theatres. *Journal of Hospital Infection* 2002; **51**: 79–84.

Emmerson M. Environmental factors influencing infection. In: Taylor EW (ed), *Infection in Surgical Practice*. Oxford: Oxford University Press, 1992: 8–17.

Gaynes RP, Culver DH, Horan TC, *et al.* Surgical Site Infection (SSI) rates in the United States, 1992–1998: the NNIS basic risk index. *Clinical Infectious Diseases* 2001; **33** (Suppl. 2): S69–S77.

Greif R, Akça O, Horn E, Kurz A, Sessler DI. Supplemental perioperative oxygen to reduce the incidence of surgical wound infection. *The New England Journal of Medicine* 2000; **342**: 161–203.

Guaschino S, De Santo D, De Seta F. New perspectives in antibiotic prophylaxis for obstetric and gynaecological surgery. *Journal of Hospital Infection* 2002; **50** (Suppl. A): S13–S16.

Hall JC, Hall JL. Antibiotic prophylaxis for patients undergoing breast surgery. *Journal of Hospital Infection* 2000; **46**: 165–170.

Holton J, Ridgway GL. Commissioning operating theatres. *Journal of Hospital Infection* 1993; **23**: 153–160.

Hospital Infection Society Working Party report. Behaviours and rituals in the Operating Theatre. *Journal of Hospital Infection* 2002; **51**: 241–255.

Hospital Infection Society Working Party Report: *Microbiological commissioning and Monitoring of Operating theater suites*, http://www.his.org.uk

Holzheimer RG, Haupt W, Thiede A, Schwarzkopf A. The challenge of postoperative infections: does the surgeon make a difference? *Infection Control and Hospital Epidemiology* 1997; **18**: 449–456.

Horan TC, Gaynes RP, Martone WJ, *et al.* CDC definitions of surgical sites infections, 1992: a modification of the CDC definitions of wound infections. *American Journal of Infection Control* 1992; **20**: 271–274.

Humphreys H, Taylor EW. Operating theatre ventilation standards and the risk of postoperative infection. *Journal of Hospital Infection* 2002; **50**: 85–90.

Humphreys H, Marshall RJ, Ricketts UE, *et al.* Theatre over-shoes do not reduce theatre floor bacterial counts. *Journal of Hospital Infection* 1991; 17–125.

Labadie JC, Kampf G, Lejeune B, *et al.* European Guidelines. Recommendations for surgical hand disinfection – requirements, implementation and need for research. A proposal by representatives of the SFHH, DGHM and DGKH for a European discussion. *Journal of Hospital Infection* 2002; **51**: 312–315.

Mangram AJ, Horan TC, Pearson ML, Silver LC, Jarvis WR. Guideline for prevention of surgical site infection, 1999. *Infection Control and Hospital Epidemiology* 1999; **20**: 250–278.

Martone WJ, Nichols RL. Recognition, prevention, surveillance and management of surgical site infections: introduction to the problem and symposium overview. *Clinical Infectious Diseases* 2001; **33** (Suppl. 2): S67–S68.

Mitchell NJ, Hunt S. Surgical masks in modern operating-rooms – a costly and unnecessary ritual. *Journal of Hospital Infection* 1991; **18**: 239–242.

Platt R, Zaleznik DF, Hopkins CC, *et al.* Perioperative antibiotic prophylaxis for herniorrhaphy and breast surgery. *The New England Journal of Medicine* 1990; **322**: 153–160.

Romney MG. Surgical face masks in operating theatre: re-examining the evidence. *Journal of Hospital Infection* 2000; **47**: 251–256.

Roy M-C. The Operating Theatre: A Special Environment Area. In: Wenzel RP (ed), *Prevention and Control of Nosocomial Infections*, 3rd edn. Baltimore: Williams & Wilkins, 1997: 515–538.

Sanga G. New perspectives in antibiotic prophylaxis for intra-abdominal surgery. *Journal of Hospital Infection* 2001; **50** (Suppl. A): S17–S21.

Scottish Intercollegiate Guidelines Network. *Antibiotic Prophylaxis in Surgery*. Edinburgh: Sign Secretariat, 2000, www.sign.ac.uk

Seropian R, Reynolds BM. Wound infections after pre-operative depilatory versus razor preparation. *American Journal of Surgery* 1971; **121**: 251.

Smyth ETM, Emmerson AM. Surgical site infection surveillance. *Journal of Hospital Infection* 2000; **45**: 173–184.

Swedish-Norwegian Consensus Group. Antibiotic prophylaxis in surgery: summary of a Swedish-Norwegian Consensus Conference. *Scandinavian Journal of Infectious Diseases* 1998; **30**: 547–557.

Traore O, Eschapasse D, Laveran H. A bacteriological study of a contamination control tacky mat. *Journal of Hospital Infection* 1997; **36**: 158.

Tunevall TG. Post-operative wound infections and surgical masks: a controlled study. *World Journal of Surgery* 1991; **15**: 383–388.

UK Department of Health. Health Building Note 26. *Operating Departments*. London: HMSO, 1991.

UK Department of Health. NHS Estates. Health Technical Memorandum 2025. *Ventilation in Healthcare Premises*. London: HMSO, 1994.

Vandenbroucke-Grauls CMJE, Kluytmans JA. Prevention of postoperative wound infections: to cover up? *Infection Control and Hospital Epidemiology* 2001; **22**: 335–337.

Wenzel RP, Perl TM. The significance of nasal carriage of *Staphylococcus aureus* and the incidence of postoperative wound infection. *Journal of Hospital Infection* 1995; **31**: 13–24.

Woodhead K, Taylor EW, Bannister G, Chesworth T, Hoffman P, Humphreys H, Zanetti G, Platt R. Guidelines for perioperative antibiotic prophylaxis. In: Abrutyn E (ed), *Saunders Infection Control Reference Service*, 2nd edn. Philadelphia: WB Saunders, 2001: 315–320.

14

Prevention of Infection Associated with Intravenous Therapy

Indwelling intravenous (IV) lines are an integral part of patient care. They provide a route for administering fluids, blood products, nutrients and IV medications, for monitoring haemodynamic function, for maintaining emergency vascular access and obtaining blood specimens. Intravascular devices are usually inserted into veins but can, on occasion, be intra-arterial (e.g. for blood pressure monitoring). Most venous catheters are short (less than 5 cm) and are inserted into smaller peripheral veins in the arms. An increasing number of central venous catheters (CVCs) are now being inserted into larger veins of the body. CVCs are usually much longer (more than 15 cm) and remain in place for longer than peripheral venous catheters. Some CVCs may be inserted via a peripheral vein site and their tip is advanced until it is situated within a central vein.

Many patients with intravascular lines have serious underlying diseases, making them more susceptible to infections. Among other complications, catheter-related sepsis is one of the most important. The *risk of infection associated with these devices can be minimized by adherence to aseptic technique during and after catheter insertion.* In addition, since the risk of infection increases with the length of time of catheterization, intravascular catheters should be used only when absolutely necessary and *must be removed when no longer needed.*

Sources of infection (Fig. 14.1)

Intrinsic: Sources of contamination may be intrinsic, where the contamination occurs before use. This contamination is due to faulty sterilization of fluids which may occur during manufacturing. Contamination of infusion solutions is rare in developed countries but more often encountered in developing countries. The microorganisms are usually Gram-negative bacteria growing in the infusate, such as *Klebsiella* spp., *Enterobacter* spp. or *Pseudomonas* spp.

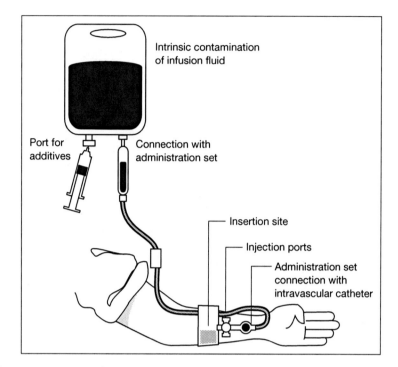

Figure 14.1 Points of access for microbial contamination in infusion therapy.

Extrinsic: The source of infection may be extrinsic (introduced during therapy) and can occur due to contamination of the intravascular catheter during the insertion, administration of the fluid or from the hands of the operator. However, the most important reservoirs of microorganisms causing catheter-related infection are the insertion site and the hub. The microorganisms are usually Gram-positive ones residing on the patient's skin, e.g. coagulase-negative staphylococci, occasionally *Staphylococcus aureus*, and less frequently diphtheroids. In addition, metastatic colonization from a distant site of infection (e.g. wound, lung, kidney) may occur.

Pathogenesis of infection

An intravascular catheter is a foreign body which produces a reaction in the host consisting of a film of fibrinous material (biofilm) on the inner and outer surfaces of the catheter (see Fig. 14.2). This biofilm may become colonized by microorganisms and will be protected from host defence mechanisms. Infection usually follows colonization of the biofilm causing local sepsis or septic thrombophlebitis. In some cases, the microorganisms grow in the biofilm on the catheter surfaces and may be released into the bloodstream causing systemic infection, e.g. bacteraemia or septicaemia.

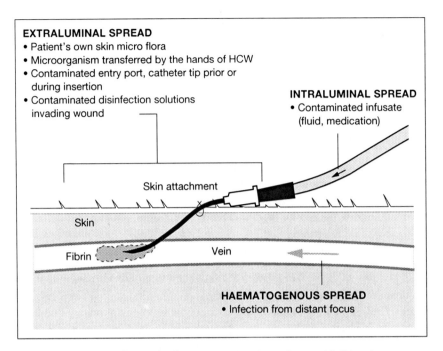

EXTRALUMINAL SPREAD
- Patient's own skin micro flora
- Microorganism transferred by the hands of HCW
- Contaminated entry port, catheter tip prior or during insertion
- Contaminated disinfection solutions invading wound

INTRALUMINAL SPREAD
- Contaminated infusate (fluid, medication)

Skin attachment

Skin

Fibrin

Vein

HAEMATOGENOUS SPREAD
- Infection from distant focus

Figure 14.2 Sources of microbial contamination in patients with IV catheter.
Reproduced with modification from Bennett JV, Brachman PS. *Hospital Infection* 3rd edn. Boston, Little Brown, 1992.

Education and training

The *intravascular catheter should be inserted by designated trained personnel with documented competence.* Adequate supervision must be provided for trainees who perform catheter insertion. Policies and procedures regarding the insertion and maintenance of intravascular access devices should be written and reviewed on a regular basis. These policies must be readily accessible.

Monitoring and surveillance of catheter-related infection

Catheter sites should be monitored visually or by palpation through on intact dressing on a regular basis for evidence of catheter-related complications (i.e. tenderness, thrombosis, swelling, or signs of inflammation or infection). The frequency of examination will depend on the clinical situation for the individual patient.

Semi-permeable adhesive dressings have the advantage of allowing inspection of the site without the removal of the dressing. If the patient has tenderness at the insertion site, fever without an obvious source, or other manifestations suggesting local or bloodstream infection, the dressing should be removed to allow thorough examination of the site. It is also important that patients should be encouraged to report any changes in their catheter site or any new discomfort.

It is essential that the surveillance of catheter-related infection should be conducted in high risk patients/areas, e.g. ICUs. The following strategies should be adopted to reduce catheter-related infections.

Intravascular catheters and parenteral solutions

Before use, intravascular catheter and parenteral solution *must be checked for expiry dates and the integrity of the packaging*. Parenteral fluid must be checked for macroscopic contamination and clarity of solution, e.g. visible turbidity, leaks, cracks, particulate matter. *Do not use any solutions if they are not clear* or if the manufacturer's expiry date has passed. *Sterile packs and parenteral solutions must be stored in a clean area and condition to avoid damage.*

Use single-dose vials for parenteral additives or medications whenever possible. If multidose vials are used, make sure that they are refrigerated after they have been opened, if recommended by the manufacturer. The access diaphragm of multidose vials should be cleaned with 70% alcohol before inserting a device into a vial. Do not touch the diaphragm after it has been disinfected. Multidose vials should be discarded if their sterility is compromised.

Selection of catheter type

Polyurethane and silicone catheters have a lower risk of complication than other types. The use of an antimicrobial/antiseptic impregnated CVC should be considered for the following adult patients who require short term (<10 days) catheterization:

- If, despite full adherence to maximum infection control precautions, there is still a high rate (>3.3/1000 catheter days) of catheter-related sepsis.

- In patients who are expected to be at high risk, e.g. patients that are receiving total parenteral nutrition, neutropenics and patients in ICU.

When prolonged IV access via a CVC is likely, catheters such as the Hickman type, which have a cuff and are tunnelled subcutaneously, should be used because they are associated with a lower rate of sepsis than standard CVCs. Totally implantable access devices should be considered for patients who require long-term, intermittent vascular access.

Single-lumen CVCs should be used unless multiple ports are essential for the management of the patient. If total parenteral nutrition is being administered, use one CVC or lumen exclusively for that purpose. Select a catheter with a smaller lumen than that of the vessel to be entered to reduce the incidence of trauma and secondary infection.

Selection of insertion site

Select the insertion site and technique with the lowest risk of complications, both infectious and non-infectious. *Do not routinely use the cutdown procedure* as a method of inserting catheters. The catheter *should not be inserted into an area of inflammation or infection.* Use of steel needles for the administration of fluids and medication should be avoided because it may cause tissue necrosis if extravasation occurs.

Peripheral intravascular lines: In adults, use an upper extremity site in preference to a lower extremity for catheter insertion. Replace a catheter inserted in a lower extremity site with one in an upper extremity site as soon as it is feasible. In paediatric patients, insert catheters into a scalp, hand or foot site in preference to a leg, arm or antecubital fossa site.

Central venous catheter (CVC): Subclavian rather than jugular or femoral sites should be selected for catheter insertion of CVCs unless medically contraindicated. Tunnelled catheters or implantable vascular access devices (e.g. Porta-A-Cath) should be used for patients who require long-term (>30 days) vascular access.

Once the catheter is inserted, it is essential that the device must be stabilized with tape to reduce catheter movement. This helps to prevent potential complications such as phlebitis, subcutaneous infiltration or sepsis. The date and time of insertion should be documented in a standardized fashion, e.g. patient's progress notes, care plans, etc.

Aseptic techniques

Adherence to aseptic techniques during catheter insertion and later during catheter manipulation is essential to reduce the risk of infection. Intravascular catheter teams should be appointed consisting of highly trained staff to ensure stringent adherence to aseptic techniques. Admix to all parenteral fluids should be carried out (preferably in the pharmacy) in a laminar-flow hood using an aseptic technique.

Hand hygiene: Hands must be disinfected prior to catheter insertion using either conventional antiseptic hand preparation or waterless alcohol-based hand disinfection. Hand hygiene must be observed before and after insertion, before and after palpation of catheter sites, as well as before and after replacing or dressing an intravascular catheter. Remember that the use of gloves does not obviate the need for hand hygiene.

Cutaneous antiseptic: Skin should be disinfected using an appropriate antiseptic before catheter insertion and at the time of dressing changes. A 2% chlorhexidine or 0.5% alcholic chlorhexidine based preparation is preferred. Alternately, tincture of iodine, an iodophor or an alcoholic povidone-iodine solution should be used for patients with a history of chlorhexidine sensitivity. Before inserting the catheter, the

Procedure for insertion of peripheral IV lines

Ensure that the patient is in a comfortable position and aware of the nature of the procedure as this will reduce anxiety. Avoid shaving the skin site; use hair clipper instead.

Procedure

- Collect all necessary equipment.

- Operator should use an alcohol rub or antiseptic detergent to disinfect hands or wash hands thoroughly for 20 s, if antiseptic is not available.

- Dry hands thoroughly on a paper towel or clean linen towel, unless alcohol is used.

- Select an appropriate site, avoiding bony prominences and joints.

- Disinfect intravascular insertion skin site with 0.5% alcoholic chlorhexidine, or 10% alcoholic povidone-iodine, or 70% isopropyl alcohol impregnated swab for at least 30 s prior to venepuncture. Allow the insertion site to dry before inserting the catheter.

- The venepuncture site should not be touched once the vein has been selected and the skin prepared. **Do not touch the shaft of the catheter with the fingers during insertion.**

- Select a catheter that will fit easily into the vein. The correct sized catheter reduces trauma and congestion of the vein.

- Insert the catheter as swiftly and as aseptically as possible using a 'no touch' technique. Do not attempt repeated insertions with the same catheter. Seek help from a senior colleage. If the first insertion is not successful the procedure should be repeated with a new catheter.

- Look out for flashback of blood and then advance the catheter slowly.

- Apply sterile dressing (gauze or equivalent, or clear semi-permeable).

- Secure catheter to avoid movement.

- Label the site with the insertion date.

- Connect up the IV administration set.

- Clean around the site with a 70% isopropyl alcohol impregnated swab.

- Ensure that all sharps are safely discarded into a sharps bin.

- Wash and dry hands.

Procedure for insertion of central venous catheter

The insertion of a CVC is an aseptic procedure. The hands must be washed with an antiseptic detergent hand wash preparation. Sterile gloves, gowns and mask should be worn. Use large sterile drapes to cover the area.

- Collect all necessary equipment.
- Wash hands using an antiseptic-detergent or an alcohol hand rub.
- Disinfect intravascular skin insertion site with 0.5% alcoholic chlorhexidine, or 10% alcoholic povidone-iodine with friction for at least 2–3 min prior to venepuncture.
- Allow the insertion site to dry before inserting the catheter.
- Surround the site with large sterile drapes.
- Insert the CVC as swiftly as possible, maintaining a 'no touch' technique throughout the procedure.
- Blood should be aspirated freely to ensure that the catheter is in a vascular space before injecting fluid. Position of CVP lines must be checked by X-ray.
- Leave the site clean and dry after insertion.
- Secure the catheter with an appropriate sterile or clear semi-permeable dressing.
- Label the site with insertion date. Record insertion date in the patient's medical notes.
- Connect up the IV administration set.
- Ensure that all sharps are safely discarded into a sharps bin.
- Wash and dry hands.

antiseptic preparation should be allowed to remain on the insertion site till it dries. If povidone iodine is used then it should remain on the skin for at least 2 min or longer if it is not yet dry before inserting the catheter. Application of organic solvent (e.g. acetone or ether) to the skin before insertion of catheters or during dressing change should be avoided.

Intravascular injection ports: Before accessing the system, intravascular injection ports should be disinfected with a 70% isopropyl alcohol impregnated swab or an iodophor. They should always be kept clean and dry. Put a cap on all stopcocks when not in use.

Catheter site dressing regimens

Sterile dressings should be used to cover the catheter site. Either a gauze or sterile transparent semi-permeable dressing should be used. If the site is bleeding or oozing, a gauze dressing is preferred. Well-healed tunnelled CVC sites may not require dressings.

The catheter site dressing should be replaced when the dressing becomes damp, loosened, or soiled, or when inspection of the site is necessary. Clean or sterile gloves must be worn when changing the dressing on intravascular catheters.

The dressing should be changed on a regular basis for adult and adolescent patients; the frequency of such changes must be determined individually depending on the circumstances. For short term CVC, the gauze dressing should be replaced every 2 days and the transparent dressings every 7 days, except in paediatric patients because in these patients, the risk of dislodging the catheter outweighs the benefit of changing the dressing. For tunnelled or implanted catheters, the dressing should be replaced no more than once per week, until the insertion site is healed. The frequency of catheter dressing change over a well-healed site is an unresolved issue.

In-line filters

In-line filters reduce the incidence of infusion-related phlebitis but there are no data to support their efficacy in preventing infections associated with intravascular therapy. Manufacturer's claim the following potential benefits of in-line filters:

- Reduce the risk of phlebitis in patients who require high doses of medication or in patients in whom infusion-related phlebitis has already occurred.

- Reduce the risk of infection from contaminated infusate or proximal contamination (i.e. introduced proximal to the filter).

- Remove particulate matter that may contaminate intravascular fluids.

- Filter endotoxin produced by Gram-negative organisms in contaminated infusate.

However, infusate-related sepsis can be minimized if most of the medications or infusates are carried out in the pharmacy under aseptic conditions. Furthermore, in-line filters may become blocked, especially with certain solutions (i.e. dextran, lipids, mannitol), thereby increasing the number of line manipulations and decreasing the availability of administered drugs. Thus, for the purpose of reducing catheter-related sepsis, the use of in-line filters is not recommended.

Antimicrobial prophylaxis

Topical antimicrobial ointments should not be used routinely prior to insertion or as part of routine catheter site care because of their potential to promote fungal infections and antimicrobial resistance. Routine use of intranasal antibiotic ointment, antibiotic lock solutions or systemic antimicrobial prophylaxis before insertion or during use of an intravascular catheter as a method to prevent catheter-related sepsis is also not recommended.

Anticoagulant flush solutions

Anticoagulant flush solutions are widely used to prevent catheter thrombosis. Since thrombi and fibrin-deposits on catheters may serve as a nidus for microbial colonization of intravascular catheters, the use of anticoagulants may have a role in the prevention of catheter-related sepsis.

Replacement of intravascular set, tubings and parenteral fluids

Administration sets, including secondary sets and add-on devices should be replaced no more frequently than at 96 h interval unless catheter-related sepsis is suspected or documented or when the integrity of the product has been compromised.

IV tubing used to administer blood, blood products, or lipid emulsions should be replaced at the end of the infusion or within 24 h of initiating the infusion. Lipid emulsion infusion should be completed within 24 h and blood within 4 h of hanging.

Replacement of catheters

The peripheral venous catheters should be removed if the patient develops signs of phlebitis (i.e. warmth, tenderness, erythema, palpable venous cord), infection, or a malfunctioning catheter. In adults, rotate peripheral venous sites every 96 h to minimize the risk of phlebitis. In paediatric patients, leave peripheral venous catheters in place until IV therapy is completed, unless a complication occurs.

Do not routinely replace CVCs or arterial catheters solely for the purpose of reducing the incidence of infection. Replacement of CVCs is necessary if the patient is haemodynamically unstable and catheter-related sepsis is suspected.

Any catheter inserted when adherence to proper asepsis is not ensured (i.e. those inserted in an emergency) should be removed and re-sited at the earliest opportunity, preferably within 48 h. Use clinical judgement to determine when to replace a catheter that could be a source of infection. Do not routinely replace catheters in patients whose only indication is fever. Venous catheters do not necessarily need to be replaced routinely in patients who are bacteraemic or fungaemic if the source of infection is unlikely to be the catheter.

Guidewire exchange

Guidewire technique to replace catheters for which there is a clinical suspicion for catheter-related infection is not recommended. If continued vascular access is required, remove the implicated catheter, and replace it with another catheter at a different insertion site.

If catheter-related infection is suspected, but there is no evidence of infection at the catheter site, remove the existing catheter and insert a new catheter over the guide wire. If catheter-related infection is confirmed, the newly inserted catheter should be removed and, if still required, a new catheter inserted at a different site.

Guidewire exchange can be used to replace a malfunctioning non-tunnelled catheter if there is no evidence of infection and the risk of inserting a new catheter into a new site is unacceptably high, e.g. due to obesity or coagulopathy. A new set of sterile gloves should be used prior to handling the new catheter when guidewire exchanges are performed.

Catheter-related infections

Blood cultures, preferably two sets from peripheral veins, should be taken. Swabs should be taken from the site of catheter insertion. If microbiological investigation proves catheter infection then the catheter should be removed and an alternative site chosen for re-insertion. *In cases of proven catheter-related sepsis, the catheter should be removed* and treated with appropriate antibiotics. The choice of antibiotic will depend on the sensitivity of the microorganisms. If the catheter is removed, then the distal end of the catheter should be sent in a sterile container for culture. If there is a strong suspicion of infection, the line should be removed. *Routine bacteriological sampling of catheter tips is not necessary.*

Device reprocessing

Intravascular devices are single-use only and must not be reprocessed. The narrow hollow lumens of catheters cannot be satisfactorily cleaned. In addition, the physical characteristics of the plastic may not withstand cleaning and sterilizing. These items, together with solution containers, are manufactured for single use only and must not be reused.

References and further reading

Abi-Said D, Raad I, Umphrey J, *et al.* Infusion therapy team and dressing changes of central venous catheters. *Infection Control and Hospital Epidemiology* 1999; **20**: 101–105.

Arnow PM, Quimosing EM, Beach M. Consequences of intravascular catheter sepsis. *Clinical Infectious Diseases* 1993; **16**: 778–784.

Cook D, Randolph A, Kemerman P, *et al.* Central venous catheter replacement: Strategies: a systematic review of the literature. *Critical Care Medicine* 1997; **25**: 1417–1424.

Crnich C, Maki DG. The promise of novel technology for the prevention of intravascular device-related bloodstream infection. II. – Long-term devices. *Clinical Infectious Diseases* 2002; **34**: 1362–1368.

Crump JA, Collignon PJ. Intravascular catheter-associated infections. *European Journal of Clinical Microbiology and Infectious Diseases* 2000; **19**: 1–8.

Dobbins B, Kite P, Wilcox MH. Diagnosis of central venous catheter related sepsis – a critical look inside. *Journal of Clinical Pathology* 1999; **52**: 165–172.

Eggimann P, Harbarth S, Constantin M-N, *et al.* Impact of a prevention strategy targeted at vascular-access care on incidence of infections acquired in intensive care. *Lancet* 2000; **355**: 1864–1868.

Elliott TSJ, Faroqui MH, Armstrong RF, Hanson GC. Guidelines for good practice in central venous catheterization. *Journal of Hospital Infection* 1994; **28**(3): 163–176.

Farr B. Preventing vascular catheter-related infections: current controversies. *Clinical Infectious Diseases* 2001; **33**: 1733–1738.

Goldmann DA, Pier GB. Pathogenesis of infection related to intravascular catheterization. *Clinical Microbiology Reviews* 1993; **6**: 176–192.

Goetz AM, Wagener MM, Miller JIM, Muder RR. Risk of infection due to central venous catheters: effect of site of placement and catheter type. *Infection Control and Hospital Epidemiology* 1998; **19**: 842–845.

Hospital Infection Control Practices Advisory Committee. Intravascular device-related infections. *American Journal of Infection Control* 1996; **24**: 262–293.

Infection Control Nurses Association. *Guidelines for preventing intravascular catheter-related infection.* UK: Infection Control Nurses Association, 2001.

Mado M, Martin CR, Turner C, *et al.* A randomized trial comparing Arglaes (a transparent containing silver ions) to Tegaderm (a transparent polyurethane dressing) for peripheral catheters and central venous catheters. *Intensive Critical Care Nursing* 1998; **14**: 187–191.

Maki DG, Weise CE, Sarafin HW. A semiquantitative culture method for identifying intravenous catheter-related infection. *New England Journal of Medicine* 1977; **296**: 1305–1309.

Maki DG. Infections due to infusion therapy. In: Bennet JV, Brachman PS (eds), *Hospital Infections*, 3rd edn. Boston: Little Brown; 1993: 849–898.

Maki DG. Pathogenesis, prevention, and management of infections due to intravascular devices used for infusion therapy. In: Bisno AL, Waldvogel FA (eds), *Infections associated with indwelling medical devises*. Washington DC: American Society for Microbiology, 1989.

Mermel LA, Farr BM, Sherertz RJ, *et al.* Guidelines for the management of intravascular catheter-related infections. *Infection Control and Hospital Epidemiology* 2001; **222**: 222–242.

Munder RR. Frequency of intravenous administration set changes and bacteremia: defining the risk. *Infection Control and Hospital Epidemiology* 2001; **22**: 134–135.

Raad I. Intravascular catheter-related infections. *Lancet* 1998; **351**: 893–898.

Raad I, Hanna HA. Intravascular catheter-related infections: New Horizons and recent advances. *Archive of Internal Medicine* 2002; **162**: 871–878.

UK Department of Health. Guidelines for preventing the infections associated with the insertion and maintenance of central venous catheters. *Journal of Hospital Infection* **47**(Suppl.): S47–S67.

Veenstra DI, Saint S, Sullivan SO. Cost-effectiveness of antiseptic impregnated central venous catheters for the prevention of catheter-related bloodstream infection. *Journal of American Medical Association* 1999; **282**: 554–560.

Ward V, Wilson J, Taylor L, Cookson B, Glynn A. Guidelines for the prevention of infection associated with central intravascular devices. In: *Preventing Hospital Acquired Infection: Clinical Guidelines*. London: Public Health Laboratory Services, 1997.

Widmer AF. Intravenous-Related Infections. In: Wenzel RP (ed), *Prevention and Control of Nosocomial Infections*, 3rd edn. Baltimore: Williams & Wilkins, 1997: 771–805.

15

Prevention of Infections Associated with Urinary Catheterization

It has been estimated that about 10% of hospitalized patients require urinary catheterization. Urinary tract infections (UTI) following catheterization or other instrumentation are the most common hospital-acquired infections, accounting for approximately 30–40% of all nosocomial infections. The risk of acquiring bacteriuria increases with time, from approximately 5% per day during the first week of hospitalization to nearly 100% in 4 weeks. It has been estimated that 1–4% of bacteriuric patients will ultimately develop clinically significant bacteraemia with a case fatality of 13–30%. Therefore, it is important that *urinary catheterization should be avoided, if possible*, and only be used when there is a clear medical indication. They *should not be used solely for the management of urinary incontinence*. Regular review should be carried out regarding the patient's clinical need for continuing urinary catheterization. *The catheter should be removed as soon as possible*, preferably within 5 days. Alternatives to indwelling catheters are intermittent catheterization with an associated infection risk ranging from 0.5–8%.

Consideration prior to catheterization

Urethral catheterization should be considered as a minor surgical procedure. Therefore *urinary catheters must be inserted using an aseptic technique and sterile equipment*. Before the procedure, efficient and effective cleaning of the area and surfaces involved should be undertaken. *Aseptic technique should be maintained throughout the procedure*. The administration of systemic antibiotics at the time of catheter insertion is not recommended (see page 278–279). Only a closed urinary drainage system should be used. It has been estimated that the risk of infection can be reduced from 97% when an open system is used to between 8–15% when a sterile, continuously closed system is employed.

Before the procedure, check the expiry dates, the integrity of containers or packaging and the correct amount of sterile water required to be inserted if the device has a balloon.

Prior to insertion, the procedure must be explained to the patients to allay any fear and anxiety they may have.

Catheter material

Choice of catheter material will depend on clinical experience, patient preference and the anticipated duration of catheterization. Latex catheters are the least expensive, but irritation and allergic reaction may occur. Silicone catheters are comfortable and may be a better choice for long-term catheterization. Silicone catheters obstruct less often than latex, Teflon, or silicone coated latex in patients prone to encrustation. Catheters coated with silver alloy (but not silver oxide) should be considered for patients at high risk of developing of catheter-associated bacteriuria. However, the particular type of catheter material does not influence the incidence of catheter-associated infection in the short term (<4 days).

Catheter size

Catheter size/gauge relates to the circumference of the catheter. Larger diameter catheters block the urethral gland and put pressure on the urethral mucosa, which may result in ischaemic necrosis. They are also resistant to bending and are more likely to cause pressure necrosis, especially in males. In general, the smallest diameter catheter (with a 10 ml balloon) that allows free flow of urine is the most desirable. The smallest size/gauge catheter is also less likely to be associated with leakage. Urological patients may require larger diameter catheters and these must be used at the advice of the urologist.

Maintenance of catheter

After insertion, regular inspection of the catheter and drainage system must be attended to and documented at least daily; the date and time of catheter changes should be documented either in nursing or medical notes.

Meatal care

Meatal cleansing should be performed at intervals appropriate for keeping the meatus free of encrustations and contamination. *Meatal cleansing with antiseptic solutions is not necessary.* Applying antimicrobial ointment to the urethral meatus has not reliably been shown to reduce the incidence of UTI. Daily routine bathing or showering is all that is needed to maintain meatal hygiene. If faecal incontinence occurs, the perineum must be cleaned and the catheter changed without delay.

Drainage bag

Reflux of urine is associated with infection. Therefore it is important that the sterile *drainage bags should be positioned in a way that prevents back-flow of urine.* The urinary drainage bags should be put on a holder attached to the bed frame or a

Procedure for urinary catheterization

Catheters must be inserted using an aseptic technique and sterile equipment. The procedure must be explained to the patient to allay fear and anxiety. Aseptic technique should be maintained throughout the procedure.

1. All equipment used must be sterile. Lay out the top of the trolley making sure all items required are open and accessible.

2. Hands must be washed thoroughly with an antiseptic hand wash preparation.

3. Sterile gloves must be worn and a 'no-touch' aseptic technique should be used. A second pair of gloves should be available should contamination occur.

4. The peri-urethral area should be thoroughly cleaned. Wiping motions should be carried out from *front to back* to avoid faecal bacteria being transported to the urinary meatus. This cleaning should be done using sterile water and saline and then dried. In a male, grasp the distal shaft of the penis and retract the foreskin. Cleanse the glans with a disinfectant/detergent preparation. In a female, separate the labia and cleanse the vulva using front to back technique. Use antiseptic solution to clean the urethral meatus prior to the insertion of the catheter.

5. Single-use sachets of sterile (water-soluble) lubricant should be used on the catheter prior to urethral insertion to reduce friction and trauma to meatus. Alternatively sterile anaesthetic (1–2% lignocaine) gel can be instilled into the urethra to minimize pain. If anaesthetic gel is used, allow 3–5 min for it to take anaesthetic effect before catheterization.

6. Gently insert the catheter and advance it by holding the inner sterile sleeve, avoiding contact with non-sterile surfaces. Ideally, the 'no-touch' technique should be used in which the operator has no contact with the sterile shaft of the catheter.

7. Inflate the balloon by instilling the manufacturer's recommended amount of sterile water. If the site is to be dressed (e.g. supra pubic) the dressings surrounding the device must be sterile.

8. Connect catheters to a sterile, closed urinary drainage system.

9. Hang drainage bag below the level of the bed to stop reflux. The bag must be supported in the drainage stand to allow free flow of urine and prevent the bag from touching the floor.

10. Secure the catheter to the patient's thigh or abdomen to prevent movement and urethral meatal ulceration.

11. Hands should be washed after gloves are removed.

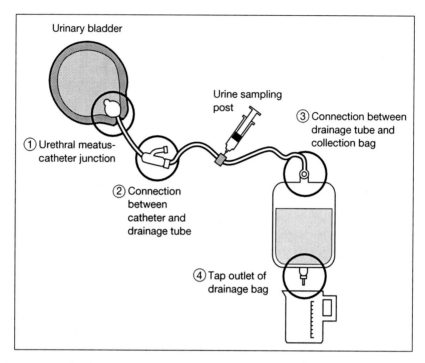

Figure 15.1 The four main sites through which bacteria may reach the bladder of a patient with an indwelling urethral catheter. The recommended measures of prevention are listed in Table 15.1.

stand to prevent contact with the floor. The *bag and tubing must at all times be below the level of the bladder* so that flow can be continuously maintained by gravity. Where dependent drainage cannot be maintained, e.g. during moving and handling, clamp the urinary drainage bag tube and remove the clamp as soon as dependent drainage can be resumed. *Routine use of antiseptics (e.g. chlorhexidine and hydrogen peroxide) in the drainage bag is not recommended,* as they do not reduce the incidence of bacteriuria.

Emptying the drainage bag

The drainage bag should be emptied regularly (i.e. 8 hourly or earlier if it fills rapidly) via the drainage tap at the bottom of the bag to maintain urine flow and to prevent reflux. The spout from the tap must be completely emptied to minimize a build-up of organisms in the stagnant urine. Extreme care must be taken when emptying the drainage bag to prevent cross-infection. *Hands must be disinfected and non-sterile disposable gloves must be worn before emptying each bag.* Alcohol impregnated swabs may be used to decontaminate the outlet (inside and outside) before and after emptying the bag. When the bag is empty, the tap should be closed securely and wiped with a tissue. If the bag does not have a tap, replace it when full

Table 15.1 Prevention of bacterial colonization/infection of the bladder in patients with indwelling urethral catheters.

Entry points for bacteria	Preventative measures
1. External urethral meatus and urethra Bacteria carried into bladder during insertion of catheter	• Pass catheter when bladder full for wash-out effect. • Before catheterization prepare urinary meatus with an antiseptic (e.g. povidone iodine or 0.2% chlorhexidine aqueous solution). • Inject single-use sterile lubricant gel (e.g. 1–2%) lignocaine into urethra and hold there for 3 min before inserting catheter. • Use sterile catheter. • Use non-touch technique for insertion.
Ascending colonization/infection up urethra around outside of catheter	• Keep peri-urethral area clean and dry. • Secure catheter to prevent movement in urethra; bladder washes and ointments are of no value. • After faecal incontinence clean area and change catheter.
2. Junction between catheter and drainage tube (when disconnected)	• Do not disconnect catheter unless absolutely necessary. • Always use aseptic technique for irrigation. • For urine specimen collection disinfect outside of catheter proximal to junction with drainage tube by applying alcoholic impregnated wipe and allow it to dry completely then aspirate urine with a sterile needle and syringe.
3. Junction between drainage tube and collection bag Disconnection	• Drainage tube should be welded to inlet of bag during manufacture.
Reflux from bag into tube	• Drip chamber or non-return valve at inlet to bag. • Keep bag below level of bladder. If it is necessary to raise collection bag above bladder level for a short period, drainage tube must be clamped temporarily. • Empty bag every 8 h or earlier if full. • Do not hold bag upside down when emptying.
4. Tap at bottom of collection bag Emptying of bag	• Collection bag *must* never touch floor. • Always wash or disinfect hands (e.g. with 70% alcohol) before and after opening tap. • Use a separate disinfected jug to collect urine from each bag. • Routine instillation of disinfectant into bag after each emptying is of no value.

Modified from Brumfitt W, Hamilton-Miller JMT, Bailey RR: *Urinary Tract Infections*. London: Chapman & Hall Medical, 1998.

using an aseptic technique. Do not reconnect a used bag. *Wash and dry hands thoroughly after touching the drainage bag.*

When emptying the drainage bag, use a separate container for each patient and avoid contact between the urinary drainage tap and the container. *Each bag should be emptied separately as required.* For the purposes of measuring urinary output, an integral measuring device is necessary. *The urine receptacle should be heat disinfected and stored dry after each use.* Single-use disposable receptacles may be used. After emptying the receptacle, gloves should be discarded and hands washed and dried thoroughly.

Bladder irrigation

Routine bladder irrigation or washout with antiseptics (e.g. chlorhexidine) or antimicrobial agents does not prevent catheter-associated infection and should not be used. Introduction of such agents causes erosion of the bladder mucosa and promotes the emergence of resistant microorganisms. They may also cause damage to the catheter. If the catheter becomes obstructed and can be kept open only by frequent irrigation, the catheter should be changed, as it is likely that the catheter itself is contributing to obstruction. However, continuous or intermittent bladder irrigation may be indicated during urological surgery or to manage catheter obstruction and should be undertaken on the advice of a urologist.

Specimen collection

Obtain urine samples from a sampling port. *Do not disconnect the drainage bag to obtain a sample* as this causes interruption to the closed drainage system and may pose a risk of infection to the patient. If a sample of urine is required for bacteriological examination, it should be obtained from a sampling port or sleeve using an aseptic technique. *Do not obtain a sample for bacteriological culture from the drainage bag.* The sampling port must first be disinfected by wiping with a 70% isopropyl alcohol impregnated swab. The sample may then be aspirated using a sterile small bore needle and syringe and transferred into a sterile container. Routine bacteriological testing is not cost-effective.

Removal of catheter

The optimal time limit for replacing catheters depends upon individual circumstances and the type of catheter used. However, urinary catheters should not be changed as long as they are functioning well. A catheter that requires frequent irrigation for recurrent obstruction should be changed and replaced.

Use of antimicrobial agents

The administration of systemic antibiotics at the time of catheter insertion may provide early benefit to prevent catheter-associated infections but it also exposes the patient to a risk of antibiotic associated toxicity and subsequent development of infections with resistant bacterial strains. Therefore, *routine administration of prophylactic antibiotic in catheterized patients is not recommended*. It may be reserved for patients who are at a high risk of developing infection.

Long-term antibiotic prophylaxis is ineffective and predisposes to infection with resistant microorganisms and fungi. Treatment of asymptomatic bacteriuria (i.e. significant bacteriuria in the absence of clinical symptoms) in patients who require continued catheterization is also not indicated. *Treat patients with antibiotics only if there is evidence of clinical infection.* Treatment of catheter-associated UTI in patients with long-term catheters may be difficult without removal or changing of the catheter because bacteria are embedded in the biofilm (or encrustation) on the surface of the catheter and may be protected from the action of antibiotics. In addition, the *use of an antibiotic in the presence of the catheter often results in infection with a more resistant strain of bacteria*. After the catheter is removed, in most patients the bacteriuria spontaneously resolves; if treatment is indicated, it is only for those cases in which the bacteriuria has persisted after catheter removal and in which there are no underlying anatomical or physiological barriers to eradication of the bacteriuria.

Routine administration of prophylactic antibiotic at the time of catheter removal is not recommended. Culturing of urine sampled after catheter removal is indicated only for patients where there is a high degree of suspicion or symptoms suggestive of infection.

Policy and staff training

Catheterization is an aseptic procedure. *Ensure that health care personnel are trained and competent to carry out urethral catheterization.* Policies and procedures regarding the insertion, maintenance and changing regimes of indwelling urinary devices should be written and reviewed and updated on a regular basis. These policies should be readily accessible.

Regular education as well as orientation programmes should be implemented to include instruction on the importance and principles of catheterization and the care of the patient with indwelling urinary devices.

Re-use of catheters

Indwelling urinary catheters have narrow hollow lumens and cannot satisfactorily be cleaned. Also, the physical characteristics of the latex or plastics may not withstand cleaning and resterilizing. *These items, together with drainage/collection systems, are manufactured for single use only and must not be reused.*

References and further reading

Ball AJ, Carr TW, Gillespie WA, Kelly M, Simpson RA, Smith PJ. Bladder irrigation with chlorhexidine for the prevention of urinary infection after transurethral operations: a prospective controlled study. *Journal of Urology* 1987; **138**: 491–494.

Burke JP, Garibaldi RA, Britt MR. Prevention of catheter-associated urinary tract infections. Efficacy of daily meatal care regimens. *The American Journal of Medicine* 1981; **70**: 655–658.

Classen DC, Larsen RA, Burke JP, Alling DW, Stevens LE. Daily meatal care for the prevention of catheter-associated bacteriuria: results using frequent applications of poly-antibiotic cream. *Infection Control and Hospital Epidemiology* 1991; **12**: 157–162.

Classen DC, Larsen RA, Burke JP, Stevens LE. Prevention of catheter-associated bacteriuria: clinical trial of methods to block three known pathways of infection. *American Journal of Infection Control* 1991; **19**: 136–142.

Davies AJ, Desai HN, Turton S, Dyas A. Does instillation of chlorhexidine into the bladder of catheterized geriatric patients help reduce bacteriuria? *Journal of Hospital Infection* 1987; **9**: 72–75.

Desautels RF, Walter CW, Graves RC, Harrison JH. Technical advances in the prevention of urinary tract infection. *Journal of Urology* 1962; **87**: 487–490.

Deckhouse KD, Garibaldi RA. Prevention of Catheter-Associated Urinary Tract Infections. In: Abrutytn E, Goldmann DA, Scheckler WE (eds), *Saunders Infection Control Reference Service*, 2nd edn. Philadelphia: WB Saunders Co., 2001: 257–262.

Falkiner FR. The insertion and management of indwelling urethral catheter-minimizing the risk of infection. *Journal of Hospital Infection* 1993; **25**: 79–90.

Garibaldi RA, Burke JP, Dickman ML, Smith CB. Factors predisposing to bacteriuria during indwelling urethral catheterization. *New England Journal of Medicine* 1974; **291**: 215–218.

Gillespie WA, Lennon GG, Linton KB, Slade N. Prevention of urinary infections in gynaecology. *British Medical Journal* 1964; **2**: 423–425.

Gillespie WA, Simpson RA, Jones JE, *et al.* Does the addition of disinfect to urine drainage bags prevent infection in catheterised patients? *Lancet* 1983; **1**: 1037–1039.

Johnson JR, Roberts PL, Olsen RJ, Moyer KA, Stamm WE. Prevention of catheter-associated urinary tract infection with a silver oxide-coated urinary catheter: clinical and microbiologic correlates. *Journal of Infectious Diseases* 1990; **162**: 1145–1150.

Kunin CM. *Urinary Tract Infections: Detection, Prevention, and Management*, 5th edn. Baltimore: Williams & Wilkins; 1997: 249–250.

Kunin CM, McCormack RC. Prevention of catheter-induced urinary tract infections by sterile closed drainage. *New England Journal of Medicine* 1966; **274**: 1155–1162.

Liedberg H, Lundeberg T. Silver alloy coated catheters reduce catheter-associated bacteriuria. *British Journal of Urology* 1990; **65**: 379–381.

Liedberg H, Lundeberg T, Ekman P. Refinements in the coating of urethral catheters reduces the incidence of catheter-associated bacteriuria. An experimental and clinical study. *European Urology* 1990; **17**: 236–240.

Nicolle LE. The SHEA Long Long-Term-Care facilities. Urinary Tract Infections in Long-Term-Care facilities. *Infection Control and Hospital Epidemiology* 2001; **167**: 167–175.

Olson ES, Cookson BD. Do antimicrobial have a role in preventing septicaemia following instrumentation of the urinary tract? *Journal of Hospital Infection* 2000; **45**: 85–97.

Pearman JW. Catheter care. In: Brumfitt R, Hamilton-Miller JMT, Baily RR (eds), *Urinary Tract Infections*. London: Chapman & Hall Medical, 1998: 303–316.

Riley DK, Classen DC, Stevens LE, Burke JP. A large randomised clinical trial of a silver-impregnated urinary catheter: lack of efficacy and staphylococcal super infection. *American Journal of Medicine* 1995; **98**: 349–356.

Saint S, Elmore JG, Sullivan SD, Emerson SS, Koepsell TD. The efficacy of sliver alloy-coated urinary catheters in preventing urinary tract infection: A meta-analysis. *American Journal of Medicine* 1998; **105**: 236–241.

Saint S, Lipsky BA. Preventing catheter-related bacteriuria. Should we? Can we? How? *Archives of Internal Medicine* 1999; **159**: 800–808.

Schneeberger PM, Vreede RW, Bogdanowicz JF, van Dijk WC. A randomised study on the effect of bladder irrigation with povidone-iodine before removal of an indwelling catheter. *Journal of Hospital Infection* 1992; **21**: 223–229.

Sedor J, Mulholland G. Hospital-acquired Urinary tact infection associated with the indwelling catheter. *Urologic Clinic of North America* 1999; **26**: 821–828.

Stamm WE. Catheter-associated urinary tract infection: epidemiology, pathogenesis and prevention. *American Journal of Medicine* 1991; **91**(Suppl. 3B): 65S–71S.

Stamm WE. Urinary Tract Infections. In: Bennett JV, Brachman PS (eds), *Hospital Infection*, 4th edn. Philadelphia: Lippincott-Raven, 1998: 477–485.

Sweet DE, Goodpasture HC, Holl K, Smart S, Alexander H, Hedari A. Evaluation of H_2O_2 prophylaxis of bacteriuria inpatients with long-term indwelling Foley catheters: a randomised controlled study. *Infection Control* 1985; **6**: 263–266.

Thompson RL, Haley CE, Searcy MA, Guenthner SM, Kaiser DL. Catheter-associated bacteriuria. Failure to reduce attack rates using periodic instillations of a disinfectant into urinary drainage systems. *Journal of the American Medical Association* 1984; **251**: 747–751.

Thornton GF, Andriole VT. Bacteriuria during indwelling catheter drainage: II. Effect of a closed sterile draining system. *Journal of the American Medical Association* 1970; **214**: 339.

UK Department of Health. Guidelines for preventing infections associated with the insertion and maintenance of short-term indwelling urethral catheters in acute care. *Journal of Hospital Infection* 2001; **47**(Suppl.): S39–S46.

Wagenlehner FME, Naber KG. Hospital-acquired urinary tract infections. *Journal of Hospital Infection* 2000; **46**: 171–181.

Ward V, Wilson J, Taylor L, Cookson B, Glynn A. *Preventing Hospital acquired infection: clinical guidelines.* London: Public Health Laboratory Services, 1997: 25–29.

Warren JW, Platt R, Thomas RJ, Rosner B, Kass EH. Antibiotic irrigation and catheter-associated urinary-tract infections. *New England Journal of Medicine* 1978; **299**: 570–573.

Wong ES, Hooton TM. Guideline for prevention of catheter-associated urinary tract infections. *American Journal of Infection Control* 1983; **11**(1): 28–36.

16

Prevention of Nosocomial Pneumonia

Nosocomial pneumonia is the second most common hospital-acquired infection and has a mortality rate of 20–50%. Ventilator-associated pneumonia refers specifically to nosocomial bacterial pneumonia that has developed in patients receiving mechanical ventilation. Compared to non-ventilated patients, the risk of pneumonia is increased at least 7–10 fold in patients following surgery or in intensive care who require mechanical ventilation. It has been estimated that nosocomial pneumonia typically lengthens a patient's hospital stay by 4–9 days and is associated with very high morbidity and mortality.

Ventilator-associated pneumonia that occurs within 48–72 h after tracheal intubations is usually termed early-onset pneumonia and often results from aspiration, which complicates the intubation process. They are usually caused by antibiotic sensitive bacteria, e.g. *Staphylococcus aureus*, *Haemophilus influenzae* and *Streptococcus pneumoniae*. Ventilator-associated pneumonia that occurs after this period is usually considered late-onset pneumonia and is usually caused by resistant bacteria, e.g. methicillin resistant *Staph. aureus* and Gram-negative bacilli, i.e. *Pseudomonas aeruginosa*, *Klebsiella pneumoniae*, *Escherichia coli*, *Serratia marcescens*, *Citrobacter* spp., *Enterobacter* spp. and *Acinetobacter* spp.

Nosocomial pneumonia can be caused by Legionella which can be acquired from hospital air conditioning systems or from water supplies, particularly in immuno-compromised patients. Other organisms responsible for hospital-acquired pneumonia are viruses and fungi, e.g. *Candida albicans*, *Aspergillus fumigatus* (acquired from building work) and *Mycobacterium tuberculosis* and other atypical mycobacteria.

Pathogenesis

The pathogenesis of ventilator-associated pneumonia usually requires two important processes to take place, i.e. bacterial colonization of the aerodigestive tract, and aspiration of contaminated secretions into the lower airway. Therefore, the

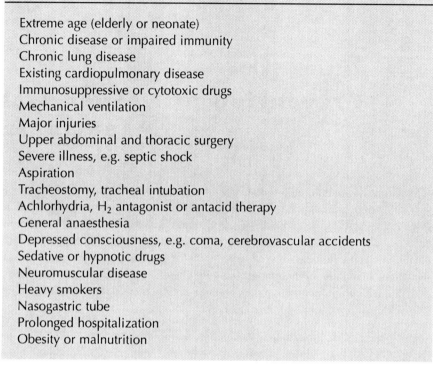

Risk factors for oropharyngeal colonization and nosocomial pneumonia

Extreme age (elderly or neonate)
Chronic disease or impaired immunity
Chronic lung disease
Existing cardiopulmonary disease
Immunosuppressive or cytotoxic drugs
Mechanical ventilation
Major injuries
Upper abdominal and thoracic surgery
Severe illness, e.g. septic shock
Aspiration
Tracheostomy, tracheal intubation
Achlorhydria, H_2 antagonist or antacid therapy
General anaesthesia
Depressed consciousness, e.g. coma, cerebrovascular accidents
Sedative or hypnotic drugs
Neuromuscular disease
Heavy smokers
Nasogastric tube
Prolonged hospitalization
Obesity or malnutrition

strategies aimed at preventing ventilator-associated pneumonia usually focus on reducing the bioburden of bacterial colonization in the aerodigestive tract, decreasing the incidence of aspiration, or both.

The presence of invasive medical devices is an important contributor to the pathogenesis and development of ventilator-associated pneumonia. This is because the presence of invasive medical devices causes mechanical and chemical injury to the ciliated epithelium of the respiratory tract. The injury promotes colonization and aspiration of bacteria from the oropharynx or stomach into the tracheobronchial tree. In addition, the presence of a foreign body, e.g. an endotracheal tube, facilitates bacterial colonization of the tracheobronchial tree. The presence of nasogastric tubes predisposes to gastric reflux and increases the potential for aspiration. Therefore, it is essential that *nasogastric or endotracheal tubes should be removed as soon as clinically feasible. Unnecessary reintubation should be avoided to prevent injury.* Adequate pressure should be maintained in the endotracheal-tube cuff.

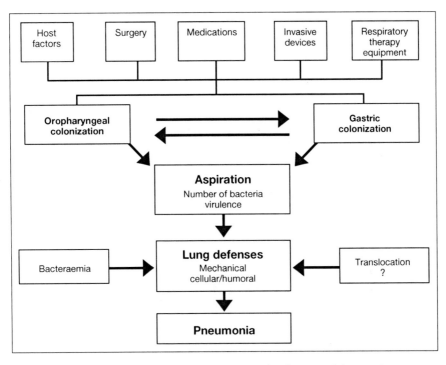

Figure 16.1 Factors influencing colonization and infection of the respiratory tract.
Reproduced with permission from Craven *et al*. Nosocomial pneumonia in the 90's: update of the epidemiology and risk factors. *Semin Respir Infect* 1990; **5**: 157–192.

Strategy for prevention

The following measures should be adopted to prevent nosocomial pneumonia in hospitalized patients:

Surveillance: Surveillance of nosocomial infection in the intensive care unit (ICU) should be introduced and infection rate should be presented to intensive care physicians on a regular basis.

Infection control programme: An infection control awareness programme should be introduced to promote hand hygiene after contact with patients and wearing of gloves for contact with the respiratory secretions, devices, or environmental surfaces and performing tracheostomy using aseptic techniques.

Education and training: Education and training of staff in cleaning, disinfection and maintenance of respiratory equipment is essential.

Ventilator circuits: Routine changing of ventilator circuit tubing is not recommended because of rapid bacterial colonization of tubing which usually occurs within 24 h of its placement. However, ventilator circuits should be changed if there is overt soiling (e.g. with vomit or blood) or mechanical malfunction. Since a high concentration of pathogenic bacteria is found in condensate fluid, it is important that *ventilator circuits should also be monitored regularly and any accumulated condensate fluid in the tubing removed.*

Nasogastric tube: A nasogastric tube for enteral feeding may erode the mucosal surface or block the sinus ducts and is responsible for causing regurgitation of gastric contents leading to aspiration. Therefore, nutritional status must be assessed on a regular basis and *removal of a nasogastric tube should be considered if clinically indicated.*

Continuous subglottic suctioning: Secretions from the respiratory tract usually pool above inflated endotracheal tube cuffs and may act as a source of aspirated material. Endotracheal tubes with a separate dorsal lumen above the cuff to suction pooled secretions from the subglottic space are now available. These specialized endotracheal tubes should be part of an organized approach to preventing ventilator-associated pneumonia and should not be used in place of such efforts. The pressure of the endotracheal tube cuff should be adequate to prevent the leakage of colonized subglottic secretions into the lower airway.

Suction catheters: There are two types of suction catheter systems available, i.e. open (single-use) and closed (multi-use). The risk of nosocomial pneumonia appears to be similar in both systems. The main advantages attributed to the closed, multi-use catheters are lower costs and decreased environmental contamination. Daily changes of in-line suction catheters are not necessary, which is another advantage of using closed, multi-use catheter systems instead of open, single-use systems, especially for patients who require prolonged ventilatory support.

Humidification with heat and moisture exchangers: Heat and moisture exchangers are attractive alternatives to heated-water humidification systems. In theory, heat and moisture exchangers reduce the incidence of ventilator-associated pneumonia by minimizing the development of condensate within ventilator circuits. However, they should be considered primarily a cost-effective method of providing humidification to patients receiving ventilation if there are no contraindications (e.g. haemoptysis, copious or tenacious secretions, or difficulty discontinuing mechanical ventilation because of increasexd airway resistance).

Respiratory filter: The use of respiratory filters in the breathing system for the prevention of ventilator-associated pneumonia is an unresolved issue.

Postural changes: Patients who are confined to bed have an increased frequency of pulmonary and non-pulmonary complications. Therefore it is important that the patient should be turned to encourage postural drainage. They *should also be encouraged to take deep breaths and cough.* The patient should be maintained in an upright position (elevate patient's head to a 30–45° angle) to reduce reflux and aspiration of gastric bacteria.

Table 16.1 Methods of prevention of nosocomial pneumonia.

Procedure/device	Intervention to decrease risk
Suctioning	• Use single-use disposable gloves and wash hands before and after the procedure. • Use sterile suction catheter and sterile fluid to flush catheter. • Change suction tubing between patients.
Suction bottle	• Use single-use disposable. Non-disposable bottles should be washed with detergent and allow to dry. Heat disinfect in washing machine or send to SSD.
Ventilator breathing circuits	• Replace mechanical ventilators circuit every 48 h or protect with filter. • Periodically drain breathing-tube condensation traps, taking care not to spill it down the patient's trachea; wash hands after the procedure.
Oxygen mask	• Change oxygen mask and tubing between patients and more frequently if soiled.
Nebulizers	• Change and reprocess device between patients by using sterilization or a high-level disinfection or use single-use disposable item. • *Fill with sterile water only.*
Humidifiers	• Clean and sterilize device between patients. • *Fill with sterile water* which must be changed every 24 h or sooner, if necessary. • Single-use disposable humidifiers are available but they are expensive.
Ventilators	• After every patient, clean and disinfect (high-level) or sterilize re-usable components of the breathing system or the patient circuit according to the manufacturer's instructions.

Surgical patients: Pre-operatively, patients should be encouraged to stop smoking and any existing infection should be treated. Post-operatively, coughing exercise and breathing techniques should be taught. *Early mobilization is essential* and post-operative pain should be controlled with judicious use of analgesics.

Stress-ulcer prophylaxis: Patients receiving mechanical ventilation are at high risk for upper gastrointestinal haemorrhage from stress ulcers. Bacterial colonization of the stomach, enhanced by the administration of pH-lowering drugs (e.g. H_2-receptor antagonists and antacids), is thought to be an important source of pathogens that can cause pneumonia. The administration of sucralfate into the stomach, which acts as a cytoprotective that does not block or significantly neutralize gastric acid secretion, has been found to prevent bleeding or stress

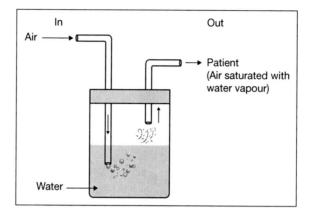

Figure 16.2 In a humidifier, gas bubbles through water, enabling it to pick up vapour but not actual droplets.

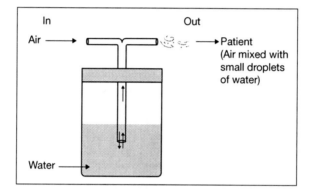

Figure 16.3 In a nebulizer, gas passes rapidly through a tube which is immersed in solution creating small droplets of fluid.

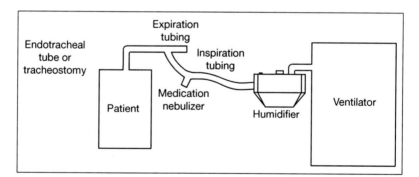

Figure 16.4 Patient on a continuous-volume ventilator, showing the location of humidifier and nebulizer.

Reproduced from Castle M and Ajemian E. *Hospital Infection Control: Principles and Practice*. New York, John Wiley & Sons, 1987.

ulcers without lowering gastric pH. Several randomized trials have found that sucralfate is associated with lower rates of ventilator-associated pneumonia than antacids or H_2-receptor antagonists.

Selective decontamination therapy: When ventilator-associated pneumonia occurs, treatment usually consists of supportive care and the administration of antibiotics. Widespread use of broad spectrum antibiotics in the ICU should be avoided. In addition, routine administration of oral or parenteral antibiotics as part of selective decontamination of the oropharynx and gastrointestinal tract in critically ill patients is controversial and should be avoided to prevent problems of widespread bacterial resistance.

References and further reading

Bonten MJM, Bergmans DCJJ. Nosocomial pneumonia. In: Mayhall CG (ed), *Hospital Epidemiology and Infection Control*, 2nd edn. Baltimore: Williams & Wilkins, 1999: 211–238.

Craven DE, Driks MR. Nosocomial pneumonia in the intubated patient. *Seminars in Respiratory Infections* 1987; **2**(1): 20–33.

Craven DE, Barber TW, Steger KA, Montecalvo MA. Nosocomial pneumonia in the 90's: update on epidemiology and risk factors. *Seminars in Respiratory Infection* 1990; **5**: 152–172.

Das I, Fraise AP. How useful are microbial filters in respiratory apparatus? *Journal of Hospital Infection* 1997; **37**: 263–272.

Harmanci A, Harmanci Ö, Akova M. Hospital-acquired pneumonia: Challenges and options for diagnosis and treatment. *Journal of Hospital Infection* 2000; **51**: 160–167.

King TA, Cooke RPD. Developing an infection control policy for anaesthetic equipment. *Journal of Hospital Infection* 2000; **47**: 257–261.

Koerner RJ. Contribution of endotracheal tubes to the pathogenesis of ventilator-associated pneumonia. *Journal of Hospital Infection* 1997; **35**: 83–89.

Kollef MH. The prevention of ventilator-associated pneumonia. *The New England Journal of Medicine* 1999; **340**(8): 627–633.

Leeming JP, Pryce-Roberts DM, Kendrick AH, Smith EC. The efficacy of filters used in respiratory function apparatus. *Journal of Hospital Infection* 1995; **31**: 205–210.

Mayhall CG. Nosocomial Pneumonia: Diagnosis and Prevention. *Infectious Disease Clinics of North America* 1997; **11**(2): 427–457.

Tablan OC, Anderson LF, Arden NH, *et al*. Guideline for prevention of nosocomial pneumonia. *Infection Control and Hospital Epidemiology* 1994; **15**: 587–627.

Ward V, Wilson J, Taylor L, Cookson B, Glynn A. *Preventing Hospital acquired infection: clinical guidelines.* London: Public Health Laboratory Services. 1997: 31–35.

Webb CW. Selective bowel decontamination in intensive care – a critical appraisal. *Reviews in Medical Microbiology* 1992; **3**: 202–210.

Wiblin RT. Nosocomial Pneumonia In: Wenzel RP (ed), *Prevention and Control of Nosocomial Infections*, 3rd edn. Baltimore: Williams & Wilkins, 1997: 807–819.

17

Hospital Support Services

FOOD AND CATERING SERVICES

Food service establishments are frequently identified as places where mishandling of food has led to outbreaks of foodborne disease. Hospitals and other health care facilities represent a special case of food service operation. The need for adequate food hygiene facilities is of paramount importance, since the consequences of an outbreak of food poisoning in a health care facility can be life threatening for patients. Therefore, particular care must be taken to minimize the risk of infection or intoxication through the food service system. Preparation of food requires attention to raw materials, personal hygiene, kitchen hygiene, and especially time/temperature control of all food-handling operations including cooking, cooling, reheating and distribution. Assuring safe food requires management and control of microbiological, chemical and physical hazards.

It is recommended that food service departments in health care establishments take the HACCP (Hazards Analysis Critical Control Point) approach to the food safety programme instead of the traditional approach based only on cooking procedures (recipe-based), as the latter may not address all the steps that a food product passes through, including receipt of goods, meal service and distribution.

The HACCP approach has been used widely in the food industry. The HACCP concept evolved at the NASA (National Aeronautics and Space Agency) laboratories with the aim of guaranteeing that the food provided for space travellers was not contaminated microbiologically, chemically, or physically in a way that would lead to either a space mission failure or catastrophe. HACCP is a powerful process which focuses control at seven points in a process which are critical to the safety of the end product. The systematic approach of HACCP helps analyze potential hazards and identify the points where hazards may occur. Once the changes are implemented, it must be reviewed periodically. An integral part of a properly constructed HACCP plan is the

Table 17.1 The commonest causes of food poisoning.

- Preparing food too long in advance.
- Storing food at ambient temperatures.
- Cooling food too slowly before placing in refrigerator.
- Not reheating food to temperatures at which food poisoning bacteria can be destroyed.
- Using contaminated food.
- Undercooking meat, meat products and poultry.
- Not thawing frozen poultry and meat for long enough.
- Cross-contamination between raw and cooked food.
- Keeping hot food below 63°C.
- Infected food handlers.

Reproduced with permission from Barrie D. The provision of food and catering services in hospital. *Journal of Hospital Infection* 1996; **33:** 13–33.

existence of good manufacturing practice throughout the food service chain. This includes factors that have become known as prerequisite or support programmes, including supplier control, cleaning and sanitation, personal hygiene and staff training. All food must comply with relevant local food safety acts and the food hygiene regulations of the country involved.

Staff health/hygiene

Although catering staff are mainly responsible for providing food in hospitals, nursing and domestic staff are also involved in distributing or serving meals to patients. Everyone who handles, prepares, processes and distributes food must understand the principles of basic food hygiene and *should be trained in personnel and catering hygienic methods.*

Cook-chill food production systems

There has been an increasing trend in health care establishments to use 'cook-chill' food service systems to extend the life of prepared food products. The time and temperature control of product chilling and subsequent storage and handling is critical in cook-chill systems because bacteria can grow in the extended time between food production and consumption. The storage temperature for cook-chill systems should be 0°C, which is lower than that required for conventional cold storage. The storage time (shelf life) also needs to be closely monitored and may vary according to the production method used as well as the storage temperature (storage below 0°C controls the growth of most pathogenic bacteria).

Table 17.2 General rules of food hygiene.

Delivery	• Accept frozen food below −18°C • Accept chilled food below +13°C • Check 'within date' code • Check state of packaging
Storage	• Practise stock rotation • Provide clean, dry, pest-free conditions • Keep at correct temperatures • Keep covered until required • Keep raw food separately from cooked items • Use separate utensils, surfaces • Wash hands between different food
Thawing	• Thaw below 15°C • Thaw completely • Cook within 24 h
Cooking	• Ensure centre of food reaches 70°C for 2 min • Cook on the day of consumption or chill rapidly and refrigerate within 1½ h. Consume within 3 days • Hold below 10°C or above 63°C
Reheating	• Avoid, if possible • Reheat rapidly • Attain 70°C (use temperature probe)
Distribution	• Hot food above 63°C • Cold food below 10°C • Check with temperature probe
Waste	• Discard unwanted food after 1 h • Always cover food waste
Cleaning maintenance	• Observe schedules for all items • Ensure good state of service and repair

Reproduced with permission from Barrie D. The provision of food and catering services in hospital. *Journal of Hospital Infection* 1996; **33**: 13–33.

Texture modified products

Texture modified meals, which are provided to people with chewing and/or swallowing problems, also have a greater risk of bacterial contamination. This includes all food that has been pureed or minced *after* cooking. Where possible, food should be pureed *before* cooking. Where this is not possible, for example with pureed fruit, particular care must be taken to minimize cross-contamination. Strict time and temperature control must also be maintained.

Food trolleys

In hospitals and large health care establishments, mechanical transport can make it easier to distribute equipment and also reduce the movement of people, thus minimizing the spread of infection. Trolleys should be of suitable height to allow good visibility during use, be appropriate for the type of transport, and should be enclosed or draped. *They should be cleaned daily or more frequently if contamination occurs.*

Refrigerators

Refrigerators used by health care workers for storage of food items should be used neither for storage of contaminated material, including clinical specimens, nor for storage of medical products such as drugs, vaccines or blood, under any circumstances. *Medications and vaccines should be stored in accordance with the manufacturer's instructions.* Vaccines (and other medications) requiring refrigeration should be stored in a refrigerator dedicated to vaccine storage. Blood and other clinical specimens requiring refrigeration should also have a dedicated refrigerator for storage.

Inspection

The catering manager has the responsibility for catering services. *Daily inspection of kitchens and all food-handling areas are necessary by catering managers* and supervisory staff with the aid of check-lists. Hospital administrators are responsible for food hygiene in hospitals and should ensure that a full inspection is carried out at least twice yearly. Full reports of these inspections should be submitted to the hospital administrator and the hospital Infection Control Committee.

Food handlers

All food handlers should complete a pre-employment questionnaire, which should be reviewed by a person competent to assess the implications of any positive answers and decide if examination of faecal specimens is necessary. Pre-employment stool testing is not generally required in the absence of a history of enteric fever. *All food handlers with infections, diarrhoea or suspected gastrointestinal infection must stop working and report to their manager.* Return to work depends on whether it is considered safe, usually by the occupational health department, but the opinion of the microbiologist or infection control doctor may also be sought.

Hospital kitchen

The kitchen should have an agreed cleaning procedure. Methods, materials and frequency should be defined. Cleaning materials should be stored in a designated area. Good practice includes the use of separate bays for each task, colour coded cloths, and satisfactory cleaning knives, preparation surfaces and chopping boards/blocks. Food stores should be generally clean, uncluttered and with good access for cleaning. Shelving should be easy to clean. Any food capable of supporting microbial growth should be stored either below 8°C or above 63°C. Cook-chilled food should be stored below 3°C. Deep frozen food should be at −18°C or below; chilled food should be between 0°C and +3°C.

Ward kitchens

Ward kitchens or food-handling areas and the staff using them should observe the same levels of food and personal hygiene as other food handlers. There should be specific written cleaning and waste disposal policies. These should comply with written codes of practice for food-handling in ward kitchens.

Ward refrigerators, dishwashers, microwave ovens and ice-making machines are used by nursing staff, domestic staff and visitors, and are often used incorrectly. *Ward kitchen refrigerators should be used solely for patients' food* and never for medicines, units of blood or pathology specimens. Ice-making machines should be purchased in consultation with the infection control team (ICT) and a planned maintenance and cleaning protocol should be drawn up.

Ice machines

Ice from contaminated ice machines has been associated with patient infection. Microorganisms may be present in ice, ice storage chests and ice-making machines. The two main sources of microorganisms in ice are the potable water from which it is made and a transfer of organisms from hands.

Currently, there are no microbiological standards for ice, ice-making machines, or ice storage equipment. However, it is important to clean ice storage chests at least monthly, with more frequent cleanings recommended for open chests. Portable ice chests and containers require cleaning and low-level disinfection before the addition of ice intended for consumption. Ice-making machines may also be contaminated via improper storage or handling of ice by patients and/or staff. Suggested steps to avoid this means of contamination include:

- Minimizing or avoiding direct hand contact with ice intended for consumption.
- Using a hard-surface scoop to dispense ice.
- Installing machines that dispense ice directly into portable containers at the touch of a control.

Culturing of ice machines is not routinely recommended but may be useful as part of an epidemiologic investigation.

If the source water for ice in a health care facility is not faecally contaminated, then ice from clean ice machines and chests should pose no special hazard for immuno-competent patients. Some waterborne bacteria found in ice could potentially be a

General steps to maintain ice machines

- Disconnect the ice machine from the power supply.
- Remove and discard the ice.
- Disassemble the removable parts of the machine that make contact with water to make ice.
- Thoroughly clean the machine and the parts.
- Check for any needed repair.
- Ensure the presence of an air space in the tubing that leads from the water inlet into the water distribution system of the machine.
- Inspect for rodent or insect infestations under the machine and treat if necessary.
- Check door gaskets (open compartment models) for evidence of leakage or dripping into the storage chest.
- Clean the ice-storage chest.
- Disinfect the machine by circulating with a diluted hypochlorite (50–100 ppm av Cl_2) solution through the ice-making and storage systems (suggested contact time: 4 h for 50 ppm av Cl_2 solution, 2 h for 100 ppm av Cl_2 solution).
- Drain the chlorine solution, and flush with fresh tap water.
- Allow the ice-storage chest to dry, and return to service.

risk to immunocompromised patients if they consume ice or drink beverages with ice. It may therefore be prudent to protect the immunosuppressed.

All ice machines must regularly be maintained. The following steps should be taken to clean and disinfect the ice machines:

- Disconnect the machine from the power supply.
- Remove and discard the ice.
- Allow the machine to warm to room temperature.
- Clean the machine with fresh water and detergent.
- Rinse with fresh tap water.
- Wipe dry with clean materials.
- Rinse with diluted hypochlorite solution (100 ppm av Cl_2).
- Air dry all surfaces before returning the machine to service.

References and further reading

Barrie D. The provision of food and catering services in hospital. *Journal of Hospital Infection* 1996; **33**: 13–33.

Bryan FL. *Hazard Analysis Critical Control Point Evaluations*. Geneva: World Health Organisation, 1992.

Richards J, Parr E, Risborough P. Hospital food hygiene: The application of hazard analysis critical points to conventional hospital catering. *Journal of Hospital Infection* 1993; **24**: 273.

Mortimore S, Wallace C. *HACCP – A Practical Approach*, 2nd edn. Maryland: Aspen publishers, 1998.

UK Department of Health. *Health Service Catering Hygiene*. London: Department of Health and Social Security, 1986.

UK Department of Health. Chilled and Frozen. *Guidelines on Cook-Chill and Cook-Freeze Catering systems*. London: HMSO, 1989.

UK Department of Health. *Management of outbreaks of food borne illness*. London: DoH, 1994.

UK Department of Health. Food handlers: *Fitness to work*. London: DoH, 1995.

UK Department of Health. NHS Management Executive. *Hospital catering – delivery of a quality service*. EL (96)37, 1996.

UK Department of Health. NHS Executive. *Management of food hygiene and food services in the National Health Service*, London: DoH, 1996.

LINEN AND LAUNDRY SERVICE

Although soiled linen may be contaminated with organisms, the risk of disease transmission is negligible if it is handled, transported and laundered in a manner that avoids dispersal. Infection in laundry workers after handling soiled linen has only rarely been reported, and is usually ascribed to improper handling practices.

Inadvertent disposal of objects (sharps and personal property) in linen is a common problem. Therefore all staff are urged to remove these objects which not only endanger staff in the laundry from sharps injuries but can cause extensive damage to expensive laundry machine.

General principles to prevent infection

Common sense, basic principles of infection control and accepted recommendations for handling and processing procedures must be adhered to to minimize the risk of infection. These recommendations must be adhered to regardless of the use of in-house or off-site contractors. Management should ensure that *all staff and laundry contractors responsible for handling or laundering linen are appropriately trained.*

The following principles should be followed for safe handling of laundry:

Laundry staff: All personnel involved in the collection, transport, sorting, and washing of soiled linen should be adequately trained and *wear appropriate personal protective equipment.* All workers must cover all lesions on exposed skin with waterproof plasters and wear appropriate gloves. Gloves used for the task of sorting laundry should be of sufficient thickness to minimize sharps injuries. They must have access to hand washing facilities.

Sorting: After removal, soiled linen must be handled with care at all times. It should be placed into bags (or other appropriate containers) at the point of generation as soon as possible. Bags must be securely tied or otherwise closed to prevent leakage. Rinsing soiled laundry at the point of generation should not be done.

Infectious linen: Only linen visibly contaminated with blood and/or body fluids should be viewed as potentially infectious. Within infectious linen, it is possible to identify a 'high risk' group where the diseases involved are transmitted through a low infectious dose of organisms, e.g. *Escherichia coli* 0157, shigellosis etc.

Infectious linen should be segregated at the point of use and care should be taken to ensure that only this type of linen is placed in the container. Bags containing infectious linen should be sealed, with an appropriate biohazard label indicating the point of origin attached, and should be of a material which either dissolves, or has stitching which dissolves, in the wash. A red plastic or other appropriately colour coded bag should be used as an impervious outer container. The plastic bag should be discarded as clinical waste immediately before the linen is placed in the wash. Alternatively a red textile bag may be used. This should be removed prior to placing the inner bag into the wash and then it should be laundered.

Laundry bags: Single bags of sufficient tensile strength are adequate for containing laundry; leak-proof containment is needed if the laundry is wet and can soak through a cloth bag. Bags containing soiled laundry should be clearly identified with labels; colour-coding should meet the local policy so that HCWs may handle these items safely, regardless of whether the laundry is transported within the facility or destined for transport to an off-site laundry service.

Transport of soiled linens: Soiled linen in bags can be transported by cart or chute. Loose, soiled pieces of laundry should not be tossed into chutes.

Transport and storage of cleaned linens: Clean laundry should be transported separately from contaminated laundry. Clean linen must be wrapped prior to transport to prevent inadvertent contamination from dust and dirt during loading, delivery, and unloading. *Clean linen should be stored in a clean area* of the ward or department until it is distributed for patient use.

Laundry contract: It is important that the ICT should be involved in the contract-setting process for laundry services. Care must be taken to ensure that any contract change occurs only after a full appraisal of the above issues.

Laundry process

Linen and clothing used in health care facilities are disinfected during laundering and generally rendered free of vegetative pathogens (hygienically clean), but they are not sterile. Washing machines in health care facilities can be either washer/extractor units or continuous batch machines. A typical washing cycle consists of three main phases, i.e. pre-wash, main wash and rinse cycle.

The antimicrobial action of the laundering process results from a combination of physical and chemical factors. Dilution and agitation in water removes significant quantities of microorganisms. Soaps and detergents loosen soil and also have some antimicrobial properties.

High-temperature wash

Hot water provides an effective means of destroying microorganisms. A temperature of at least 71°C (160°F) for a minimum of 25 min is commonly recommended for hot-water washing. Water of this temperature can be provided by steam jet or separate booster heater. Chlorine bleach provides an extra margin of safety. A total available chlorine residual of 50–150 ppm is usually achieved during the bleach cycle. The last action in the washing process is the addition of a mild acid to neutralize any alkalinity in the water supply, soap, or detergent. The rapid shift in pH from approximately 12 to 5 may also inactivate some microorganisms.

Chlorine bleach is a cheap broad-spectrum chemical disinfectant that enhances the effectiveness of the laundering process. However, chlorine bleach is not an appropriate laundry additive for all fabrics. Bleach was not recommended in the past for laundering fire-retardant fabrics, linen and clothing because its use diminished the flame-retardant properties of the treated fabric. Some modern flame-retardant fabrics can now tolerate chlorine bleach and chlorine alternatives such as activated oxygen-based laundry detergents.

Low-temperature wash

Although hot-water washing is an effective laundry disinfection method, the cost can be significant. Laundries are typically the largest users of hot water in hospitals, consuming between 50–75% of the total hot water. Several studies have shown that lower water temperatures can satisfactorily reduce microbial contamination when the cycling of the washer, the wash-detergent, and the amount of bleach are carefully monitored and controlled.

Low-temperature laundry cycles rely heavily on the presence of chlorine or oxygen-activated bleach to reduce the levels of microbial contamination. Regardless of whether hot or cold water is used for washing, the temperatures reached in drying and especially during ironing provide additional significant microbiocidal action.

Dry cleaning

The dry cleaning process involves organic solvents such as perchloroethylene for soil removal and use for linen that might be damaged in conventional water and detergent washing. A number of studies have shown that dry cleaning alone is relatively ineffective in reducing the numbers of microorganisms on contaminated linen. Although a number of microorganisms are significantly reduced when dry cleaned articles are heat pressed, *dry cleaning should not be used routinely*. It should be *reserved only for fabrics which cannot be safely cleaned with water and detergent.*

Microbiological sampling

In the absence of agreed standards, routine *microbiological sampling of cleaned linen is not recommended*. Sampling may be used as part of an outbreak investigation if epidemiological evidence suggests linen or clothing as a vehicle for disease transmission.

Hygienically clean linen is suitable for neonatal intensive care units. The use of sterile linen in burns units remains unresolved.

Staff uniforms

Uniforms without blood or body substance contamination presumably do not differ appreciably from street clothes in the degree and microbial nature of soilage.

Home laundering would be expected to remove this level of soil adequately. However, if health care facilities require the use of uniforms, it would seem reasonable that they provide workers with clean uniforms.

Mattresses and pillows

Standard mattresses and pillows can become contaminated with body substances during patient care. *Mattress covers should be replaced when torn.* The practice of *sticking needles into the mattress should be avoided.* Visibly stained mattresses should be replaced.

Wet mattresses, in particular, can be a significant environmental source of micro-organisms. Infection and colonizations due to *Acinetobacter* spp., methicillin-resistant *Staphylococcus aureus* (MRSA), and *Pseudomonas aeruginosa* have been described, especially among burn patients.

Air-fluidized beds

Air-fluidized beds are used for the care of patients immobilized for extended periods of time, e.g. decubitus ulcers, burns. These specialized beds consist of a base unit filled with microsphere beads fluidized by warm, dry air flowing upward from a diffuser located at the bottom of the unit. A porous, polyester filter sheet separates the patient from direct contact with the beads but allows body fluids to pass through to the beads. Moist beads aggregate into clumps which settle to the bottom where they are removed as part of routine bed maintenance. Because the beads become contaminated with the patient's body substances, concerns have been raised about the potential for these beds to serve as an environmental source of pathogens. Pathogens such as *Enterococcus* spp., *Serratia marcescens*, *Staph. aureus*, and *Streptococcus faecalis* have been recovered either from the microsphere beads or the polyester sheet after cleaning.

Reports of cross-contamination of patients, however, are few. Nevertheless, *routine maintenance and between-patient decontamination procedures are important to minimize potential risks to patients.* Regular removal of bead clumps, coupled with the warm, dry air of the bed can help minimize bacterial growth in the unit. Beads are decontaminated between patients by high heat (range 45–90°C [113–194°F]), depending on the manufacturer's specifications for at least 1 h; this is especially important for the inactivation of *Enterococcus* spp. which are relatively resistant to heat. It is essential that the bed is thoroughly cleaned and disinfected, especially between patients. The polyester filter sheet requires regular changing.

References and further reading

Barrie D. How hospital linen and laundry services are provided. *Journal of Hospital Infection* 1994; **27**: 219–239.

Department of Health NHS Executive. *Hospital laundry arrangements for used and infected linen*. Heywood: Health Publications Unit, 1995.

McDonald LL, Pulgiese G. Textile processing service. In: Mayhall CG (ed). *Hospital epidemiology and infection*, 2nd edn. Baltimore, MD: Williams and Wilkins, 1999: 1031–1034.

NHS Executive. HSG (95)18. *Hospital laundry arrangements for used and infected linen*. London: 1995.

Standeert SM, Hutcheson RH, Schaffner W. Nosocomial transmission of salmonella to laundry workers in a nursing home. *Infection Control and Hospital Epidemiology* 1994; **15**: 22.

MANAGEMENT OF CLINICAL WASTE

The most practical approach to clinical waste management is to identify wastes that represent a sufficient potential risk of causing infection during handling and disposal and for which some precautions appear prudent. It is essential that *all health care facilities should have clearly defined guidelines* to ensure the safe identification, packaging, labelling, storage, transport, treatment and disposal of waste, from the point of generation to the point of final disposal. Management of clinical and related wastes must conform to the appropriate national and international guidelines.

It is essential that all employees who are required to handle and move clinical waste should be adequately trained in safe procedures. They must be provided with appropriate protective equipment e.g. water-repellent clothing, heavy-duty gloves and protective footwear. Spillages and other incidents must be dealt with according to written protocols. All accidents and incidents involving clinical waste, particularly those resulting in injury to or contamination of handlers, must be dealt with according to local policy.

Definition and categorization of clinical waste

The definition and categorization of clinical or medical waste varies from country to country. Terms such as 'hospital waste', 'clinical waste', 'infectious waste', 'medical waste', 'biomedical waste' and 'biohazard waste', have been used synonymously and often inappropriately in many situations.

Clinical waste: Clinical waste has been defined as all types of waste (clinical, related and general) arising from medical, nursing, dental, veterinary, pharmaceutical or similar practices and waste produced in hospitals or other facilities during the investigation or treatment of patients and in research projects.

Non-clinical: Non-clinical or household waste is defined as other waste not in the categories of either clinical waste or special waste. It is non-toxic, non-infectious or its basic nature is unlikely to prove a health hazard or give offence in its existing form.

Special waste: Special waste is defined as waste that is dangerous to life and difficult to dispose of by its nature. Some clinical waste is also classified as 'special waste', and is subject to control under the special waste regulations. This waste includes waste originating from patients with Hazard Group 4 biological agents (e.g. viral haemorrhagic fevers), which has not been autoclaved.

Categorization of clinical waste

Group A: Includes the following items: identifiable human tissue,* blood, animal carcasses and tissue from veterinary centres, hospitals or laboratories. Soiled surgical dressings, swabs and other similar soiled waste. Other waste materials, for example from infectious disease cases, excluding any in Groups B–E.

Group B: Discarded syringe needles, cartridges, broken glass and any other contaminated sharp instruments or items.

Group C: Microbiological cultures and potentially infected waste from pathology departments and other clinical or research laboratories.

Group D: Drugs or other pharmaceutical products.

Group E: Items used to dispose of urine, faeces and other bodily secretions or excretions that do not fall within Group A. This includes used disposable bed pans or bed pan liners, incontinence pads, stoma bags and urine containers.**

*All identifiable human tissue, whether infected or not, may only be disposed of by incineration.
**Where the risk assessment shows there is no infection risk, Group E wastes are not clinical waste as defined.
Adapted from UK Health and Safety Commission. *Safe disposal of clinical waste.* Norwich: HMSO, 1999.

Methods for safe handling of clinical waste

Clinical waste should be disposed of in a plastic bag (yellow with a black biohazard symbol). The thickness should meet the appropriate local standard. It is recommended that the clinical waste bag should be a minimum gauge of 225 (55 μ) if high density, or a minimum gauge of 100(25 μ) if low density. Plastic bags should be secured in a foot-operated lidded bin or carrier frame.

- Clinical waste should be placed into the plastic waste bag at the point of generation.

- Bags should be replaced daily or when three-quarters full. Bags should be securely closed by tying or sealed by plastic closures or heat sealers, purpose-made for clinical waste bags. Staples must not be used as they do not provide secure closure. They may puncture the bag and/or cause a sharps injury to the handler.

- Bags should be suitably identified with the name of the health care facility and the department concerned, which clearly identifies their point of origin. Closing the bag with pre-printed coded clips should be considered.

- Bags should be handled by the neck only and kept upright. To avoid injuries, the hand should not be put underneath the waste bag while lifting.

- Waste should be stored in a neat fashion within a designated collection area of each ward or department, which should be secured against unauthorized access and must be removed from clinical areas daily or more frequently if necessary. The area should be cleaned when necessary and kept dry.

- Bulk waste transport vehicles are the responsibility of the transport manager. Loaded vehicles leaving the health care facility or hospital site must be properly secured. Spillage should be dealt with safely. Vehicles should have a regular cleaning and disinfection schedule.

- Central collection or storage points should be secured from unauthorized access, the elements, pests or rodents.

- *All employees who are required to handle and move clinical waste should be adequately trained* in safe procedures and in dealing with spillages or other incidents in their area of work. A record of training should be kept.

- Staff who regularly have to handle, transfer, transport or incinerate clinical waste containers *must be provided with appropriate protective equipment,* i.e. heavy-duty gloves, appropriate footwear, and industrial apron or leg shields, waterproof clothing, face visors or respiratory equipment as required.

- Spillages of waste should be treated according to the local policy.

- All accidents and incidents involving clinical waste, particularly those resulting in injury to or contamination of handlers, must be reported without delay to the line manager.

Methods for safe use, handling and disposal of sharps

The safe handling and disposal of needles and other sharp instruments form part of an overall strategy of clinical waste disposal to protect staff, patients and visitors from exposure to blood-borne pathogens.

Sharps are any medical items or devices, which are contaminated with blood, tissues and high risk body fluids that can cause laceration or puncture wounds. Examples include discarded hypodermic needles, instruments used in invasive procedures (e.g. blood sampling, surgery and dentistry, acupuncture, ear-piercing and tattooing).

In clinical settings, sharps injuries are predominantly caused by needle devices and associated with venepuncture, administration of medication via intravascular lines and recapping of needles.

Contaminated sharps represent the major cause of accidents involving potential exposure to blood-borne diseases, and must be handled with care at all times. Health care facilities should provide documented operating procedures for safe handling of sharps, and ensure that health care workers are fully trained in the recommended handling techniques.

General principles for handling and use of sharps are:

- *Avoid sharps usage wherever possible.*

- Handling should be kept to a minimum. Needles should not be bent or broken by hand, removed from disposable syringes or otherwise manipulated by hand. *Sharps must not be passed directly from hand-to-hand.*

- Never leave sharps lying around; dispose of them carefully.

- Do not keep syringes, needles or any other sharps object in pockets. Many needlestick injuries happen during re-sheathing, therefore *used needles must not be re-sheathed unless there is a safe means available for doing so.* Syringes/cartridges and needles should be disposed of intact. However in certain situations, where re-sheathing of needles is necessary, it is essential that a safe method is used i.e. one-handed scoop technique (see Fig. 17.1). A mechanical device for holding or disposing of needles should be considered. Alternatively, the needle can be destroyed at the point of use using a mechanical device.

- Do not use needles or any sharps if there is any suspicion of a broken seal or other indication that it may have been used previously.

Sharps disposal: It is the *personal responsibility of the individual using a sharp to dispose of safely as soon as possible after use.* Where the specific clinical procedure prevents the user from doing this, the user still retains overall responsibility for ensuring the safe disposal of used sharps.

If a sharp has been accidentally dropped, it must be recovered and disposed of properly. If the search is unsuccessful, the individual should ensure that other people using the area are informed so that they can take care. It is particularly important to notify cleaning staff of the possible danger. The person in charge of the area should be notified and a record kept until the sharp has been found and properly disposed of.

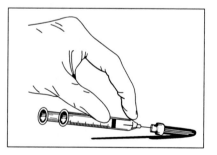

Figure 17.1 Never recap needle by hand. However, recapping of needle is required in certain situations. To recap needle safely, place the needle horizontally, on a flat surface. Using one hand, insert the needle into the cap, as shown. Then, use your other hand to pick up the cap and tighten it to the needle hub.

Where possible, needles and syringes should be discarded as a single unit into a designated sharp box. Glass slides, glass drug ampoules, razors, disposable scissors and IV cannulae must be discarded into a sharps box.

When syringes containing arterial blood are to be sent to the laboratory, needles should be removed and the nozzles of the syringes sealed by means of a luer rubber cap or a blunt hub on the syringe nozzle.

Used needles and syringes must not be disposed of in domestic waste. Health care staffs who treat patients at home should place any sharps and syringes that they generate in appropriate containers for disposal through their employer's clinical waste disposal system or via collection as appropriate.

When an injury occurs with a contaminated sharp, bleeding should be encouraged and the site should be washed under running water. The injury must be reported to the line manager without delay and should be dealt with according to the written protocols.

Use of sharps boxes: All sharps boxes must be correctly assembled and used according to the manufacturer's instructions. They must be puncture resistant and should comply with appropriate standards (e.g. British Standard BS 3720, UN 3291). They *should be kept in a location that excludes injury to patients, visitors and staff.* To avoid damage by heat, sharps boxes should not be placed near radiators or in direct sunlight.

They should be readily available wherever blood samples are taken. The person in charge of the ward or department is responsible for ensuring safe handling and disposal of sharps within their own area.

Sharps containers should be closed securely when three-quarters full and placed at a designated secure collection point. The *sharps container must never be overfilled* since used sharps protruding from overloaded containers constitute a very significant hazard to those who have to handle them. The lid of the sharps box must not be used as a means of ensuring that the needle and syringe 'fit' inside the box.

Used sharps boxes must be suitably marked for identification from wards or departments of the hospital or the health care facility. This enables the exact location and responsibility for any offending container to be determined.

Do not use sharps boxes for any other purpose e.g. storage of ward items, etc.

In the ward, sharps boxes must be securely stored whilst awaiting collection. The staff responsible for the transport of the boxes must take special care and should wear heavy-duty gloves when collecting sharps containers.

Particular attention should be paid for the needs for the provision of sufficient sharps boxes in a number of areas where use of sharps is high e.g. operating theatres, accident and emergency and out-patients departments.

Management and disposal of clinical waste

Of all the categories comprising clinical medical waste, microbiological waste and sharps pose the greatest risk for injuries and infections. On-site incineration should be considered for microbiological, pathological and anatomical waste, provided the incinerator is engineered to completely burn these wastes and stay within local emissions standards. Improper incineration of waste with high moisture and low energy content (e.g. pathology waste), can lead to emission problems. Contaminated sharps and related waste should be disposed of by incineration.

Some clinical waste may be considered for disinfection and subsequent transfer to landfill. Waste known or likely to contain Hazard Group 3 and 4 pathogens (see table 17.3) should be made safe either by autoclaving within the laboratory or in the case of an autoclave malfunction, should be packaged in accordance with the approved requirements for carriage, and transferred to an incinerator as soon as possible. Laboratory waste should not be allowed to accumulate for more than 24 h.

The contents of disposable items in group E wastes, such as excreta, may be discharged to the sewer via the sluice, WC or purpose-built disposal unit. These items do not normally fall within the definition of infectious waste for transport purposes and therefore do not have to be packaged in UN type approved containers.

Household waste is disposed of by landfill and may be compacted. Clinical waste must not be compacted prior to disposal. Pathological waste (e.g. human tissue, limbs, placentae) must be disposed of by incineration.

Treatment methods

Clinical waste is treated or decontaminated to reduce the microbial load and to render the by-products safe for further handling and disposal by landfill. Historically, treatment methods involved steam-sterilization (autoclaving), incineration, or interment (for anatomical wastes). Alternative treatment methods developed in recent years include, (but are not limited to) chemical disinfection, grinding/shredding/disinfection methods, energy-based technologies (e.g. microwave or radiowave treatments) and disinfection/encapsulation methods.

Table 17.3 Categorization of biological agents according to hazard and categorizes of containment.*

	Group 1	Group 2	Group 3	Group 4
European Community (EC)	One that is unlikely to cause human disease.	One that can cause human disease and might be a hazard to workers; it is unlikely to spread in the community; effective prophylaxis or treatment usually available.	One that can cause severe human disease and presents a serious hazard to workers; it may present a risk of spreading to the community but effective prophylaxis or treatment is usually available.	One that causes severe human disease and is a serious hazard to workers; it may present a high risk of spreading to the community; no effective prophylaxis or treatment is usually available.
UK (Advisory Committee on Dangerous Pathogens [ACDPI])	A biological agent unlikely to cause human disease.	A biological agent that can cause human disease and may be a hazard to employees; it is unlikely to spread to the community and there is usually effective prophylaxis or effective treatment available.	A biological agent that can cause severe human disease and presents a serious hazard to employees; it may present a risk to the community, but there is usually effective prophylaxis or treatment available.	A biological agent that causes severe human disease and is a serious hazard to employees; it is likely to spread to the community and there is usually no effective prophylaxis or treatment available.
USA**	Agents that offer no or minimal hazard under ordinary conditions of handling.	Agents of ordinary potential hazard, including those that may produce disease of varying degrees of severity as a result of accidental laboratory infections.	Agents that offer special hazards to laboratory workers.	Agents that are extremely hazardous to laboratory workers or cause more serious epidemic disease.
World Health Organisation (WHO)	An organism unlikely to cause human disease.	Moderate individual risk, low community risk: a pathogen that can cause human or animal disease but is unlikely to be a serious hazard to laboratory workers, the community, livestock or the environment. Laboratory exposures may cause serious infection, but effective treatment and preventive measures are available and the risk of spread of infection is limited.	High individual risk, low community risk: a pathogen that usually causes serious human or animal disease but does not ordinarily spread from one infected individual to another. Effective treatment and preventive measures are available.	High individual and community risk: a pathogen that usually causes serious human or animal disease and which may be readily transmitted from one individual to another, directly or indirectly. Effective treatment and preventive measures are not usually available.

*All the systems differ in their wording but agree in general principles.
**The USA uses 'Classes' while others use 'Groups'. USA subsumed its classes into biosafety levels.

Reference and further reading

Association of Operating Room Nurses. Regulated medical waste definition and treatment: a collaborative document. *AORN Journal* 1993; **58**: 110–114.

Ayliffe GAJ. Clinical waste: how dangerous is it? *Current Opinion in Infectious Diseases* 1994; 7: 499–502.

British Medical Association. *The Safe Use and Disposal of Sharps.* London: BMA, 1993.

Blenkharn JI. The disposal of clinical wastes. *Journal of Hospital Infection* 1995; **30** (Suppl.): 514–520.

Collins CH, Kennedy DA. *The Treatment and Disposal of Clinical Waste.* Leeds: H and H Scientific Consultants Ltd, 1993.

Collins CH, Kennedy DA. Microbiological hazards of occupational needlestick and 'sharps' injuries. *Journal of Applied Bacteriology* 1987; **62**: 385–402.

Collins AH and Kennedy DA. *Laboratory–acquired infections: History, incidence, causes and prevention.* 4th edn. Oxford; Butterworth Heinemann, 1999.

Daschner F. The hospital and pollution: role of the hospital epidemiologist in protecting the environment. In: Wenzel RP (ed). *Prevention and Control of Nosocomial Infections,* 3rd edn. Baltimore: Williams & Wilkins; 1997, 595–605.

Daschner F. Unnecessary and ecological cost of hospital infection. *Journal of Hospital Infection* 1991; **18** (Suppl. A): 73–78.

Department of the Environment, Scottish and Welsh Office. Waste management: The duty of care, a code of practice. London: HMSO, 1992.

Gwyther J. Sharps disposal containers and their use. *Journal of Hospital Infection* 1990; **15**: 287–294.

Gordon JG and Denys GA. Infectious Waste: efficient and effective management. In: Block SS (ed). *Disinfection, Sterilization and Preservation.* 5th edn. Baltimore: Lippincott Williams & Wilkins; 2001, 1139–1157.

Gordon JD, Reinhardr PA, Denys GA, Alvarado CJ. Medical waste management. In: Mayhall CG (ed). *Hospital Epidemiology and Infection Control,* 2nd edn. Philadelphia: Lippincott Williams & Wilkins; 1999, 1387–1397.

London Waste Regulation Authority (LWRA). Guidelines for the segregation, handling, transport and disposal of clinical waste. 2nd edn. London: LWRA, 1994.

NHS Executive. Health Guidance Note. Safe disposal of clinical waste whole hospital policy guidance. London: HMSO, 1995.

Phillips G. Microbiological aspects of clinical waste. *Journal of Hospital Infection* 1999; **41**: 1–6.

Pruess A, Townend WK. Teacher's Guide: *Management of Wastes from Health-care Activities*. Geneva, World Health Organization, 1998. WHO/EOS/98.6.

Rutala WA, Mayhall CG. SHEA position paper: Medical Waste. *Infection Control and Hospital Epidemiology* 1992; 13: 38–47.

Taylor LJ. Segregation, collection and disposal of hospital laundry and waste. *Journal of Hospital Infection* 1998; 11 (Suppl. A): 57–83.

UK Department of the Environment. *Waste management: The duty of care, a code of practice*. London: HMSO, 1992.

UK Department of Health. Expert Advisory group on AIDS and the Advisory group on Hepatitis. *Guidance for clinical health care workers: Protection against infection with blood borne viruses*. London: DoH, 1998.

UK Health and Safety Commission. *Safe disposal of clinical waste*. Norwich: HMSO, 1999.

UK Advisory Committee on Dangerous Pathogens (ACDP). Categorisation of biological agents according to hazard and categorises of containment. 4th edn. Sudbury: HSE, 1995.

PEST CONTROL

Cockroaches, flies and maggots, ants, mosquitoes, spiders, mites, midges and mice are among the typical arthropod and vertebrate pest populations found in health care facilities. Insects can serve as agents for the mechanical transmission of micro-organisms, or as active participants in the disease transmission process by serving as vectors. Arthropods recovered from health care facilities have been shown to carry a wide variety of pathogenic microorganisms.

Apart from the possibility of disease transmission, food may be tainted and spoiled, fabric and building structure damaged. *Pharaoh's ants have been responsible for the penetration of sterile packs* and the invasion of patient's dressings, including those in use on a wound. Cockroaches can carry Gram-negative bacilli and spoil food. Cockroaches, in particular, have been known to feed on fixed sputum smears in laboratories. Insects need to be kept out of all areas of the health care facility, but this is especially important for the operating rooms and any area where immunosuppressed patients are located.

Hospital kitchens, boiler rooms, ducts and drains provide warmth, water, food and shelters for cockroaches, pharaoh's ants and other pest. In addition, insects also feed on food scraps from kitchens/cafeterias, foods in vending machines, discharges on dressings either in use or discarded, medical wastes, human wastes, and routine solid waste. Both cockroaches and ants are frequently found in the laundry, central sterile supply departments, or anywhere in the facility where water or moisture is present (e.g. sink traps, drains, cleaning staff closets).

Every effort must be made to achieve a reasonable level of control or the eradication of pests. Hospital management is responsible for ensuring that the premises are free from pests. Each health care facility should have a pest control programme. This may be contracted to an approved pest control contractor.

From a public health and hygiene perspective, it is reasonable to *control and eradicate arthropod and vertebrate pests from all indoor environments*, including health care facilities. Modern approaches to institutional pest management usually focus on:

1. Eliminating food sources, indoor habitats, and other conditions that attract pests.

2. Excluding pests from the indoor environments.

3. Applying pesticides as needed.

Sealing windows in modern health care facilities helps to minimize insect intrusion. It is essential that older buildings should be of sound structure and well maintained. Cracks in plaster and woodwork, unsealed areas around pipe work, damaged tiles, badly fitted equipment and kitchen units are all likely to provide excellent points of entry or refuge for pests. The drains should be covered, and any leaking pipe work repaired.

Close-fitted windows and doors, fly screens and bird netting will help to exclude pests from hospitals and other health care facilities. When windows need to be opened for ventilation, ensuring that screens are in good repair and closing doors to the outside can help with pest control.

Pests require food, warmth, moisture, refuge, and a means of entry; hospital staff should be encouraged to keep food covered, to remove spillage and waste, and to avoid accumulations of static water.

References and further reading

Barker LF. Pests in hospitals. *Journal of Hospital Infection* 1981; **2**: 5–9.

UK Department of Health. *Pest Control Management for the Health Services*. UK Department of Health; London: HMSO, 1992. [HSG(92)35].

Infection Control
Information Resources

INTERNET RESOURCES

Journals	Websites
American Journal of Infection Control	http://www.mosby.com/ajic
Canada Communicable Disease Report	http://www.hc-sc.gc.ca/main/lcdc/web/
Communicable Disease Review (CDR)	http://www.phls.co.uk/publications/CDR
Emerging Infectious Diseases	http://www.cdc.gov/ncidod/EID/index.htm
Eurosurveillance	http://www.eurosurv.org
Infection Control and Hospital Epidemiology	http://www.slackinc.com/general/iche
Journal of Hospital Infection	http://www.elsevierhealth.com/journals/jhin
Morbidity and Mortality Weekly Report (MMWR)	http://www.cdc.gov/mmwr/
WHO weekly Epidemiology Record	http://www.who.int/wer/

Organizations and regulatory bodies	Websites
Association for Professionals in Infection Control and Epidemiology (APIC), USA	http://www.apic.org
Association of Preoperative Nurse (AORN), USA	www.aorn.org
Center for Disease Control and Prevention (CDC), USA	http://www.cdc.gov
Communicable Disease Surveillance and Response (WHO)	http://www.who.int/emc
Community and Hospital Infection Control Association (CHICA), Canada	http://www.chica.org

Organizations and regulatory bodies	Websites
European Operating Room Nurses Association (EORNA)	www.eorna.org
Department of Health, England, UK	http://www.doh.gov.uk/dhhome.htm
Food and Drug Administration (FDA), USA	http://www.fda.gov
Health Canada Disease Prevention and Control Guidelines	www.hc-sc.gc.ca/
Hospital Infection Society, UK	http://www.his.org.uk
Hospital in Europe Link for Infection Control through Surveillance (HELICS)	http://helics.univ-lyon1.fr
Infection Control Nurses Association (ICNA), UK	http://www.icna.co.uk
Infectious Diseases Societies Worldwide	http://www.idlinks.com/
Infectious Diseases Society of America	http://www.idsociety.org/index.htm
International Federation Infection of Infection Control (IFIC)	http://www.ific.narod.ru
International Health Care Worker Safety Centre, USA	www.med.virginia.edu/~epinet/
International Society of Infectious Diseases	www.isid.org
John Hopkins University-Infectious Diseases, USA	http://www.hopkins-id.edu/index_id_linls.html
Medical Devices Agency (MDA), UK	http://www.medical-devices.gov.uk
National Disease Surveillance Centre, Republic of Ireland	http://www.ndsc.ie
National Foundation for Infectious Diseases, (USA)	www.nfid.org/
National Institute for Public Health Surveillance, France	http://www.rnsp-sante.fr/
National Nosocomial Surveillance System, (CDC), USA	http://www.cdc.gov/ncidod/hip/Surveill/nnis.htm
Public Health Laboratory Services (PHLS), UK	http://www.phls.co.uk
Robert Koch-Institut, Germany	http://www.rki.de/index.htm
Scottish Centre for Infection and Environmental Health (SCEIH)	http://www.show.scot.nhs.uk/scieh/
Société Francaise d'Hygiène Hospitalière, France (SFHH)	http://sfhh.univ-lyon1.fr/
Society for Healthcare Epidemiology of America (SHEA), USA	http://www.shea-online.org
World Health Organization (WHO)	http://www.who.int/

BOOKS

1. Association for Professionals in Infection Control and Epidemiology. *APIC Infection Control and Applied Epidemiology: Principles and Practice*. St Louis: Mosby, 2000.

2. American Institute of Architects: *Guidelines for Design and construction of Hospital and Health Care Facilities*. Washington DC: The American Institute of Architects, 2001.

3. Arias KM. *Quick Reference to Outbreak Investigation and Control in Health Care facilities*. Gaithersburg: Aspen Publication, 2000.

4. Abrutyn E, Goldmann DA and Schecler WE (eds). *Saunders Infection Control Reference Service*, 2nd edn. Philadelphia: WB Saunders, 2001.

5. Ascenzi JM. *Handbook of Disinfectants and Antiseptics*. New York: Marcel Dekker Inc, 1996.

6. Altemeier WA, Burke JF, Pruitt BA, Sandusky WR (eds). *Manual on Control of Infection in Surgical Patients*. Philadelphia, PA: Lippincott, 1984.

7. Ayliffe GAJ, Coates D, Hoffman PN. *Chemical disinfection in hospitals*, 2nd edn. London: Public Health Laboratory Service, 1993.

8. Ayliffe GAJ, Babb JR, Taylor LJ. *Hospital-acquired infection. Principles and prevention*, 3rd edn. London: John Wright, 1999.

9. Ayliffe GAJ, Fraise AP, Geddes AM, Mitchell K. *Control of Hospital Infection – a practical handbook*, 4th edn. London: Arnlod, 2000.

10. Bartzokas CA, Williams EE, Slade PD. *A Psychological Approach to Hospital Acquired Infections*. New York: The Edwin Mellen Press, 1995.

11. Bennett JV, Brachman PS. *Hospital infections*, 4th edn. Boston, MA: Little Brown, 1998.

12. Block SS. *Disinfection, sterilization and preservation*, 5th edn. Philadelphia: Lippincott, Williams & Wilkins, 2001.

13. Chin J. *Control of communicable disease manual*, 17th edn. Washington: American Public Health Association, 2000.

14. Collins CH, Kennedy DA. *Laboratory-acquired infections. History, incidence and preventions*, 4th edn. Oxford: Butterworth-Heinemann, 1999.

15. Cudy KR, Kleger B, Hinks E, Miller LA. *Infection Control: Dilemmas and Practical Solutions*. New York: Plenum Press, 1988.

16. Cafferkey MT. *Methicillin-Resistant Staphylococcus aureus: Clinical management and Laboratory aspects*. New York: Marcel Dekker, 1992.

17. Castle M, Ajemian E. *Hospital Infection Control*, 2nd edn. New York: John Wiley & Sons, 1987.

18. Damani NN. *Manual of Infection Control Procedures*. London: Greenwich Medical Media, 1997.

19. Davies EG, *et al. Manual of Childhood infections*, 2nd edn. London: WB Saunders, 2001.

20. Donowitz LG. *Hospital acquired infection in the Paediatric patient*. Baltimore: Williams & Wilkins, 1988.

21. Donowitz LG. *Infection Control in Child Care Center and Preschool*, 5th edn. Philadelphia: Lippincott, Williams & Wilkins, 2002.

22. Ducel G, Fabry J and Nicolle L. *Prevention of Hospital acquired infections: A Practical Guide*. 2nd edn. Geneva: World Health Organization, 2002.

23. Dunitz M. *Infection Control in Dental Environment effective procedure*. London: The University Press, 1991.

24. Emmerson AM, Ayliffe GAJ (eds). *Surveillance of Nosocomial Infections. Bailliere's clinical infectious diseases*, Vol 3. London: Bailliere Tindall, 1996.

25. Gardner JF, Peel MM. *Sterilization, Disinfection and Infection Control*, 3rd edn. Edinburgh: Churchill Livingstone, 1998.

26. Giesecke J. *Modern Infectious Disease Epidemiology*, 2nd edn. London, Arnold, 2002.

27. Gruendemann BJ, Mangum SS. *Infection Prevention in surgical settings*. Philadelphia: WB Saunders, 2001.

28. Hobbs BC, Roberts D. *Food Poisoning and Food Hygiene*, 6th edn. London: Edward Arnold, 1995.

29. Herwaldt LA. *A Practical Handbook for Hospital Epidemiologists*. New Jersey: Slack Incorporated, 1998.

30. Health Care Professional Guides. *Safety and Infection Control*. Pennsylvania: Springhouse Corporation, 1998.

31. Horton R, Parker L. *Informed Infection Control Practice*. 2nd edn. London: Churchill Livingstone, 2002.

32. Hawker J, Begg N, Weinberg J, Blair I, Reintjes R. *Communicable Disease Control Handbook*. London: Blackwell Science, 2001.

33. Humphreys H, Willats S, Vincents J-C. *Intensive Care infections*. London: WB Saunders, 2000.

34. Jennings J, Manian FA. *APIC Handbook of Infection Control*, 2nd edn. Washington DC: APIC Publication, 1999.

35. Jenson HB. *Pocket Guide to Vaccination and Prophylaxis*. Philadelphia: WB Saunders Company, 1999.

36. Kaplan C. *Infection and Environment*. Oxford: Butterworth, Heinemann, 1997.

37. Lynch P, Jackson M, Preston GA, Soule BM. *Infection Prevention with Limited Resources*. Chicago: ETNA Communications, 1997.

38. Lennan WJ, Watt B, Elder AT. *Infections in elderly patients*. London: Edward Arnold, 1994.

39. Mandell GL, Bennett JE, Dolin R. *Principles and Practice of Infectious Disease*, 5th edn. Edinburgh: Churchill Livingstone, 2000.

40. Maurer IM. *Hospital hygiene*, 3rd edn. London: Edward Arnold, 1985.

41. Mayhall CG (ed.). *Hospital Epidemiology and Infection Control*, 2nd edn. Philadelphia: Lippincott, Williams & Wilkins, 1999.

42. McCulloch J (ed.). *Infection Control: Science, management and practice*. London: Whurr Publishers, 2000.

43. McLaughlin AJ. *Manual of Infection Control in Respiratory Care*. Boston: Little Brown, 1983.

44. Meakins JL (ed.). *Surgical Infections: Diagnosis and treatment*. New York: Scientific American, Inc., 1994.

45. Meers P, McPherson M, Sedgwick J. *Infection: Control in Healthcare*. Cheltenham: Stanley Thornes, 1997.

46. Mercier C. *Infection Control: Hospital and community*. Cheltenham: Stanley Thornes, 1997.

47. Mehtar S. *Hospital Infections Control: Setting up a Cost-effective Programme with Minimal Resources*. Oxford: Oxford Medical Publications, 1992.

48. Moi Lin L, Ching Tai Yin P, Wing Hong S. *A Handbook of Infection Control for the Asian Healthcare Worker*. Hong Kong: Excerpta Medica Asia Ltd, 1999.

49 Nicolle L. *Infections control programmes to control antimicrobial resistance*. Geneva: World Health Organization, 2001. WHO/CDS/CSR/DRS/2001.7.

50. Nixon RG. *Communicable Diseases and Infection Control for EMS*. New Jersey: Practice Hall Inc, 2000.

51. Philpott-Howard J, Casewell M. *Hospital Infection Control: Policies and Practical Procedures*. London: Saunders, 1994.

52. Plamer MB. *Infection Control: A Policy & Procedure Manual*. Philadelphia: WB Saunders Company, 1984.

53. Poland GA (ed.). *Immunizing Healthcare Workers: A Practical Approach*. New Jersey: Slack Incorporated, 2000.

54. Pearse J. *Infection Control Manual.* Houghton: Jacana Education, 1997.

55. Reichert M, Young JH. *Sterilization Technology for the Health Care Facility,* 2nd edn. Maryland: An Aspen Publication, 1997.

56. Rello J, Valles J, Kollef M (eds). *Critical Care Infectious Diseases Textbook.* Boston: Kluwer Academic Publishers, 2001.

57. Russell AD, Hugo WB, Ayliffe GAJ (eds). *Principles and practice of disinfection, preservation and sterilization,* 3rd edn. Oxford: Blackwell Science, 1999.

58. Schaffer SD, Garzon LS, Heroux DL, Korniewicz DM. *Infection Prevention and Safe Practice.* St. Louis: Mosby, 1996.

59. Soule BM, Larson EL, Preston GA. *Infections and Nursing Practice: Prevention and Control.* St Louis: Mosby, 1995.

60. Smith PH. *Infection Control in Long-term Care Facilities.* New York: John Wiley & Sons, 1984.

61. Sim AJW, Jefferies DJ. *Aids and Surgery.* London: Blackwell Scientific Publications, 1990.

62. Taylor EW (ed.). *Infection in Surgical Practice.* Oxford: Oxford Medical Publications, 1992.

63. UK NHS Estates. *Infection Control in the build environment.* Norwich: The Stationary Office, 2002.

64. Van Saene HFK, Silvestri L, de la Cal MA (eds). *Infection Control in Intensive Care.* Milan: Springer Verlag, 1998.

65. Verghese A, Berk SL. *Infections in Nursing Homes and Long-term Care Facilities.* Basel: Karger, 1990.

66. Wenzel RP (ed.). *Prevention and Control of Nosocomial Infections,* 3rd edn. Baltimore, MD: Williams & Wilkins, 1997.

67. Wenzel R, Brewer T, Butzler J-P (eds). *A Guide to Infection Control in the Hospital,* 2nd edn. Hamilton: B C Decker, 2002.

68. Weinstein RA, Bonten M (ed.). *Infection Control in the ICU Environment.* Boston: Kluwer Academic Publishers, 2002.

69. Wilson J. *Infection Control in Clinical Practice,* 2nd edn. London: Bailliere Tindall, 2001.

70. Worsley MA, Ward KA, Parker L, Ayliffe GAJ, Sedgwick JA. *Infection control: guidelines for nursing care.* London: Infection Control Nurses Association, 1998.

71. Wood PR. *Cross infection Control in Dentistry: a Practical Illustrated Guide.* London: Wolfe, 1992.

COMPUTER SOFTWARE

CD-ROM

- *Bloodborne Viruses and Infection Control: a Guide to Health Care Professionals.* London: BMA Board of Science & Education, 1998.

- *Hospital Infection Control: Principles and Practice.* EA Partnership and the Infection Control Nurses Association, 2000.

- *Infection Control Training and Policies for Hospital.* Howard JP, Casewell M, Desi N. London: WB Saunders Company, 1998.

Epi Info

Epi Info is a software programme developed by the Centers for Disease Control and Prevention to manage and analyse data collected during an epidemiologic investigation. Epi Info also calculates statistical test use in an outbreak situation. The Epi Info can be downloaded from the CDC web site, www.cdc.gov free of charge.

EPINet

The Exposure Prevention Information Network (EPINet) system collect data about precutaneous injuries among health care workers. Run by the International Health Care Workers Safety Centre at the University of Virginia Health Sciences Centre, EPINet also standardizes reporting of information pertaining to such injuries as well as contact with patient's blood and body fluids. Hospitals can use the EPINet system to share and compare information and to identify successful injury-prevention measures. EPINet can be reached at its web site www.med.virginia.edu/~epinet/

WHOCARE

WHOCARE was developed by the WHO. It comes in two versions: the Basic version, published 1989 which was designed for surveillance of surgical sites infections, and comprehensive version which treats other kind of nosocomial infection. It is available from the WHOCARE distribution centre in Copenhagen, Denmark (Fax: 45 32 68 38 77).

epinet InCONTROL

The package is designed by Public Health Laboratory Services in Wales to assist infection control nurses in the routine management and surveillance of hospital acquired infections. It helps monitor alert organisms and conditions within their hospital. It is available free to Infection Control Practitioners working in the UK National Health Service. Web site address: www.hospitalacquiredinfection.net The programme can be downloaded from www.phls.wales.nhs

Index

A

Absolute risk, 43
Acid alcohol-fast bacillus (AAFB), 112
Acinetobacter spp., 283
Acquired immunodeficiency syndrome
   (AIDS), 104
  See also HIV infection
Actinomycosis, 104
Air borne precautions, 96–97
Air borne transmission, 5
Air conditioning, 23
Air fluidized beds, 301
Airways and endotracheal tube, 81
Alcohol, 59, 62, 63
Alchololic hand rub, 99
Aldehydes
  formaldehyde, 66
  glutaraldehyde, 66
Amoebiasis, 104
Ampoule, 81
Anesthetic tubing
  See ventilatory tubing
Anthrax, 104
Antibiotic
  lock therapy, 269
  prophylaxis surgical, 250–251
Antibiotic associated diarrhoea
  See Clostridium difficile infection
Antiseptics, 56
  alcohols, 59, 62
  antimicrobial activity (*Table*), 62
  chlorhexidine, 62, 64
  hexachlorophane, 62, 65
  iodine compounds
    iodophores, 62, 64

  quaternary ammonia compounds, 62,
    64
  triclosan, 62, 65
Aprons and gowns, 100, 141–142
Arm splint, 81
Ascariasis, 104
Aspergillosis, 24, 104
Attack rate, 43
Auroscope tips, 81
Auto-infection, 2
Autoclave, 56–57

B

Baby feeding bottles and teats, 81
Bacillus cereus, 156
Barrier precautions, 7, 8
Bath water, 81
Baths, 81
BCG (Bacilli Calmette-Guérin) vaccine,
  144–145
Bed-frames, 82
Bedpans and urinals, 82, 101
Bedpan washers, 101
Beds, 20
  See also Linen
Bias
  information bias, 45
  selection bias, 44
Bilharziasis, 111
Biological agents
  categorisation of, 178
Birthing pool, 82
Bladder irrigation, 280
Bleach
  See Chlorine-based disinfectant

Blinds, 19
Blood-borne (viral) infections
    infection control precaution, 191
    procedure after death, 199
    protection to newborn, 198
    responsibility of health care, 193
    risk of acquiring, 206–207
    risk to HCWs from patients, 192
    risk to patients from HCWs, 192
    routes of transmission, 190
    surgical procedures, 194–198
Blood and body fluids
    precautions, 78
Blood spills
    management of, 77
Bloodstream infection, 28
Bone marrow transplant patients, 21
Botulism, 104, 156
Bowls, 82
Breast pump, 82
Brucellosis, 104
Building work, 24

C

Campylobacter gastroenteritis, 104, 158
Candidiasis, 104
Carpets, 19, 83
Case-control studies, 40–41
Catering services
    cook-chill food production systems, 292
    causes of food poisoning, 295
    food handlers, 294
    food trolleys, 293
    general rules of food hygiene, 293
    HACCP, 291
    hospital kitchen, 294
    ice machines, 284, 295–296
    inspection, 294
    refrigerators, 294
    staff health/hygiene, 292
    texture modified products, 293
    ward kitchens, 295
Cardiac monitor, 83
Cefotaxime, 161
Ceftriaxone, 162
Ceilings, 18
Central venous catheter
    See Intravenous catheters

Chain of infection
    causative agent, 1
    mode of transmission, 5
    portal of entry, 6
    portal of exit, 4
    reservoir of infection, 3
    susceptible host, 6
Chlorine-based disinfectants, 59–60, 63
Cheatle forceps, 83
Chemical disinfectants
    See Disinfectants
Chickenpox, 165
    See also Varicella/herpes zoster
Chi-square test, 49
Chlamydia trachomatis, 104
Chlorhexidine, 62, 64, 125
Chlorine-based disinfectants, 59–60, 63
Cholera, 104
Ciprofloxacin, 161
Cleaning, 55
    See also Environmental cleaning
Clinical waste
    categorization, 304
    definition, 303
    disposal of sharps, 305
    handling of clinical waste, 304–305
    safe handling of sharps, 305
    sharps boxes, 307
    treatment methods, 308
Clostridium botulinum, 115, 156
Clostridium difficile infection, 105, 157
    clinical features, 147
    control of antibiotic usage, 148
    infection control measures, 148–149
    management, 147
    patients discharge, 149
    risk factors, 147
Clostridium perfringes, 105, 156
Cohort studies, 39–40
Commodes, 83
Confidence intervals, 51–52
Confounders, 45
Conjunctivitis, 105
Construction and renovation, 24
Contact isolation, 96
Contact precautions, 97, 102
Contact transmission, 5
Cooling towers, 23–24
Coxiella burnetti (Q fever), 111
Creutzfeldt-Jakob Disease, 105, 169–172

childbirth, 173
clinical manifestations, 169
diagnosis, 170
distribution of tissue infectivity in the
    body, 171
infection control precautions, 170
methods of decontamination, 171–172
mode of transmission, 169
occupational exposure, 173
post-mortem, 172
surgical procedures, 170
Critical items, 57
Cross-infection, 3
Cross sectional studies, 41–42
Crockery and cutlery, 83, 100
Cryptococcus, 105
Cryptosporidiosis, 105
Curtains & blinds, 19
Cytomegalovirus, 105, 212, 218, 219

D

Decontamination procedure
    airways and endotracheal tube, 81
    ampoules, 81
    arm splint, 81
    arthroscope, 84
    auroscope tip, 81
    babies feeding bottles and teats, 81
    bath water, 81
    baths, 81
    bed frames, 82
    bedpans and urinals, 82
    beds and cots, 82
    birthing pool, 82
    bowls, 82
    breast pumps, 82
    cardiac monitors, 83
    carpets, 83
    cheatle forceps, 83
    cleaning equipment, 83
    commodes, 83
    crockery and cutlery, 83
    drains, 84
    drip stands, 84
    duvets, 84
    enuresis monitors, 81
    endoscopes, 84
        See also Endoscopes

enteral feeding lines, 84
fixtures and fittings, 84
floors, 84
furniture and ledges, 85
haemodialysis machines, 85
hoist, 85
humidifiers, 85
hydrotherapy pools, 85
infants incubators, 85
laryngoscope blade, 86
lockers top, 86
mattresses and pillows, 86
methods prior to inspection, service
    and repair, 70
mops, 86
nail brushes, 86
neurological test pin, 86
nebulizers, 86
oxygen tents, 86
pillows, 86
proctoscope, 86
razors, 87
rhino/laryngoscope, 87
scissors, 87
shaving brushes, 87
sheepskins, 87
sigmoidoscope, 84
splints and walking frames, 87
speculae, 87
stethoscope, 87
suction equipment, 80, 88
thermometers, 88
toilet seats, 88
tooth mugs, 88
toys, 88
trolleys, 89
tubing, anaesthetic/ventilator,
    89
ultrasound, 89
urinals, 89
ventilators, 89
wash hand basins/sink, 89
wheel chairs, 89
X-ray equipment, 89
Diarrhoea, 105
    See also Gastrointestinal infection
Diphtheria, 105, 220, 224
Disinfection, 55
Disinfection procedure, 81
    See also Decontamination procedure

Disinfectants (chemical)
  alcohols, 59, 62–63
  aldehydes, 66
  antimicrobial activity, 63
  chlorine-based, 59–60, 63
  formaldehyde, 66
  glutataldehyde, 63, 67
  hydrogen peroxide, 67–68
  ortho-phthaladehyde, 67–69
  peracetic acid, 63, 66–68
  peroxygen compounds, 63
  phenolic, 60–64
  properties and use, 58–59
Drains
  surgical, 130, 247, 249, 255
Drip stands, 84
Droplets precautions, 97, 102
Droplets transmission, 5
Duvets, 84
Dysentery
  amoebic, 106
  bacillary, 106

E

Ebola virus, 106
  See also Viral haemorrhagic fevers
Echinococcosis, 106
Ectoparasites
  fleas, 181
  lice, 180–181
  scabies, 181–182
Encephalitis & encephalomyelitis,
  106
Endogenous infection, 2
Endoscopes, 69
  arthroscope, 69, 84
  automatic washer/reprocessor system,
    72–73
  cleaning and disinfection, 71–72
  cystoscopes, 69
  endoscopic unit, 70
  laparoscope, 69
  microbiological quality of water, 73
  problems due to inadequate
    decontaminations, 72
  proctoscope, 84
  renewal of disinfectant, 73
  sigmoidoscope, 84

Endoscopic Unit, 70
Endogenous infection, 2
Enteric (typhoid) fever,
  paratyphoid, 106
  typhoid, 106
Enteric pathogens
  See Gastrointestinal infections
Enterobacter spp., 261
Epidemiology
  case-control study, 40
  epidemic curve, 33–34
  experimental study, 39
  cohort study, 39–40
  nosocomial infection, 42
  risk ratio & odds ratio, 43–44
  surveillance, 39
Environment cleaning, 73–76, 78,
  101
  cleaning equipment, 83, 86
  terminal cleaning of room, 75
Epidemic curve, 34
Epiglottis, 106
Epi info, 45–46, 321
Equipment
  cleaning and disinfect in, 78–79
  decontamination prior to service and
    repair, 79
Error
  type I (alpha) error, 49
  type II (beta) error, 49
Escherichia coli 0157, 157
Ethylene oxide, 69
Exogenous infection, 2–3
Exposure prone procedures, 193–194
Exogenous infection, 2, 3
Experimental studies, 39
Eye wear, 240

F

Face mask
  See Mask
Fibreoptic endoscopes
  See Endoscopes
Fisher exact test, 49–50
Fixtures and fittings, 19, 84
Fleas, 181
Floors, 18–19, 84
Food handlers, 294

Food and catering service
    See Catering services
Food poisoning, 155–159
Formaldehyde, 66
Furniture, 19

G

Gas gangrene, 106
Gastrointestinal infections, 155–159
    incubation periods, 155
    infection control precautions, 155
    notification, 155
    risk groups, 155
German measles, 106
Glandular fever, 108
Gloves, 100, 237–239
    donning technique, 236
    glove materials, 237
    glove removal technique, 236
    latex allergy, 237
    types of gloves, 240
Glutaraldehyde, 63, 66–67
Gonococcal infections, 107
Gowns
    See Aprons and gowns
Gram-negative bacilli, multi-resistant
    risk factors for colonisation, 134
    infection control measures, 134–135
Glycopeptide resistant enterococci
    See Vancomycin resistant enterococci
Gut decontamination
    See Selective gut decontamination

H

Haemophilus influenzae, 109, 115
Hand hygiene
    areas most frequently missed, 26
    compliance, 234
    facilities, 20
    hand care products, 234
    hand cleaning preparations, 232
    hand drying, 231
    hygienic hand disinfection, 230
    hygienic hand rub, 230–231
    methods of hand decontamination, 228
    nail brushes, 233

parts frequently missed, 231
routine handwashing, 228
surgical (scrub) and disinfection, 231,
    254–255
technique, 229
wash hand basin, 20, 231
Health Care Workers
    health status, 205
    immunization against hepatitis, 72,
        107
    measures to protect, 204
    occupational risks, 206
    post-exposure counselling, 213
    post exposure prophylaxis, 213
        diphtheria, 223
        hepatitis A virus, 222
        hepatitis B virus, 210, 212
        hepatitis C virus, 213
        human immunodeficiency virus,
            210–211
        meningococcal infection, 162, 223
        pertussis, 223
        varicella zoster, 222
    pre-employment assessment, 204
    pregnant staff,
        cytomegalovirus, 216
        hepatitis B, 216
        parvovirus B18, 218
        rubella, 215
        varicella-zoster, chickenpox, 217
    protection against tuberculosis, 213
    responsibility of HCW, 193
    restrictions of work, 219–222
    screening for tuberculosis, 214
Heat sterilization, 56
Hepatitis B immunoglobulin (HBIG),
    198
Hepatitis viral
    hepatitis A, 107
    hepatitis B, 107, 185–187
    hepatitis C, 107, 186–188
    hepatitis D, 187–188
    hepatitis E, 107
    hepatitis G, 188
    incubation periods, 114
    infection control precautions, 191
    interpretation of serological makers,
        187
    protection of newborn, 198
    risk to health care worker from, 192

Hepatitis viral (continued)
  risk to patients from health care worker,
    192–193
  routes of transmission, 190
Herpes simplex, 107
Herpes zoster (shingles), 107
Hexachlorophane, 62, 65, 125
Hoist, 85
Hookworm, 108
Hospital waste
  See Clinical Waste
Host defense mechanisms, 6–7
Human immunodeficiency virus (HIV)
    infection
  clinical features, 188–189
  consent & pre-test discussion, 189–190
  infected health-care worker, 192–193
  infection control precautions, 107, 191
  laboratory diagnosis
    CD4 count, 190
    HIV serology, 190
    HIV viral load, 190
  post exposure prophylaxis, 210
  routes of transmission, 190
  window period, 190
Humidifiers, 85, 287, 298
Hydrogen peroxide, 67, 68
Hydrotherapy pool, 85
Hypochlorite
  See Chlorine-based disinfectant
Hypothesis
  error of hypothesis testing, 49
  testing, 49

I

Ice machines, 295–296
Impetigo, 108
Incidence rates, 42
Incubation periods, 114–118
Incubators, infants, 85
Immunocompromised patients,
  96–97
Infection control
  link nurses, 12
  risk assessment, 18
  risk management, 14
  strategies to control, 7
Infection Control Committee, 11

Infection Control Doctor, 9
Infection Control Link Nurse, 12
Infection Control Manual, 13
Infection Control Nurse, 10
Infection Control Team, 11
Infectious mononucleosis, 108
Infestation
  with ectoparasites, 180–182
Influenza, 108
  virus, 97, 116
Internet resources, 315–316
Intravenous catheter
  anticoagulant flush solutions, 269
  antimicrobial prophylaxis, 269
  aseptic techniques, 265
  catheter dressing regimens, 268
  dressing, 268
  education and training, 263
  guidewire exchange, 270
  in-line filters, 268
  monitoring and surveillance, 263
  pathogenisis, 262
  parenteral solutions, 264
  points of access for microbial
    contamination, 262
  procedure for insertion of central
    venous catheter, 267
  procedure for insertion of peripheral
    line, 266
  replacement of catheters, 269
  selection of catheter type, 264
  selection of insertion site, 265
  sources of infection, 261–262
  sources of microbial contamination,
    263
  surveillance, 263
Iodine & Iodophors, 62, 64
Isolation
  categories of, 95–96, 102
  precautions
    airborne isolation, 96–97, 102
    droplets, 97, 102
    protective isolation, 87, 95
    source isolation, 95
    standard isolation, 96
  rooms, 20
    protective isolation room, 21
    source isolation room, 20–21
Isopropyl alcohol (isopropanol), 59
  See also Alcohol

K

Kitchen, Food and Catering Service
 See Catering Service
Klebsiella spp., 228

L

Laboratory specimens, 102–103
Laryngoscope blades, 86
Lassa fever, 108
 See also Viral Haemorrhagic Fever
Latex allergy, 237
Laundry Services
 See Linen and Laundry Service
Legionnaires' disease
 case definition, 152
 clinical features, 151
 cooling towers, 23–24
 diagnosis, 152
 incubation period, 151
 investigation, 153
 prevention, 152–154
 risk factors, 151
 source of infection, 151
 surveillance and notification, 154
Leprosy, 108
Leptospirosis, 108
Lice (Pediculosis)
 body louse, 180
 control measures, 180–181
 head louse, 180
 pubic or crab louse, 180
Linen and laundry service
 air-fluidized beds, 301
 dry cleaning, 300
 general principles to prevent infection,
  298
 high temperature wash, 299
 infectious linen, 298
 laundry bags, 299
 laundry contract, 299
 laundry process, 299
 laundry staff, 298
 low temperature wash, 300
 mattresses and pillows, 301
 microbiological sampling, 300
 staff uniforms, 300–301
 transport of linen, 299

Link Nurse, 12
Listeriosis, 108
Locker top, 86
Look back investigations, 35
Lyme disease, 108

M

Malaria, 108
Marburg disease, 108
 See also Viral Haemorrhagic Fever
  (VHF)
Mask, 100, 241
Mattresses and pillows, 86
Measles, 108
Measures of association, 43–44
Measures of central tendency, 46
Measures of disease frequency, 42
Measures of dispersion, 48
Meningitis, 109
 coliforms, 109
 Haemoplilus influenzae type b,
  109
 Listeria monocytogenes, 109
 meningococcal *(Neisseria meningitides)*,
  109
 pneumococcal, 109
 tuberculous, 109
 viral, 109
Meningococcal disease, 109, 160–164
 chemoprophylaxis, 161
 clinical symptoms, 160
 diagnosis, 161
 emergency action by medical
  practitioner, 160
 health care worker, 162
 household contact, 162
 immunization of contacts, 163
 incubation period, 160
 management in hospital, 161
 management of contacts, 162–163
 notification, 161
 transmission, 160
Methicillin resistant *Staph. aureus*
  (MRSA), 109, 121
 ambulance transportation, 126
 clearance of carriage, 126
 decolonization therapy, 125
 health care worker, 127

Methicillin resistant *Staph. aureus* (MRSA) (continued)
    infection control measures, 109, 122–124
    microbiological clearance, 126
    mode of transmission, 122
    screening, 126
    source of infection, 121–122
    transfer of patients, 124, 126
    treatment of carriage, 125
    visit to other department, 124
Mops, 86
MRSA
    See Methicillin resistant *Staph. aureus*
Multi-resistant Gram-negative bacilli
    See Gram-negative bacilli
Mumps, 109
Mupirocin (*Bactroban*), 125
Mycobacterium spp., 73
    atypical, 73
    M. chelonei, 91
    M. tuberculosis, 61, 78
Mycoplasma, 110

N

NaDCC (Sodium dichloroisocyanurate), 59
Nail brushes, 233
Nebulizers, 86, 288–289
Needlestick injury
    See Sharps injuries
Neurological test pins, 86
Nocardia, 110
Non-critical items, 58
Nosocomial pneumonia
    See Pneumonia, nosocomial
Nosocomial infections
    bloodstream infections, 28
    incidence of (various), 27
    respiratory tract infections, 27
    surgical site infections, 28
    surveillance, 28–29
    urinary tract infection, 27

O

Observational studies, 39
Occupational Health Department
    pre-employment screening, 204
    role and responsibility, 203

Odds Ratio, 44
Operating Theatres
    conventional ventilated theatre, 22
    environmental cleaning, 257
    microbiological monitoring, 256
    staff movement, 255
    theatre wear, 253
    ultra clean theatre, 22–23
Operation, surgical
    pre-operative shaving, 251
    skin disinfection, 254
    surgical technique, 255
Operative patient care, 248
    antibiotic prophylaxis, 250
    patient's risk factor, 249
    pre-operative hospitalization, 251
    pre-operative showers, 248
    pre-operative shaving, 251
Orf, 110
Ortho-phthaladehyde, 67, 69–70
Outbreak control
    communication, 34
    definition, 30
    management, 30, 32
    outbreak control plan, 34
    recognition, 32
    summary of outbreak investigation, 33
Overshoes, 240
Oxygen tents, 86

P

P value, 50
Parovirus B19, 219
Pathology specimens, transport of, 103
Patient isolation
    See Isolation of patients
Pediculosis (Lice infestation), 180–181
Peracetic acid, 63, 66, 67–68
Peroxygen compounds, 63
Personal protective equipment
    aprons & gowns, 100, 102, 196, 239–240
    face protection, 102, 196, 239
    footwear, 196
    gloves, 100, 237–239
    masks, 196, 241
    overshoes, 240
    theatre wear, 253

Pertussis (Whooping cough), 110
Pest control, 312
Pharaoh's ants, 312
Phenolics, 60–62, 64
Pillows, 86
Pinworm infection, 110
Plague, 110
Plastic overshoes, 240
Pneumonia, nosocomial
    factors influencing colonization,
        285
    humidification with heat and moisture
        exchangers, 286
    pathogenesis, 285–286
    postural changes, 286
    respiratory filter, 286
    risk factors, 286
    strategy for prevention, 285–287
    suction catheters, 286
Pneumonias, 110
Pneumocystis carinii, 116
Poliomyelitis, 110
Pontaic fever, 151
Post exposure prophylaxis (PEP)
    diphtheria, 223
    hepatitis A virus, 222
    hepatitis B virus, 210, 212
    hepatitis C virus, 213
    human immunodeficiency virus,
        210–211
    meningococcal infection, 223
    pertussis, 223
    varicella zoster, 222
Povidone iodine
    See Iodine and Iodophores
Predictive value, 52
Pre-employment screening, 204
Pregnant health care workers
    cytomegalovirus, 216
    hepatitis B, 216
    parvovirus, 218
    rubella, 216
    varicella-zoster virus (chickenpox and
        shingles), 217
Pre-operative skin disinfection, 254
Prevalence rate, 42
Prevalence survey, 41–42
Prion diseases
    See Creutzfelt-Jakob disease
Proctoscope, 84

Protective isolation, 96
Pseudomembranous colitis, 147
Pseudomonas aeruginosa, 61, 73
Psittacosis (Q fever), 111
Pulmonary tuberculosis
    See Tuberculosis

Q

Q fever, 111
Quaternary ammonium compounds, 62,
    64–65

R

Rabies, 111, 179
Razors, 87
Relative risk, 43
Resident organisms, 227
Resistant organisms, 109, 119
Rhino/laryngscope, 87
Rifampicin, 106, 109
Ringworm, 111
Risk management, 14
Risk ratio, 43
Rubella, 106, 111

S

Salmonellosis, 111, 158
Scabies, 111, 181–182
Schistosomiasis, 111
Scissors, 87
Selective decontamination therapy, 289
Semi-critical items, 57
Sensitivity and specificity, 52
Sharps
    injury and management, 205–209
    boxes, 307
    safe handling and disposal, 307
Shaving brushes, 87
Sheepskins, 87
Shiglellosis, 111, 158
Shingles
    See herpes zoster
Sigmoidoscope, 84
Soap, 234

Sodium dichlorocyanurate
    (NaDCC), 59
Source isolation, 95
Sources of infection, 4
Spillages
   management of blood spills, 77
   management of infectious spills, 78
Staff health
   See Health Care Workers
Standard precautions, 96
Staphylococcal infection
   food poisoning, 111, 156
   See also MRSA
Sterilizer, 56–57
Sterilization
   dry heat, 56
   moist heat, 56
Stethoscope, 87
Streptococcal (β haemolytic) infection,
   111
Suction catheter, 80, 286
Suction equipment, 80
Surgical hand scrub, 252–253
Surgical prophylaxis, 250
Surgical site infection
   definitions, 246–247
   incidence, 28
   microbiology, 248
   operative factors
     draping, 255–256
     duration of operation, 255
     skin disinfection, 254
     staff movement, 255
     surgical hand scrub, 252, 253
     surgical technique, 255
     theatre wear, 254–255
     wound drains, 255
   pre-operative factors
     risk factors, 248
   postoperative factors
     antibiotic prophylaxis, 251
     pre-operative shaving, 251
     pre-operative showers, 248
     wound dressing, 256
   surveillance of SSI, 245
   wound classification, 249
Surveillance
   advantages and disadvantages, 31
   methods, 29, 31
Syphilis, 111

T

Tacky mats, 256
Terminal cleaning of room, 75
Tetanus, 112
Theatre
   See operating theatre
Theatre wear, 253
Thermometers, 88
Threadworms, 112
Toilet seats, 88
Toxocara, 112
Toxoplasmosis, 112
Toys, 88
Tooth mugs, 88
Transplant patients
   infection in, 98, 114
Transient microorganisms, 229–230
Transmission
   mode of
     airborne transmission, 5, 96
     contact transmission, 5, 97
     droplet transmission, 5, 97
Trichomoniasis, 112
Trichuriasis, 112
Triclosan, 62, 65, 125
Trolleys, 89
Tuberculosis, 112
   atypical mycobacteria, isolation, 141
   clinical manifestations, 137
   contact tracing, 144–145
   duration of isolation, 140
   incubation period, 139
   infection control precautions,
     140–142
   mode of transmission, 138
   multi-drug resistant tuberculosis, 143
   negative pressue isolation room, 21
   pre-employment screening, 213–215
   risk factors, 139
   treatment, 139
Tubing, anaesthetic/ventilator, 89
Two-by-two contingency table, 44
Typhoid and paratyphoid fever, 112

U

Ultrasound equipment, 89
Urinals, 89

Urinary catheterization
  antibiotic, prophylactic and treatment, 279
  bladder irrigation, 278
  catheter material, 274
  catheter size, 274
  drainage bag, 274
  emptying the drainage bag, 276
  incidence of, 27
  meatal care, 274
  policy and staff training, 279
  prevention of bacterial colonization, 277
  procedure for urinary catheterization, 275
  removal of catheter, 278
  specimen collection, 278
  use of antimicrobial agents, 278–279

V

Vancomycin resistant enterococci (VRE)
  infection control measures, 130–131
  mode of transmission, 130
  risk factors, 130
  screening of patients, 132
  source of infection, 130
Varicella\herpes zoster
  clinical features, 165
  infection control measures, 166
  neonates, 167
  period of infectivity, 165
  pregnant women, 167
  pregnant staff, 217–218
  susceptible patients, 166–167
  transmission, 165
Varicella zoster immunoglobulin (VZIG), 166–167
Ventilation and air conditioning, 23
Ventilators, 89, 289
Vibrio cholerae, 157
Vibrio parahaemolyticus, 157
Vincent's angina, 112

Viral haemorrhagic fevers, 175
  clinical manifestations, 175
  diagnosis, 175
  incubation period, 176
  infection control precautions, 177
  laboratory investigation, 177
  management, 177
  mode of transmission, 177
  notification, 175–176
  risk categories, 176
  source of infection, 176
Viral hepatitis
  See Hepatitis

W

Walls and ceilings, 18
Ward kitchen, 295
Wash basin/sink, 89
Waste disposal
  See Clinical waste
Wheel chairs, 89
Whipworm, 112
Whooping cough, 112
Wound infection
  See surgical site infection

X

X-ray equipment, 89

Y

Yellow fever, 112, 118
Yersinia enterocolitica, 115

Z

Z score, 49
Ziehl-Nielsen Stain, 139

Printed in the United Kingdom
by Lightning Source UK Ltd.
130264UK00001B/64-69/A